BLUEPRINTS IN MEDICINE

Blueprints: USMLE Steps 2 & 3 Review Series

General Series Editor:

Bradley S. Marino, MD, MPP
Department of Pediatrics
Johns Hopkins Hospital
Baltimore, Maryland

CURRENT BOOKS IN THE SERIES:

Blueprints in Obstetrics and Gynecology
Blueprints in Pediatrics
Blueprints in Psychiatry
Blueprints in Surgery

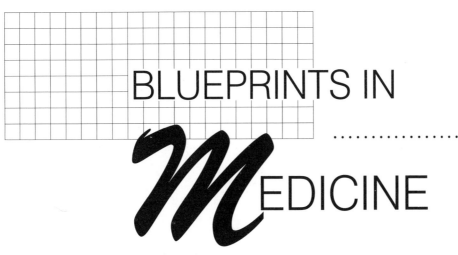

BLUEPRINTS IN

MEDICINE

Vincent B. Young, MD, PhD
Postdoctoral Fellow
Division of Toxicology
Massachusetts Institute of Technology
Cambridge, Massachusetts
Fellow
Infectious Diseases
Massachusetts General Hospital
Boston, Massachusetts

William A. Kormos, MD
Clinical and Research Fellow in Medicine
Harvard Medical School
Massachusetts General Hospital
Boston, Massachusetts

Allan H. Goroll, MD
Associate Professor of Medicine
Harvard Medical School
Associate Physician
Massachusetts General Hospital
Boston, Massachusetts

b

**Blackwell
Science**

Blackwell Science

Editorial Offices:
350 Main Street, Malden, Massachusetts 02148, USA
Osney Mead, Oxford OX2 0EL, England
25 John Street, London WC1N 2BL, England
23 Ainslie Place, Edinburgh EH3 6AJ, Scotland
54 University Street, Carlton, Victoria 3053, Australia

Other Editorial Offices:
Blackwell Wissenschafts-Verlag GmbH Kurfürstendamm 57, 10707 Berlin, Germany
Blackwell Science KK, MG Kodenmacho Nihombashi
   Chuo-ku Tokyo 104, Japan

Distributors:
USA
   Blackwell Science, Inc.
   Commerce Place
   350 Main Street
   Malden, Massachusetts 02148
   (Telephone orders: 800-215-1000
   or 781-388-8250; Fax orders: 781-388-8270)
Canada
   Login Brothers Book Company
   324 Saulteaux Crescent
   Winnipeg, Manitoba
   Canada, R3J 3T2
   (Telephone orders: 204-224-4068)

Australia
   Blackwell Science Pty., Ltd.
   54 University Street
   Carlton, Victoria 3053
   (Telephone orders: 03-9347-0300;
   Fax orders: 03-9349-3016)
Outside North America and Australia
   Blackwell Science, Ltd.
   c/o Marston Book Services, Ltd.
   P.O. Box 269, Abingdon
   Oxon OX14 4YN
   England
   (Telephone orders: 44-01235-465500;
   Fax orders: 44-01235-465555)

Acquisitions: Joy Ferris Denomme
Production: Karen Feeney
Manufacturing: Lisa Flanagan
Typeset by Publication Services
Printed and bound by Capital City Press
©1998 by Blackwell Science, Inc.
Printed in the United States of America

   00   5

Library of Congress Cataloging-in-Publication Data

Goroll, Allan H.
   Blueprints in medicine: USMLE steps 2 & 3 review series / Allan H. Goroll,
Vincent B. Young, William A. Kormos.
      p.   cm.—(The blueprints series)
   Includes bibliographical references and index.
   ISBN 0-86542-537-X (pbk.)
   1. Internal medicine—Outlines, syllabi, etc. I. Young, Vincent B.
II. Kormos, William A. III. Title. IV. Series.
   [DNLM: 1. Internal Medicine—examination questions.
WB 18.2 G672b 1997]
RC59.G67   1997
616'.0076—dc21
DNLM/DLC
for Library of Congress   97-6519
                                                              CIP

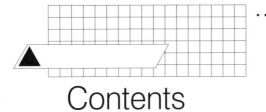

Contents

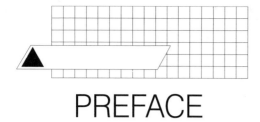

PREFACE

$\mathcal{F}$ourth-year medical students, interns, and residents are chronically sleep deprived, have little time to study due to their clinical duties, and have a low tolerance for medical literature that is not clear and to the point. All too often as a medical student, and now as a resident, I have heard my colleagues bemoan the fact that there is no succinct, clinical text on each of the core subjects tested on the USMLE Steps 2 & 3. These trainees need review materials they can digest quickly, perhaps a subject in a weekend, which will enable them to answer correctly the majority of questions in each discipline. This attitude is especially evident for the USMLE Step 3, for example, where surgical residents are tested on pediatrics although they have not completed a clinical rotation in the discipline for two years.

Our goal in writing *Blueprints in Medicine* was to enable the reader to review the core material quickly and efficiently. The topics were chosen after analyzing over 2,000 review questions, which we believed were representative of the internal medicine questions on the USMLE Steps 2 & 3 exams. This book is not meant to be comprehensive, but rather it is composed of the "high-yield" topics that consistently appear on these exams.

The questions on the USMLE Steps 2 & 3 are now crafted into clinical vignettes. To assist you in studying for this new format, the material in this book is presented either as the workup of a symptom or as a discussion of a particular disease or pathological process. Although this series is designed for the medical student or resident reviewing for the USMLE, we believe the books will be equally useful to all medical students during their clerkships or subinternships.

We hope that you find *Blueprints in Medicine* informative and useful. We welcome any feedback you may have about this text or any others in the Blueprints series.

Bradley S. Marino, MD, MPP
Blueprints Series Editor
c/o Blackwell Science, Inc.
Commerce Place
350 Main Street
Malden, MA 02148

▲ PART I
....

Cardiovascular

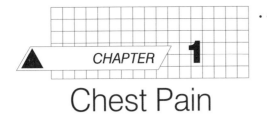

Chapter 1

Chest Pain

*I*n diagnosing the patient with chest pain, it often helps to categorize the pain by its pathophysiology. Inflammation of serosal surfaces leads to **pleuritic pain,** characterized by increased pain with inspiration or cough. This pain may also be aggravated by movement or position. Pleuritic pain is most often seen in pulmonary etiologies, pericarditis, and musculoskeletal disorders. **Visceral pain,** such as in myocardial ischemia and esophageal disease, often presents as dull, aching, tight, or sometimes burning pain that is poorly localized.

The most important decision for the physician is to distinguish life-threatening causes, such as myocardial ischemia, pulmonary embolus, and aortic dissection, from non-life-threatening causes. The key to identifying the etiology of the pain lies in the patient's history.

▶ RISK FACTORS

In evaluating the patient with chest pain, certain risk factors may increase the suspicion for coronary artery disease (CAD). Risk factors for CAD include:

▲   diabetes mellitus

▲   smoking

▲   hypertension

▲   hyperlipidemia

▲   family history of CAD

Patients with chest pain and many cardiovascular risk factors require further workup for CAD, even if the story is atypical. CAD is uncommon (but not unheard of) before age 40, and men are at greater risk than women until about age 65. Cocaine abuse is an important consideration, especially in younger patients with no other cardiac risk factors.

▶ CLINICAL MANIFESTATIONS
History

The following diseases often present with the sharp pleuritic type of pain. **Pneumothorax** has an acute onset and is pleuritic and associated with dyspnea. This occurs mostly in young patients (spontaneous) or those with underlying lung disease (secondary to blebs). **Pulmonary embolism** is similar to pneumothorax with pleurisy and dyspnea. Risk factors should be taken into account (see Chapter 15). **Pericarditis** is pleuritic and positional in nature and is classically relieved with sitting forward. Substernal pain may radiate to shoulder/trapezius (due to diaphragmatic/phrenic nerve irritation).

In contrast, other diseases may present with a more visceral type of pain, aching and poor localization. **Myocardial ischemia** often presents with a squeezing or pressure sensation and possibly a burning sensation. Located substernally, the pain classically radiates to the ulnar aspect of the left arm but may also go to jaw, shoulders, epigastrium, or back. Brought on by exertion or emotional stress, it usually lasts only minutes. Worrisome features include prolonged pain (>30 minutes) with myocardial infarction and rest pain with unstable angina. **Aortic dissection** presents with abrupt pain that is most intense at onset, which distinguishes this "must not miss" diagnosis. Pain is often tearing and radiates to back. In **gastrointestinal disease** (such as reflux and esophageal spasm), symptoms may be relieved with antacids, are related to food intake, and are worsened in supine position. Esophageal spasm may share many similar qualities with angina.

Finally, other conditions may have a component of both types of pain. In musculoskeletal disorders, pain is more easily localized and worsened with movement or palpation. Pain ranges from darting, lasting seconds, to a prolonged dull ache for days. In herpes zoster, because pain may precede rash by several days, a burning sensation in a dermatomal distribution is a key feature. With anxiety, pain is often atypical and prolonged, and workup reveals no other cause.

Physical Examination

Remember that ischemic heart disease may present (and often does) with a *completely normal* physical examination. However, some physical findings may lead to the correct diagnosis.

▲   Unequal blood pressures between arms is an important feature for aortic dissection. Tachypnea is seen in pulmonary causes such as pneumothorax and pulmonary embolism.

▲ Reproduction of the chest pain by palpation is a key feature of musculoskeletal causes. This is not the case in angina, pulmonary embolus, aortic dissection, or true pleuritic disease.

▲ Cardiac findings include a fourth heart sound (ischemia), an apical holosystolic murmur (ischemic mitral regurgitation), a blowing diastolic murmur (aortic regurgitation due to aortic dissection involving the valve root), and a pericardial rub (pericarditis).

▲ Pulmonary findings of a pneumothorax include hyper-resonance to percussion, decreased fremitus, and tracheal deviation to the affected side. A pleural rub may indicate pulmonary infarction or pneumonia.

▶ DIAGNOSTIC EVALUATION

The initial history and physical examination should guide the diagnostic workup. If the chest pain appears cardiac in nature, an electrocardiogram (ECG) should be obtained. Furthermore, in those patients with a high probability of underlying CAD (older, smoker, etc.), an ECG should be checked even if the story is atypical. Some helpful findings are listed in Table 1-1.

In patients with pleuritic pain and dyspnea as predominant symptoms, a chest x-ray should be the initial step to rule out pneumothorax, pulmonary infiltrates, or rib fractures. A widened mediastinum on chest x-ray may be seen with aortic dissection. Specific chest x-ray findings for pulmonary embolism can be found in Chapter 15.

TABLE 1-1
Electrocardiogram

---

1. Q waves in two or more leads = previous myocardial infarction
2. ST depression > 1 mm = ischemia
3. ST elevation = acute myocardial infarction or pericarditis (the latter often has involvement of all leads and associated PR depression)
4. Left bundle branch block = suggests underlying heart disease (ischemic, hypertensive)
5. Right bundle branch block = may be indicative of right heart strain (as in pulmonary embolus)
6. T wave inversions and nonspecific ST changes = seen in both normals and many diseases (therefore, not useful)

Note: A normal ECG does not rule out ischemia or serious disease, especially when taken in the absence of pain. Right bundle branch block and early repolarization may be seen in young healthy normal individuals.
Occlusion of the right coronary artery by an aortic dissection may present with inferior ST elevation. This is a vital distinction to make.

In the case of suspected musculoskeletal pain in the low-risk patient, a trial of nonsteroidal anti-inflammatory drugs is appropriate.

Other important diagnostic tests include the **aortogram**, in which patients with worrisome stories for aortic dissection should be further evaluated regardless of chest x-ray (CXR) or ECG. Transesophageal echocardiogram is a minimally invasive method of making the diagnosis. The V/Q scan is used in patients with pleuritic pain and normal chest x-ray who may need further workup. A normal V/Q scan rules out the diagnosis of pulmonary embolus, whereas a high probability scan confirms the diagnosis when accompanied by a high clinical suspicion. This is further detailed in Chapter 15. The exercise stress test is used in patients with a chronic stable pattern of pain; this may be the appropriate next step (see Chapter 3).

In chest pain of esophageal origin, pain induced by esophageal reflux may be confirmed by the Bernstein test (acid instillation in esophagus, reproducing pain), 24-hour esophageal pH monitoring, or an empiric trial of antacids or H2 blockers.

▶ KEY POINTS

1. Patients with good stories for serious causes of chest pain (ischemia, dissection, embolus) deserve further evaluation even if physical examination, chest x-ray, and ECG are normal.

2. Certain chest pain syndromes have very typical patterns such as the acute tearing pain of aortic dissection, the dermatomal distribution of herpes zoster, or the positional pleuritic pain of pericarditis (relieved with sitting forward).

3. Risk factors are important to determine probability of CAD in a patient with chest pain. These include age, sex, diabetes mellitus, hypertension, hyperlipidemia, smoking, and family history.

4. The ECG is a key test in patients with a suspected cardiac origin of chest pain. The findings of Q waves, ST elevation, or ST depression all signify cardiac ischemia. A notable exception is pericarditis, which has diffuse ST elevation often with associated PR depression.

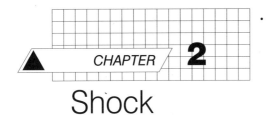

CHAPTER 2

Shock

*S*hock is a term used to describe decreased perfusion and oxygen delivery to the body. Shock presents with a decrease in blood pressure and may result from either a decrease in cardiac output (CO) or a decrease in systemic vascular resistance (SVR). This is best defined by the following equation:
Blood Pressure = CO × SVR.

The three main syndromes leading to shock (i.e., hypovolemia, cardiogenic, and sepsis) are defined by their effect on the CO or SVR. An additional clinical feature is the volume status, best assessed at the bedside by the jugular venous pressure (JVP) and in the intensive care unit by the postcapillary wedge pressure (PCWP). The syndromes and their features are defined in Table 2-1.

The low CO seen in cardiogenic shock may also be seen in syndromes resulting in right heart failure (such as **massive pulmonary embolism**), decreased venous filling of the heart (**tension pneumothorax**), and obstruction of outflow (**cardiac tamponade**). The low vascular resistance that occurs in sepsis may be mimicked by **adrenal crisis** (insufficiency) or **anaphylaxis.** CO varies in these conditions depending on severity and volume status.

Although often defined as a systolic blood pressure less than 90 or mean arterial pressure less than 60, shock is truly defined by its **effect on other organ systems.** Failure of other organs is evidence of insufficient blood pressure regardless of the actual value. Manifestations of inadequate perfusion include:

▲ renal dysfunction (decreased or no urine output)

▲ central nervous system dysfunction (worsening mental status)

▲ tissue hypoxia (lactic acidosis)

TABLE 2-1

Definitions of Shock Syndromes

	CO	SVR	JVP/PCWP
Hypovolemia	Decrease	Increase	Decrease
Cardiogenic	Decrease	Increase	Increase
Sepsis	Increase	Decrease	Decrease

▶ CLINICAL MANIFESTATIONS

History

History is usually not helpful because the patient often has a clouded sensorium due to decreased perfusion. However, the following findings may be helpful:

▲ recent use or discontinuation of corticosteroids (adrenal crisis)

▲ ingestion of certain foods/drugs or occurrence of beesting (anaphylaxis)

▲ history of chest pain (pleuritic: pulmonary embolism or tension pneumothorax; nonpleuritic: ischemia)

Physical Examination

Vital signs are essential to evaluating the patient with shock. **Tachycardia** is almost always present; failure to increase the heart rate in the presence of hypotension suggests a primary cardiac conduction disturbance (see Chapter 6). **Pulsus paradoxus** is seen in cardiac tamponade; this is defined as a decrease in systolic blood pressure of greater than 10 mm Hg with inspiration.

JVP provides a rough bedside estimate of central venous pressure. Shock due to a cardiopulmonary etiology (see below) will present with increased JVP. Systemic causes of shock are caused by either systemic vasodilation or decreased volume; JVP is decreased or undetectable in these patients.

Absence of breath sounds on one side and **tracheal deviation** to the opposite side are findings of a tension pneumothorax. Pulmonary examination may also reveal rales in cardiogenic shock or wheezing in anaphylaxis.

▶ DIFFERENTIAL DIAGNOSIS

Cardiac

1. Low output heart failure;
2. Cardiac tamponade.

Pulmonary

1. Tension pneumothorax;
2. Massive pulmonary embolism.

Systemic

1. Sepsis;
2. Hypovolemia;
3. Adrenal crisis;
4. Anaphylaxis.

▶ DIAGNOSTIC EVALUATION AND TREATMENT

The hypotension present in shock is easily diagnosed, and efforts are directed at discerning the correct etiology of shock. This always begins with treating the hypotension itself. The initial approach is based on the volume status, often using the JVP as a guide. For patients with **shock due to systemic etiology (with decreased JVP)**, treatment should begin with intravenous fluids (normal saline or Ringer's lactate) while evaluating the cause of the hypotension. The patient should be examined for possible causes of hypovolemia including blood loss, dehydration, and third-spacing of fluid (as in pancreatitis). An acute onset after ingestion of a food (especially nuts) or drug suggests an anaphylactic reaction and 0.3 mg epinephrine subcutaneously should be given immediately. The diagnosis of **adrenal insufficiency** is suggested by:

▲ hyponatremia

▲ hyperkalemia

▲ hypoglycemia

▲ eosinophilia

▲ mild hypercalcemia

Adrenal insufficiency is then confirmed by a suboptimal response to corticotropin (ACTH) (see below). However, the emergent nature of adrenal crisis requires treatment with intravenous steroids (**100 mg hydrocortisone IV**) while waiting for the test results to return. Patients with possible sepsis should have blood cultures drawn and **empiric antibiotic therapy** directed at the most likely pathogens.

Shock due to cardiopulmonary etiologies (increased JVP) requires specific treatment aimed at the underlying cause. In cardiogenic shock, intravenous fluids (IVF) are likely to be more harmful; IVF may be temporizing measures in pulmonary embolism or tamponade. An electrocardiogram (ECG) should be obtained to look for an acute myocardial infarction.

Along with the clinical examination and empiric treatment, the **chest x-ray** is a useful first test in hypotension with increased JVP. A chest film may show bilateral alveolar infiltrates (pulmonary edema), an enlarged cardiac silhouette (tamponade or cardiomyopathy), or a pneumothorax with mediastinal shift to the opposite side. Chest x-ray is often normal in pulmonary embolism, but certain findings may be present (see Chapter 15).

An **ECG** may show acute myocardial ischemia, with either ST segment elevation or depression. Old Q waves may suggest past myocardial injury and a predisposition to cardiogenic shock. In pulmonary embolism, the **ECG** may show evidence of right heart strain, such as right bundle branch block.

Although a chest x-ray can confirm the diagnosis of tension pneumothorax, the emergent nature of the problem may demand immediate treatment. In a patient at risk for pneumothorax with typical findings (absent breath sounds, tracheal deviation, increased JVP), decompression of the affected side must be accomplished immediately. **Insertion of a chest tube** is the optimal treatment, but if not readily available, a large gauge needle should be inserted in the midclavicular second intercostal space of the affected side.

In the patient with hypotension and increased JVP, an **echocardiogram** may help determine the underlying cause. For example, echocardiographic findings seen in pericardial tamponade include moderate to large pericardial effusion and diastolic collapse of the right atrium or ventricle. In addition, the echocardiogram may reveal diffuse hypokinesis (cardiogenic shock), right-sided heart failure (pulmonary embolism), or valvular or septal wall rupture.

Invasive monitoring may be necessary to evaluate and treat the patient with shock. In the patient whose etiology is unclear or in whom treatment is ineffective, a **Swan-Ganz (pulmonary artery) catheter** should be placed. This can be used to obtain a PCWP, which is a proxy for left atrial filling pressures. The PCWP is only elevated in cardiac etiologies of shock. In cardiac tamponade, equalization of pressures may occur. This is when the right atrial pressure is equal to the right ventricular diastolic pressure and the left atrial pressure.

CO may also be measured with a pulmonary artery catheter; the output is then divided by the patient's body size to yield a cardiac index. Normal values for cardiac index are 2 to 4 liters/min/m^2. CO is decreased in cardiopulmonary etiologies and increased in early (warm) sepsis. In late sepsis, CO may decline (cold sepsis).

The **ACTH stimulation test** involves measurement of a basal cortisol level (preferably at its morning peak, 8 to 9 a.m.), followed by a cortisol measurement 1 hour after administration of ACTH. Basal or post-stimulation values greater than 20 μg/dL rule out adrenal insufficiency. However, because stress increases cortisol levels, some authorities have recommended increasing this cutoff to 25 µg/dL in the acutely ill patient.

▶ KEY POINTS

1. Shock, manifested by decreased blood pressure, is the result of decreased cardiac output (CO) or decreased systemic vascular resistance (SVR).

2. Shock due to cardiopulmonary etiologies is due to decreased CO and presents with increased jugular venous pressure (JVP). Hypovolemia may also decrease CO but the JVP is undetectable.

3. Unilateral absence of breath sounds, increased JVP, and tracheal deviation suggests tension pneumothorax. Immediate decompression is required.

4. Hyponatremia and hyperkalemia in the patient with hypotension may suggest adrenal crisis. Treatment with intravenous hydrocortisone is indicated. Diagnosis may be confirmed by a suboptimal ACTH stimulation test.

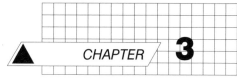
Coronary Artery Disease

► EPIDEMIOLOGY

Coronary artery disease (CAD) is the leading cause of death in people over the age of 45 in the United States. An estimated 5 million people in the United States have CAD. Many more have conditions that predispose to its development. CAD is responsible for an estimated 400,000 to 500,000 deaths each year, but overall the death rate has been declining over the past 20 to 30 years. This is believed to be due to improvements in the management of CAD, including prevention of CAD progression, treatment of myocardial ischemia, and management of acute myocardial infarction (AMI).

► ETIOLOGY AND PATHOGENESIS

The formation of an **atherosclerotic plaque** within a coronary artery proceeds through a number of stages. In the first stage, formation of a "fatty streak"—a longitudinal accumulation of lipid with surrounding smooth muscle proliferation—occurs. This can occur quite early in life (during the second decade). In the second stage, low-density lipoprotein (LDL) enters the endothelium in the area of the fatty streak. The LDL becomes oxidized, attracting **macrophages** that ingest the LDL ("foam cells"). These macrophages release factors that recruit more macrophages, fibroblasts, and other inflammatory cells. In the final stage, proliferating smooth muscle cells, connective tissue (produced by infiltrating fibroblasts), and lipids (cholesterol, cholesterol esters, triglycerides, and phospholipids) become incorporated into the maturing plaque. At this point, the formation of a "fibrous cap" results in narrowing of the artery lumen. Areas of cell necrosis and calcification within the plaque may occur.

Myocardial ischemia occurs in the setting of coronary artery atherosclerosis. The narrowing of the coronary artery lumen by an atherosclerotic lesion reduces blood flow to the distal myocardium. As the lesion continues to grow, oxygen supply becomes increasingly limited, and under conditions of increased demand (e.g., exercise, emotional stress) myocardial ischemia occurs. At this stage, the cross-sectional area of artery is generally less than 30% of normal.

Progressive luminal compromise can lead to the expansion of **collateral circulation**, alternate distal vessels that can increase blood supply to the compromised area. In some cases, complete occlusion of the diseased artery can result in little or no myocardial damage due to extensive distal collateralization.

► RISK FACTORS

Patient characteristics that predispose to the development of coronary artery disease include:

▲ hypercholesterolemia (elevated LDL)

▲ low high-density lipoprotein (HDL) levels

▲ smoking

▲ hypertension

▲ male sex

▲ diabetes mellitus

▲ family history of CAD (especially early AMI)

► CLINICAL MANIFESTATIONS
History

The typical manifestation of symptomatic CAD is **angina pectoris**, characterized as a substernal pressure, heaviness, burning, squeezing, or choking. The discomfort is rarely well localized or described as sharp pain. Radiation to the jaw, shoulder, back, or arms can occur.

In so-called **stable angina pectoris**, attacks are brought on by exertion or emotion. The pain will increase over several minutes and is relieved by rest in several minutes. **Unstable angina pectoris** is defined as angina that occurs at rest or a significant change in the pattern of existing chronic angina.

It is important to note that not all patients will describe typical anginal pain during periods of myocardial ischemia. Patients with **atypical angina** may manifest with isolated symptoms such as jaw pain or dyspnea. This is particularly true in patients with underlying diabetes. Patients with **silent ischemia** can be completely asymptomatic.

In some patients with angina who have underlying compromise of ventricular function or have severe widespread ischemia, angina can be accompanied by symptoms of **heart failure** (dyspnea, orthostatis).

Physical Examination

CAD patients often have a normal physical examination, particularly if they are not symptomatic at the time of examination. They may have findings due to predisposing conditions or due to atherosclerosis outside of the coronary arteries:

▲ retinal vascular changes (e.g., A-V nicking and/or "copperwire" changes due to hypertension)

▲ fourth heart sound (hypertension)

▲ arterial bruits (peripheral atherosclerosis)

▲ absent or diminished peripheral pulses (peripheral atherosclerosis)

▲ xanthomas (hyperlipidemia)

Examination during an anginal attack can reveal a fourth heart sound (due to decreased compliance of the ischemic myocardium) or signs of left ventricular failure (third heart sound, single S2, pulmonary edema, elevated jugular venous pressure).

▶ DIFFERENTIAL DIAGNOSIS

The differential diagnosis of chest pain is discussed in Chapter 1. The important diseases to consider include:

▲ myocardial infarction

▲ pulmonary embolism

▲ aortic dissection

▲ gastrointestinal disease (cholecystitis, esophageal spasm, pancreatitis)

▲ pneumonia

▶ DIAGNOSTIC EVALUATION

The resting electrocardiogram (ECG) is normal in about half of patients with angina pectoris. Some may have evidence of old myocardial infarction (Q-waves, inverted T-waves). The typical ECG change seen during actual ischemia is ST-segment depression, defined as a >1 mm depression of the ST segment from baseline in at least two contiguous leads.

The suspected diagnosis of CAD can be confirmed with an **exercise stress test.** During a stress test, the patient exercises on a treadmill or bicycle ergometer. The workload is increased in a standardized progressive manner, and symptoms, vital signs, and ECG are monitored. This test is much more sensitive than a resting ECG for detecting CAD. The test is discontinued for chest pain, dizziness, severe dyspnea, greater than 2 mm ST-segment depression, fall in systolic blood pressure of >15 mm Hg, or ventricular tachyarrhythmias. Development of diagnostic ST-segment depression is considered to be a positive test. In patients who are unable to exercise due to orthopedic problems or severe deconditioning, stress testing can be done with the administration of **persantine.** Persantine acts as a vasodilator of normal but not atherosclerotic coronary vessels and thus can cause shunting of blood flow away from diseased vessels, resulting in ischemia.

The sensitivity of stress testing (exercise and persantine) can be improved (especially in patients with an abnormal resting ECG) by the use of **radiolabeled tracers** (e.g., thallium 201) to determine regional myocardial perfusion. Images are recorded immediately after exercise and then after a several hour rest period to identify areas that have decreased blood flow after exercise but normal or increased flow after rest. Infarcted areas of myocardium lack perfusion at both time points. This technique is semiquantitative, estimating the amount of ischemic or infarcted myocardium by the size of the defect seen on the images.

The precise coronary anatomy can be determined by the technique of **coronary arteriography.** Although this technique can be used to make the diagnosis of CAD, it is generally used to determine whether mechanical revascularization (bypass or angioplasty) is possible and to guide this therapy.

▶ TREATMENT

The initial treatment of angina pectoris is usually medical. Goals of therapy are:

▲ to control symptoms

▲ to stop or limit the progression of disease

▲ to avoid myocardial injury (i.e., infarction)

Secondary prevention by removing or treating underlying risk factors for CAD is a key element in treatment. This includes:

▲ smoking cessation

▲ treatment of hyperlipidemia

▲ treatment of hypertension

▲ control of diabetes

▲ weight loss

▲ improvement in physical conditioning (through regular exercise)

▲ reduction of physical and emotional stress

Secondary prevention has been shown to limit progression and symptoms and reduce the risk of infarction and coronary death. Lipid management has been shown to result in partial resolution of atherosclerotic lesions.

The **drug therapy** of angina pectoris involves several classes of agents; **nitrates** (nitroglycerine, isosorbide dinitrate) are the most widely used agents. They act by causing **systemic venodilation,** which relieves cardiac workload by decreasing ventricular wall tension. They also cause coronary arterial dilation, increasing myocardial blood flow. They are used in sublingual form for relief of acute ischemia and also in long-acting form (via transdermal patches or slow release oral formulations) for limiting frequency and severity of attacks. Intravenous nitroglycerine can be used for severe acute attacks. **Side effects** (most prominent with sublingual and intravenous administration) are hypotension, lightheadedness, and headache.

Aspirin is given daily in CAD to limit platelet aggregation. Platelet activation and thrombosis can occur both as a result of acute atherosclerotic plaque rupture and statis due to vessel obstruction. **Beta-adrenergic blocking agents** (propranolol, metoprolol, atenolol, etc.) reduce myocardial workload by limiting adrenergic increases in heart rate and contractility. This effect is most prominent in the response to stress or exercise. The goal is to balance limitation of angina with the **side effects** of fatigue, impotence, bradycardia, and the development or worsening of heart failure. **Calcium channel antagonists** (diltiazem, verapamil, nifedipine, etc.) are coronary vasodilators. They also have variable peripheral vasodilatory and negative ionotropic/chronotropic activity.

The medical management of CAD involves careful titration of medicine based on monitoring of symptoms and side effects. For patients who are refractory to medical management alone, mechanical revascularization is an option. Consideration of this is generally done in consultation with a cardiologist and cardiac surgeon. Selection of which procedure (angioplasty or bypass surgery) is based on a number of variables:

▲ number of vessels involved

▲ coexisting illness

▲ patient age and functional status

▲ severity/nature of symptoms

▶ KEY POINTS

1. CAD is the leading cause of death in the United States.

2. The development of coronary atherosclerotic lesions is a stepwise process progressing from fatty streaks to lipid-filled fibrotic plaques.

3. Occlusive plaques limit coronary blood flow to areas of myocardium under conditions of increased demand leading to myocardial ischemia.

4. Myocardial ishemia generally manifests as exertional chest discomfort.

5. Treatment of myocardial ischemia involves reduction of cardiac work and increasing blood flow either through pharmacologic and/or mechanical interventions.

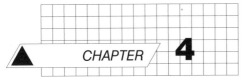

Myocardial Infarction

► EPIDEMIOLOGY

Acute myocardial infarction (AMI) is a common manifestation of coronary artery disease (CAD). Each year, approximately 1 million people suffer an AMI in the United States. Of these, about 10 to 15% will die within several days and another 10 to 15% will die within 1 year of an AMI.

► ETIOLOGY/PATHOGENESIS

Most myocardial infarctions occur in the setting of underlying CAD. The formation of an **atherosclerotic plaque** within a coronary artery is a multistep process (outlined in Chapter 3).

Spontaneous **fissuring and rupture** of a coronary atherosclerotic plaque may occur, exposing a highly thrombogenic surface. Platelet aggregation and fibrin formation result. If the resulting **thrombus** is large enough, it can cause complete occlusion of the coronary artery. Occlusion results in ischemia and eventually necrosis of the myocardium previously supplied by the occluded vessel. Necrosis occurs throughout the entire thickness of the affected area of myocardium. This results in a so-called **transmural** or **Q-wave infarction.**

A **non-Q-wave** or **subendocardial** infarction can occur as the result of transient occlusion with a thrombus, followed by spontaneous lysis before the occurrence of full-thickness myocardial death. It can also occur in the setting of vessel occlusion with extensive distal collateralization.

Although rupture of an atherosclerotic plaque with thrombus formation is responsible for most AMIs, there are other mechanisms by which coronary blood flow and/or oxygen supply can be acutely compromised, leading to myocardial ischemia and infarction:

▲ coronary artery dissection (often in the setting of a dissecting aortic aneurysm)

▲ coronary vasospasm (either idiopathic or drug induced, e.g., cocaine)

▲ in situ thrombus formation (in setting of a hypercoagulable state)

▲ coronary embolism

▲ vasculitis (e.g., Kawasaki's disease)

▲ carbon monoxide poisoning

Early death (within the first month) from AMI can be due to a number of complications:

▲ arrhythmias (ventricular fibrillation/tachycardia, complete heart block)

▲ heart failure (cardiogenic shock)

▲ ventricular rupture (peak incidence within 3 to 5 days of AMI)

▲ other mechanical complications (ventricular septal defect, mitral papillary rupture)

Death occuring more than 1 month after an AMI can be caused by reinfarction, progressive heart failure, or sudden arrhythmias.

► CLINICAL MANIFESTATIONS
History

Patients suffering an acute myocardial infarction will most often complain of **retrosternal chest pain.** The pain generally reaches a maximum over several minutes and then is prolonged and persistent. It may radiate to the back, neck, arms, or jaw. Administration of nitrates may provide some relief but generally not resolution of the pain. Other **associated symptoms** can include:

▲ diaphoresis

▲ anxiety

▲ dyspnea

▲ nausea

▲ vomiting

In some cases, patients will present shortly after an AMI with new onset heart failure (see Chapter 5).

Some patients may not present with chest pain. The elderly (particularly patients with dementia), diabetics, and postoperative patients (on analgesics) may not give a history of chest pain. These patients may present with nonspecific symptoms such as fatigue, syncope, or shortness of breath.

Physical Examination

The physical examination can be entirely normal in the setting of an AMI. A fourth heart sound (due to decreased compliance of the ischemic myocardium) is common. Certain findings can be suggestive of complications of the AMI:

▲ hypotension

▲ pulmonary edema

▲ confusion

▲ mitral regurgitation murmur (from papillary muscle dysfunction)

▶ DIFFERENTIAL DIAGNOSIS

For a detailed discussion of the differential diagnosis of chest pain, see Chapter 1. The important diseases to consider include:

▲ angina

▲ pulmonary embolism

▲ aortic dissection

▲ gastrointestinal disease (cholecystitis, esophageal spasm, pancreatitis)

In a patient with known CAD, especially one with chronic stable angina, the distinction between worsening ischemia (unstable angina) and an AMI is often difficult to make. The pain of an AMI is often described as more severe, unrelenting, not responsive to usual doses of nitrates, and more likely to be accompanied by associated symptoms (diaphoresis, dyspnea, etc.) than typical anginal pain.

▶ DIAGNOSTIC EVALUATION

The electrocardiogram (ECG) is important in the evaluation of possible AMI. It should be checked early in the evaluation and rechecked frequently during the workup. The typical **evolution of the ECG** in the setting of a Q-wave infarct is as follows:

1. Increase in amplitude of the T wave (first several minutes after vessel occlusion);
2. ST segment elevation (minutes to hours);
3. Development of Q waves (hours to days);
4. Resolution of ST segment elevation (hours to days).

In the setting of a non-Q-wave infarct, the ECG manifestations are more variable in the acute setting. Often there are only nonspecific ST- and T-wave changes (isolated ST depressions or elevations, inverted or flattened T waves). Hours after a non-Q-wave infarct, stable T-wave inversions in the affected region may develop.

The confirmation of myocardial infarction is generally done by **serial determinations of the serum creatine phosphokinase (CK)** and the CK-MB isoenzyme levels. The highest concentration of CK-MB is found in myocardium and is released by necrotic myocardial cells. Release of CK occurs within 3 hours and levels peak within 12 to 24 hours. Both an elevation in the absolute CK level and the percentage of CK-MB is required to make the diagnosis. The absolute elevation of CK provides an indirect estimate of infarct size, but this is dependent on a large number of variables, including reperfusion, cardioversion, and the performance of cardiac catheterization.

Cardiac echocardiography (both transthoracic and transesophageal) can reveal regional wall motion abnormalities indicative of ischemic or infarcted myocardium. It can also detect structural defects such as aneurysms, septal defects, pericardial effusions, valvular abnormalities, and mural thrombi. Assessments of segmental wall motion and global left ventricular function can also be made.

A **chest radiograph** can detect the presence of heart failure, cardiac enlargement, and other causes of chest pain such as pneumonia, aortic dissection, and pneumothorax.

Coronary angiography can identify the precise location of a thrombus and detect other atherosclerotic lesions. It is usually performed in the setting of AMI with the goal of mechanical revascularization (see below).

▶ TREATMENT

An AMI is a medical emergency. Prompt institution of therapy can limit the size of an infarct and preserve ventricular function postinfarct. The main **goals of therapy** are:

▲ relief of pain

▲ reduction of myocardial oxygen demand

▲ improvement/restoration of myocardial perfusion

▲ recognition and treatment of complications

When a patient presents with a possible AMI, the following steps should be taken:

1. Rapid clinical assessment with vital signs, history, and physical;
2. Obtain a 12-lead ECG and chest radiograph;
3. Administration of oxygen;
4. Institute pain treatment with nitrates and opiates (see below).

Relief of pain is an important initial intervention. It results in decreased adrenergic tone and thus decreases myocardial oxygen demand. Opiates, in particular morphine, are useful because they provide pain relief and anxiolysis and also improve hemodynamics by lowering heart rate and blood pressure. Oxygen administration can provide pain relief by increasing myocardial oxygen delivery and should be administered promptly.

A number of therapeutic agents have been shown to be useful for the acute treatment of myocardial infarction. Aspirin, presumably through its antiplatelet effects, has been shown to decrease mortality in AMI. Beta-adrenergic blocking agents lower myocardial oxygen consumption and have antiarrhythmic effects. They also have been shown to lower mortality. Bradycardia and hypotension are contraindications to their use. Nitrates (sublingual and intravenous nitroglycerine) can improve hemodynamics, reduce cardiac work, and improve myocardial oxygen delivery. Again, hypotension is of concern. Heparin is administered to prevent progression of thrombus and in the setting of thrombolysis (see below).

Other adjunctive agents are useful in selected instances, but their routine use is not generally accepted. Calcium-channel antagonists may lower the incidence of reinfarction in the setting of a non-Q-wave myocardial infarction. A number of studies have failed to show a clear benefit for their use in transmural infarcts. In fact, there is some evidence that their use is contraindicated in the setting of extensive, anterior wall, transmural infarctions. Lidocaine was previously given prophylactically to all patients with AMI but was subsequently shown to increase mortality. However, in patients who present with ventricular fibrillation/tachycardia or have frequent or multiform premature ventricular complexes, it can be useful.

Patients who have continued pain after the administration of oxygen, aspirin, nitrates, opiates, and beta-blockers and who have continued ST segment elevation should be considered for thrombolytic therapy with tissue plasminogen activator or streptokinase. Clinically, both have been shown to decrease mortality and preserve left ventricular function after myocardial infarction.

Studies have shown that the earlier that thrombolytic therapy is given after the onset of chest pain in AMI, the greater the benefit. After several hours, the benefits fall off, but some physicians treat patients up to 24 hours after the onset of pain, particularly if the pain has been of a stuttering nature.

The major toxicity of thrombolytic therapy is bleeding; therefore, absolute contraindications to thrombolytic therapy include:

▲ uncontrolled hypertension on intravenous vasodilators (systolic > 180)

▲ recent stroke

▲ recent major surgery

▲ active gastrointestinal bleeding

▲ concurrent trauma

▲ intracranial mass

Some patients with an acute myocardial infarction who are not candidates for thrombolysis can be treated by primary percutaneous transluminal coronary angioplasty (PTCA). There is evidence that prompt primary PTCA is at least as effective as thrombolysis and may be associated with fewer complications and shorter hospitalizations. Prompt access to the available facilities limits how many patients with AMI can be treated in this manner. PTCA can also be used in the setting of unsuccessful thrombolysis, so-called rescue PTCA.

Once therapy for an AMI has been initiated, including pharmacologic or mechanical revascularization, the patient will require close monitoring in an intensive care unit setting. Monitoring for and treating complications (arrhythmias, heart failure, mechanical complications) are the main priority. Two to 3 days after an uncomplicated AMI, patients can be transferred to a less acute care setting.

Initiation of therapy with angiotensin-converting enzyme inhibitors within the first several days after an AMI has been shown to decrease mortality and morbidity (mainly decreased incidence of heart failure). This is particularly true in patients who have a depressed ejection fraction.

One week after an uncomplicated AMI, patients will usually undergo a symptom-limited submaximal exercise test (see Chapter 3). This is done to look for areas of residual ischemia that could prompt coronary angiography and mechanical intervention. Results help predict prognosis. In addition, this exercise test can provide important psychological benefit for the patient.

After discharge, patients gradually increase activity over 6 weeks, avoiding maximal activity. Enrollment in a cardiac rehabilitation program and counseling can help guide activity levels. Six to 8 weeks after the AMI, the patient undergoes a maximal exercise test before resuming normal activities.

During the period of recuperation, attention is paid to identification and modification of risk factors. Smoking cessation, weight loss, lipid reduction, and exercise are all considered. Again, formal patient education is important in this intervention.

▶ KEY POINTS

1. Myocardial infarctions are a major cause of morbidity and mortality in patients with CAD.

2. Infarction generally occurs by occlusion of a coronary artery by a thrombus that forms as a result of the spontaneous rupture of a preexisting atherosclerotic plaque.

3. Most patients present with substernal chest pain. ECG is critical in initial evaluation and measurement of serial serum CK levels is used to confirm the diagnosis.

4. A number of therapeutic agents including aspirin, beta-adrenergic blocking agents, nitrates, oxygen, and thrombolytics are used in treatment. Major goals of early therapy are pain relief, reduction of myocardial oxygen demand, and improvement of myocardial perfusion.

5. Postmyocardial infarct therapy involves monitoring for complications, institution of secondary prevention, assessment/treatment of residual atherosclerotic disease, and physical rehabilitation.

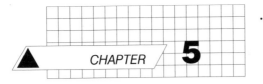

CHAPTER 5

Heart Failure

$\mathcal{H}$eart failure can be defined as the inability of the heart to pump blood at a rate that meets metabolic demands. Heart failure can be **classified** according to:

▲ the hemodynamic state of the cardiovascular system (congestive versus high output)

▲ the predominance of the ventricle affected (left versus right)

▲ the predominant form of myocardial dysfunction (systolic or diastolic)

▲ the time course (acute or chronic)

Various combinations can exist such as chronic congestive left-sided failure.

▶ EPIDEMIOLOGY

The overall prevalence of heart failure in the United States is 1% but approaches 10% among persons older than 70 years of age. About a half million individuals are diagnosed with heart failure each year.

The overall 5-year mortality is 60% for men and 45% for women. When considering patients with the greatest degree of heart failure (i.e., those with symptoms at rest), the 1-year mortality approaches 50%. The major **risk factors** for developing congestive heart failure (CHF) are:

▲ hypertension

▲ coronary artery disease (CAD)

▲ valvular heart disease

▲ pericardial disease

▲ cardiomyopathy (infiltrative, e.g., amyloid; toxic, e.g., drugs; idiopathic)

In the United States, 50 to 75% of individuals with CHF have it on the basis of CAD.

▶ PATHOPHYSIOLOGY

Cardiac output is determined by an interrelationship between three variables that reflect the state of both the heart and the rest of the circulatory system: preload, contractility, and afterload. **Preload** (also referred to as the left-ventricular end-diastolic pressure [LVEDP] or the left ventricular filling pressure) is defined as the pressure that is required to distend the ventricle a given end-diastolic volume. The relationship between pressure and volume defines the compliance of the ventricle.

Contractility refers to the stroke work that the heart will generate at a given preload. As such, it describes the **functional state** of the myocardium. Normally, as preload is increased, the stroke work that is generated also increases. The relationship between these two variables defines the **Frank-Starling law of the heart** and can be graphically displayed by plotting LVEDP against stroke work. The curve generated describes the **inotropic state** of the heart.

Afterload is the dynamic resistance against which the heart contracts. It is generally reflected in the systolic blood pressure, which is the most clinically useful measure of afterload.

Systolic dysfunction describes the situation where the inability to meet the required cardiac output is due to an inability of the myocardium to generate sufficient work. As such, this is a reflection of **decreased contractility** or a **lowered inotropic state.** This can be due to loss of viable myocardium attributable to myocardial infarction or dysfunction of the individual myofibrils attributable to conditions such as myocarditis and ischemia.

For a given level of preload, a decrease in inotropic state (or an increase in afterload) will result in a decrease in ventricular function, which can be measured clinically as a decrease in ejection fraction. Decreases in ejection fraction increase the end-diastolic volume, which in turn results in an increase in the end-diastolic pressure (i.e., the preload) and restoration of ventricular function. There is a limit to which preload can increase to compensate for decreased inotropy or increased afterload. Once the preload exceeds the pulmonary capillary oncotic pressure, fluid will pass into the alveolar space resulting in pulmonary congestion.

In the face of falling cardiac output, a number of **extracardiac responses** are seen, including **activation of the renin-angiotensin system** and the **sympathetic nervous system.** These result in systemic vasoconstriction and increased afterload, which further impair systolic function in a vicious cycle.

Another compensatory change is the **accumulation of salt and water.** The expansion of the intravascular volume increases preload. This excess fluid tends to leak from the intravascular space into the intracellular spaces, resulting in conditions such as peripheral edema.

In **diastolic dysfunction,** the main abnormality is a **decrease in the compliance** of the ventricle. In contrast to systolic dysfunction, **contractile function is usually normal** or even increased in compensatory fashion.

Decreased compliance can be due to abnormalities in the active relaxation of the myocardium during diastole or abnormalities in the elastic properties of the heart itself (or surrounding tissues). Conditions that cause these abnormalities include:

▲ hypertension (resulting in concentric hypertrophy that can slow relaxation and increase passive chamber stiffness)

▲ amyloidosis, hemochromatosis (infiltrative cardiomyopathies that increase passive chamber stiffness)

▲ hypertrophic cardiomyopathy (a familial condition associated with idiopathic hypertrophy of the myocardium)

▲ myocardial ischemia (acutely interferes with relaxation and over the long term can increase passive chamber stiffness)

Decreased compliance results in a higher than normal LVEDP for a given end-diastolic volume. This higher pressure in turn is transmitted across the pulmonary capillaries. If an increased demand is placed on the heart, for example, during exercise, still higher pressures are required to produce the greater ventricular filling necessary to meet the increased output demand. As with systolic dysfunction, once the filling pressures exceed the oncotic pressure of the pulmonary capillaries, fluid will move into the alveolar space, and again pulmonary congestion results.

As compared with systolic dysfunction, avid salt and water retention and prominent vasoconstriction is not commonly encountered in pure diastolic dysfunction.

▶ CLINICAL MANIFESTATIONS
History

Most **symptoms** due to heart failure are pulmonary in nature due to increased LVEDP that result in pulmonary venous and capillary congestion, including:

▲ dyspnea (uncomfortable breathing that initially occurs with exertion but then also at rest)

▲ orthopnea (dyspnea in the recumbent position)

▲ paroxysmal nocturnal dyspnea (sudden onset of dyspnea usually occurring about 2 to 3 hours after falling asleep in the recumbent position)

▲ cough

▲ wheezing

Other symptoms can be due to systemic fluid overload (peripheral edema, weight gain), long-standing low cardiac output (fatigue), and underlying cardiac pathology (chest pain).

Physical Examination

Physical findings generally appear once compensatory mechanisms begin to fail and significant pulmonary congestion arises. They can also give clues as to whether systolic or diastolic failure is present. Cardiovascular findings include:

▲ laterally displaced and/or enlarged point of maximal impulse (more in systolic dysfunction)

▲ ventricular heave

▲ sinus tachycardia

▲ accentuated second heart sound (due to pulmonary hypertension)

▲ third heart sound (systolic dysfunction)

▲ fourth heart sound (hypertension and diastolic dysfunction)

▲ jugular venous distention

Pulmonary findings include:

▲ fine pitched inspiratory crackles ("rales")

▲ dullness at bases (due to the presence of pleural effusions)

Peripheral findings include:

▲ pitting edema

▲ ascites

▲ hepatic congestion

▲ cyanosis

▶ DIFFERENTIAL DIAGNOSIS

In a patient with known cardiovascular disease, the diagnosis of heart failure is generally made clinically. Other possible etiologies of the presenting symptoms include:

▲ pneumonia/bronchitis

▲ pulmonary embolism

▲ acute myocardial infarction (which may present with subsequent heart failure)

▲ myocarditis

▶ DIAGNOSTIC EVALUATION

The presumptive diagnosis of heart failure can be confirmed by a number of invasive and noninvasive tests, including the chest radiograph (enlarged cardiac silhouette, pulmonary edema-manifested as Kerley B lines, pleural effusions); intravascular pressure measurements, usually through use of pulmonary artery catheter (elevated pulmonary capillary wedge pressure, elevated pulmonary artery pressures, elevated central venous pressure); and echocardiography (to assess valve function and overall ventricular function).

Echocardiography is useful in determining whether systolic or diastolic dysfunction predominates. In systolic dysfunction, echocardiography will reveal a decreased ejection fraction and cardiomegaly. In diastolic dysfunction, ejection fraction will generally be normal, and ventricular wall thickening without dilatation will be present.

▶ TREATMENT

A patient may present with both systolic and diastolic dysfunction or primarily with one or the other. The clinical picture is similar, but treatment can differ between the two, making it important to determine whether one or the other process predominates.

Given the pathophysiology of systolic dysfunction, therapy can be divided into:

▲ control of the accumulation of salt and water

▲ reduction of cardiac workload

▲ augmentation of cardiac contractility

Regulation of salt and water should begin by closely monitoring dietary sodium intake. With mild CHF, dietary sodium restriction (to less than 2 or 3g/day) will often result in significant improvement in symptoms. This level of reduction can be achieved by avoiding salt-rich foods and not adding salt after food preparation. In more severe cases of CHF, sodium should be restricted to less than 1g, which requires significant alteration of diet (often difficult to do while maintaining palatability). Water intake does not need to be restricted except in the most severe cases of CHF, where impaired excretion of water results in hyponatremia.

When sodium restriction alone proves insufficient, the next step is the addition of a **diuretic.** There are a variety of diuretic agents, differing in site of action and relative potency: thiazides (hydrochlorothiazide, chlorothiazide) inhibit sodium and chloride reabsorption in the distal convoluted tubule and are of modest potency; loop diuretics (furosemide, bumetanide, ethacrynic acid) inhibit sodium, potassium, and chloride reabsorption in the thick ascending limb of the loop of Henle and are the most potent; and spironolactone, a competitive inhibitor of aldactone, which blocks sodium/hydrogen exchange and sodium/potassium exchange in the distal tubules and collecting ducts. It is low in potency, but unlike the other two classes does not cause renal potassium loss.

Generally, thiazides are prescribed initially, and if not sufficient, a loop diuretic is substituted or added. Spironolactone is generally not used alone but added to the others where it may potentiate their actions. Diuretic therapy is titrated to eliminate excess fluid, but because fluid retention is part of a compensation for decreased systolic function, care must be taken not to remove too much fluid.

Reduction of cardiac work can be accomplished by reduction of physical activity and emotional stress. Additionally, pharmacologic **reduction of afterload** with vasodilators will further reduce cardiac work. **Vasodilators** fall into several classes:

1. Angiotensin-converting enzyme (ACE) inhibitors (lisinopril, captopril, enalapril, and others) cause both arterial and venous dilation;

2. Hydralazine and prazosin are primarily arterial vasodilators;

3. Nitrates (nitroglycerine, isosorbide dinitrate) are primarily venodilators. Nitrates also have the added benefit of limiting ischemia due to coronary artery disease, itself a major cause of systolic failure;

4. Calcium channel blockers (nifedipine, verapamil, diltiazem, and others) are peripheral arterial dilators. Their routine use in heart failure has been questioned because of a negative ionotropic effect that can have a deleterious effect in heart failure.

For treatment of acute decompensation of CHF, intravenous medicines such as nitroglycerin are useful. For long-term outpatient treatment, oral drugs such as ACE inhibitors are commonly used. ACE inhibitors have been shown to reduce the rate of progression of systolic dysfunction and to improve survival.

The final class of therapeutic agents that are commonly used in the treatment of CHF are drugs that augment cardiac contractility (**ionotropic agents**). The **cardiac glycosides** (e.g., digitalis) are agents that inhibit the cardiac muscle Na/K ATPase and subsequently elevate intracellular Ca levels, which results in an increase in contractility. Digitalis is generally used in the treatment of outpatient CHF because it is an oral medicine. The therapeutic index of digitalis is small, however, requiring monitoring of levels. The signs and symptoms of **digitalis toxicity** are both cardiac and noncardiac:

▲ anorexia

▲ nausea

▲ vomiting

▲ mental status changes (generally with chronically elevated levels)

▲ altered visual perception (generally a yellow tint)

▲ cardiac rhythm disturbances (premature ventricular beats, atrioventricular block of varying degrees, paroxysmal and nonparoxysmal atrial tachycardia)

Of the various sympathomimetic amines, the ones that have the most use in the treatment of CHF are **dobutamine** and **dopamine**. Dopamine in lower doses (1–2 μg/kg/min) can dilate renal and mesenteric blood vessels, which can aid in the action of diuretics. At higher levels, stimulation of the myocardial beta receptors (resulting in increased contractility) and eventually the alpha-adrenergic receptors occurs. The latter may be deleterious because it results in elevation of arterial resistance and thus afterload. Dobutamine (via stimulation of mostly beta$_1$ and beta$_2$ with some alpha receptor activity) increases cardiac contractility and produces peripheral vasodilatation, both of which can improve myocardial function.

The main disadvantages of these two drugs are that they require continuous intravenous infusion and that tachyphylaxis (loss of responsiveness) occurs, probably due to down regulation of the adrenergic receptors. Their main utility is in managing acute exacerbations of heart failure.

The therapy of **diastolic dysfunction** is limited. Because systolic function is generally preserved, inotropic agents are not required. Decreases in afterload do not result in a significant increase in cardiac output. Salt and water elimination may relieve symptoms due to pulmonary congestion, but because the noncompliant ventricle is dependent on increased preload for filling, aggressive diuresis can result in a major decrease in cardiac output.

Given the pathophysiology of diastolic dysfunction, therapy needs to be directed at improving the relaxation characteristic of the ventricle. Unfortunately, there are only limited therapeutic options. Calcium-channel blockers can, in some patients, increase the compliance of the ventricle by facilitating the active relaxation of the myocardium. They have little effect on conditions where the primary abnormality is an increase in passive chamber stiffness. Beta blockers and other agents that slow the heart rate can help by prolonging diastole, allowing improved ventricular filling.

Diastolic dysfunction often appears in patients with long-standing hypertension. Control of hypertension may result in some resolution of ventricular hypertrophy over time, improving diastolic filling. The available clinical data is limited at this time, however.

Overall, treatment of symptoms in diastolic dysfunction is more problematic. The afterload and preload reduction that is the cornerstone of the management of symptoms in systolic dysfunction often serves to exacerbate problems in diastolic dysfunction.

The long-term treatment of patients with heart failure involves monitoring changes in cardiac function and adjusting therapy as necessary. It is important to note that clinical deterioration can indicate a worsening of the underlying condition (e.g., worsening of coronary artery disease) and can also be a sign of a complication of therapy (e.g., digitalis toxicity or overdiuresis and resultant hypovolemia). Careful revaluation is required.

Many patients with systolic dysfunction progress to the point that outpatient treatment with diuretics, vasodilators, and cardiac glycosides fails. Hospitalization with more aggressive volume treatment and the use of more powerful intravenous vasodilators and ionotropic agents may allow for enough recovery of the myocardium that outpatient treatment can be resumed.

Patients who continually fail maximal outpatient medical treatment and continue to have severe symptoms at rest can be considered for referral to centers that offer cardiac transplantation. Given the shortage of organs and the commitment for continued aggressive medical monitoring and treatment, this is an option for only a few patients with advanced systolic heart failure.

As noted earlier, patients with refractory diastolic dysfunction have few therapeutic options.

► KEY POINTS

1. Heart failure is the inability of the heart to pump blood at a rate that can meet metabolic demands.

2. Heart failure can be on the basis of systolic dysfunction where there is an abnormality in the force generation (contractility) of the myocardium or diastolic dysfunction where there is decreased ventricular compliance.

3. Most symptoms of heart failure are related to increased left ventricular end-diastolic pressures and are pulmonary in nature.

4. The treatment of systolic heart failure involves regulation of fluid and electrolyte accumulation, reduction of cardiac workload, and augmentation of cardiac contractility.

5. The treatment of diastolic heart failure is limited to trying to improve the diastolic filling of the ventricle. Unfortunately, there are few therapeutic maneuvers that are able to accomplish this.

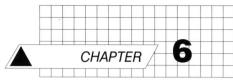

CHAPTER 6

Bradyarrhythmias

The normal pacemaker of the heart is the **sino-atrial node,** located in the right atrium. Its impulse conducts through the atria to the **atrioventricular (AV) node,** where the electrical impulse is normally slowed (0.12 to 0.20 seconds). The impulse then travels to the **bundle of His,** which branches into three separate bundles (right, left anterior, left posterior). The sinus node normally generates 60 to 100 impulses per minute. This rate may be increased by sympathetic stimulation or decreased by cholinergic (vagal) stimulation.

Bradyarrhythmias, or abnormally slow heart rates, are generally defined as heart rates less than 60 beats per minute (bpm) that are also symptomatic. A slow heart rate itself is not necessarily a concern; many professional athletes have heart rates in the 40 bpm range without any difficulty or evidence of disease. In general, bradyarrhythmias arise by one of two mechanisms:

▲ impulse formation

▲ conduction

▶ ETIOLOGY

Bradyarrhythmias may arise from a specific cardiac disease or as a general response to systemic disease, resulting in a delay in impulse formation or conduction. **Systemic causes** include:

▲ hypoxia

▲ increased intracranial pressure

▲ hypothermia

▲ hypothyroidism

Cardiac diseases associated with bradyarrhythmias are infiltrative heart disease (sarcoid, amyloid), degenerative disease of the cardiac conduction system, ischemic heart disease, Lyme disease, and rheumatic heart disease.

Degenerative disease of the conduction system is seen most often in the elderly. It may be isolated to the conduction system (Lenegre's disease) or represent generalized calcification of the cardiac skeleton, that includes aortic and mitral valve involvement (Lev's disease).

Commonly used cardiac drugs slow cardiac conduction and may result in bradyarrhythmias:

▲ beta blockers

▲ calcium channel blockers

▲ digoxin

▶ CLINICAL MANIFESTATIONS

History

The presence of symptoms with an associated bradyarrhythmia often determines the extent of treatment. Symptoms, which may be the result of cardiac or central nervous system hypoperfusion, include:

▲ syncope

▲ near syncope or light-headedness

▲ congestive heart failure

▲ angina pectoris

Nonspecific symptoms, such as fatigue, must not be overinterpreted in the setting of bradycardia.

Physical Examination

Vital signs determine the severity of the bradyarrhythmia and assist in identifying the cause. Hypotension (systolic blood pressure < 90) is evidence of hemodynamic instability and requires emergency treatment when associated with symptoms.

▶ DIFFERENTIAL DIAGNOSIS

The differential diagnosis of a bradyarrhythmia may be classified by the regularity of the heart rate. Regular rate:

▲ sinus bradycardia

▲ complete heart block

▲ sinus arrest with escape rhythm

▲ "regularized" slow atrial fibrillation

Irregular rate

▲ sick sinus syndrome (sinus node dysfunction)

▲ second degree AV block (first or second degree)

▲ slow atrial fibrillation

▶ DIAGNOSTIC EVALUATION

An **electrocardiogram** is the first diagnostic test. One should first look for the presence of P waves. The absence of a P wave may indicate **incomplete SA block.**

The entire PQRST complex is usually absent (Fig. 6-1). Complete absence of P waves may be seen in atrial fibrillation or sinus arrest. In **regularized atrial fibrillation,** complete heart block is present at the AV node and a lower pacemaker begins to fire (resulting in a rate of 40 to 60 bpm). This particular rhythm is seen in digoxin toxicity. This pattern of absent P waves with a regular escape rhythm (junctional or ventricular) is also seen in sinus arrest. Uncontrolled atrial fibrillation usually results in irregular heart rates of 80 to 140 bpm, but intrinsic AV node disease or nodal agents (beta blockers, calcium channel blockers) may slow the rate to 40 to 60 bpm.

The PR interval should be measured for each beat. In second degree AV block, a QRS complex fails to follow a P wave. In **type I (Wenckebach) second degree block,** the PR intervals progressively lengthen each beat before a P wave fails to conduct (Fig. 6-2). This usually represents AV nodal disease. In **type II second degree block,** the dropped beat occurs suddenly without warning, signifying infranodal disease (Fig. 6-3). Type II block has a higher risk of progression to complete heart block than type I block. If there is no relationship between the P waves and the QRS complex (variable PR interval), then **complete heart block** is likely to be present (Fig. 6-4). P waves, firing at a certain rate, fail to conduct to the ventricles and a slower pacemaker begins to fire. Both atrial and ventricular rates are regular but are unrelated to each other.

▶ TREATMENT

Treatment of the bradyarrhythmias consists of treating the underlying cause, if possible (ischemia, infection, drugs, metabolic causes), and correcting the rhythm with medication or extrinsic pacemaker. In treating the underlying cause, patients with evidence of cardiac ischemia should be treated with appropriate medications. Drugs that increase AV nodal block should be discontinued, and a digoxin level obtained in patients taking this medication. If hemodynamically stable (normal blood pressure, no congestive heart failure or central nervous system dysfunction), patients may be observed for resolution of the bradyarrhythmia.

Emergent treatment with atropine is indicated in the patient with:

▲ bradycardia causing hypotension

▲ congestive heart failure

▲ syncope

Atropine 0.5 mg should be given in emergent situations (see above). The drug may be given intravenously or delivered through an endotracheal tube. It is most effective in bradyarrhythmias caused by increased vagal tone.

Pacemakers may be either temporary or permanent. If the aggravating factor is reversible (e.g., cardiac ischemia), then a temporary pacemaker may be inserted. Permanent pacemakers are used for patients who have degenerative conduction disease that will not improve.

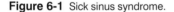

Figure 6-1 Sick sinus syndrome.

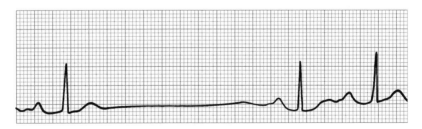

Figure 6-2 Type I second degree block.

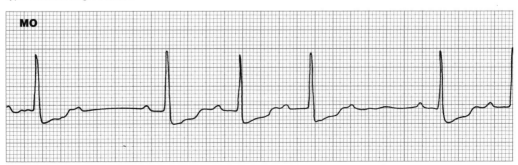

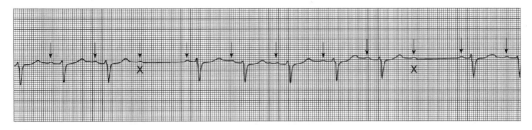

Figure 6-3 Type II second degree block.

The indications for a pacemaker are often debated. The more accepted indications for pacemaker placement include:

▲ complete heart block with symptoms

▲ sinus node dysfunction with symptoms

▲ bifasicular block within intermittent type II second degree AV block

Other indications for a pacemaker are situation dependent. For example, type II second degree AV block in the setting of an **anterior myocardial infarction** generally requires a pacemaker because progression to CHB is common.

Pacemakers are **not indicated** for asymptomatic type I second degree AV block or asymptomatic sinus node dysfunction.

Patients with asymptomatic bradyarrhythmias should avoid drugs that may exacerbate the condition. Patients who develop symptoms should be considered

for a pacemaker. Some patients may benefit from electrophysiologic studies (EPS) to determine whether the conduction disturbance is at or below the AV node. These patients include those with 2:1 AV block (Fig. 6-5), where it is impossible to classify the disturbance as type I or type II. Syncope with bundle branch block and complete heart block are other conditions that may benefit from EPS.

▶ KEY POINTS

1. A bradyarrhythmia is defined by the heart rate (<60) and the hemodynamic consequences (symptoms, hypotension).

2. Digoxin toxicity should be considered in patients presenting with atrial fibrillation and a regular ventricular response.

3. Type I second degree block has progressively increasing PR intervals before a dropped QRS complex. This block often represents underlying AV nodal disease.

4. Pacemakers should not be inserted in patients with asymptomatic sinus node dysfunction.

Figure 6-4 Complete AV block.

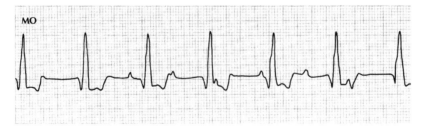

Figure 6-5 Patients with 2:1 AV block.

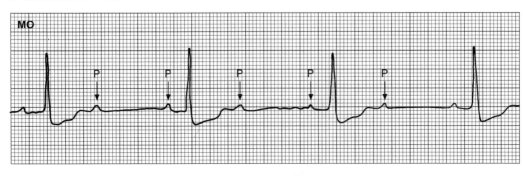

CHAPTER 7

Tachyarrhythmias

7achyarrhythmias are defined as heart rates exceeding 100 beats per minute (bpm). These rhythm disturbances are best divided into narrow complex tachycardias (QRS duration < 0.10 seconds) and wide complex tachycardias. This classification determines the treatment approach.

▶ ETIOLOGY

Two mechanisms explain tachyarrhythmias: impulse formation (enhanced automaticity or triggered activity) and impulse propagation (re-entry). **Re-entry** is considered to be the most common cause of tachyarrhythmias. The re-entry loop requires two paths with different conduction speeds and different recovery periods. The impulse is blocked in one arm of the loop, descends the other arm, and then returns up the loop in a retrograde fashion (Fig. 7-1). Treatments to interrupt this re-entry loop terminate the tachycardia abruptly.

Tachycardias may arise from the atria, ventricles, or atrioventricular (AV) node (junctional). The different types of tachycardias are discussed below. Two tachycardias with unique features are discussed here.

AV re-entrant tachycardia with an accessory pathway has a re-entrant loop with the AV node as one arm and an accessory pathway between atria and ventricles as the other arm. The most common type of accessory pathway can conduct both anterograde and retrograde, which results in a pre-excitation pattern on the electrocardiogram (ECG) (Fig. 7-2). This tachycardia is called the Wolff-Parkinson-White (WPW) syndrome. The term WPW will be used in place of AV re-entrant tachycardia throughout the chapter.

Torsades de pointes (French for "twisting of the points") is a polymorphic ventricular tachycardia. It has a characteristic appearance (Fig. 7-3) and may spontaneously stop or progress to ventricular fibrillation. Torsades is almost always associated with a prolonged QT interval. **Causes of prolonged QT interval** are:

▲ type IA and III antiarrhythmics (Table 7-1)

▲ phenothiazines

▲ tricyclic antidepressants

▲ hypokalemia

▲ hypomagnesemia

▲ hypocalcemia

▶ RISK FACTORS

Atrial fibrillation may be seen in the patient with:

▲ hyperthyroidism

▲ mitral valve stenosis or insufficiency

▲ hypertension

Nonparoxysmal junctional tachycardia is associated with:

▲ digitalis toxicity

▲ inferior myocardial infarction

▲ myocarditis

▲ mitral valve surgery

Paroxysmal atrial tachycardia with 2:1 block is most commonly caused by digitalis toxicity. **Multifocal atrial tachycardia** often occurs in the patients with an exacerbation of chronic obstructive pulmonary disease.

Figure 7-1 Mechanism of re-entry.

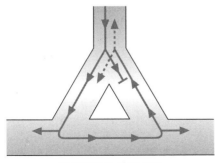

Mechanism of reentry

TABLE 7-1		
Examples of Antiarrhythmics		
Type IA	Type IC	Type III
Procainamide	Flecainide	Sotalol
Quinidine	Encainide	Amiodarone
Disopyramide	Propafenone	

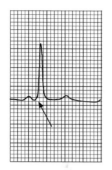

Figure 7-2 Wolff-Parkinson-White syndrome (arrow pointing to Delta wave).

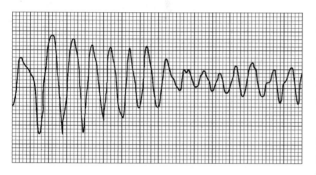

Figure 7-3 Torsades de pointes.

▶ CLINICAL MANIFESTATIONS
History

The patient wth a tachyarrhythmia usually presents with:

▲ dizziness or syncope

▲ palpitations

▲ diaphoresis

These symptoms are not specific for a particular etiology and therefore do not help to distinguish the cause.

Physical Examination

Blood pressure should be measured immediately. **Hypotension** indicates hemodynamic instability and requires prompt electrical cardioversion (except in sinus tachycardia, which will not respond). **Signs of AV dissociation,** cannon A waves and variable first heart sounds, may help identify ventricular tachycardia; AV dissociation is rarely present in supraventricular tachycardias.

DIFFERENTIAL DIAGNOSIS

The differential is categorized by width of the QRS on ECG and regularity of the rhythm (classification used in the diagnosis section as well).

Regular narrow complex tachycardia

▲ sinus tachycardia

▲ atrial tachycardia

▲ AV nodal re-entrant tachycardia

▲ WPW syndrome

▲ atrial flutter

▲ junctional tachycardia

Irregular narrow complex tachycardia

▲ atrial fibrillation

▲ multilocal atrial tachycardia

▲ atrial flutter with variable block

Wide complex tachycardia

▲ ventricular tachycardia (VT)

▲ torsades de pointes

▲ supraventricular tachycardia (SVT) with aberrant conduction

▶ DIAGNOSTIC EVALUATION
Electrocardiogram
Regular Narrow Complex Tachycardia

Once the tachyarrythmia is classified as regular narrow complex, the **P waves** should be identified if possible. P waves that **precede** the QRS complex are seen in sinus tachycardia and atrial tachycardia. P waves **will not be visible** or **will follow** the QRS complex in AV nodal re-entrant tachycardia (AVNRT), WPW syndrome, and junctional tachycardia. The P waves of atrial flutter are described as "sawtooth," are seen best in leads VII and II, and occur at a rate of 250 to 350 bpm (Figure 7-4).

When tachycardia is not present, the ECG in WPW shows a short PR interval (<0.12 seconds) and a delta wave, an upward deflection immediately before the QRS complex (see Fig. 7-2).

Irregular Narrow Complex Tachycardia

This tachycardia also) requires identifying the P waves. Flutter waves, at 300 bpm, may be conducted with

Figure 7-2 Atrial flutter

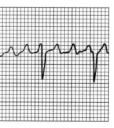

variable (3:1 or 4:1) AV block. **P waves of three different morphologies** defines multifocal atrial tachycardia. Absence of P waves with an irregular ventricular response is consistent with atrial fibrillation.

Wide Complex Tachycardia

The appearance of torsades de pointes is characteristic and associated with hemodynamic instability if prolonged. Differentiating between VT and SVT with aberrancy is difficult, and several rules have been developed to distinguish the two tachycardias (not discussed here). The presence of AV dissociation on ECG (P waves with no relation to QRS complex) is diagnostic for VT. In the patient with known heart disease, the rhythm is most often VT. In general, it is best to err on the side of treating for VT when in doubt.

Other Laboratory Studies

Underlying exacerbating conditions, such as **hypokalemia** or **hypomagnesemia**, should be excluded. A **digoxin level** should be ordered for patients taking this drug, especially when the rhythm is atrial tachycardia with 2:1 block or nonparoxysmal junctional tachycardia. **Thyroid-stimulating hormone** may be sent in patients with AF to exclude hyperthyroidism.

▶ TREATMENT

Synchronized countershock is indicated in all patients who are unstable (hypotension, congestive heart failure, chest pain, decreased level of consciousness). For regular rhythms (atrial flutter, AVNRT), 50 joules is the appropriate level of energy. For AF and VT with a pulse, the starting level is 100 joules. The exception to use of cardioversion is torsades de pointes, where **external pacing** to override the rhythm is the treatment of choice.

Vagal maneuvers include Valsalva maneuver and carotid artery massage. By blocking AV conduction, they unmask or terminate many supraventricular tachycardias. It is generally recommend to try vagal maneuvers in SVT before pharmacotherapy if the patient is stable.

Adenosine (see below) is often used as a diagnostic (and therapeutic) agent for narrow complex tachycardias. Tachycardias that use a re-entry mechanism through the AV node (AVNRT, WPW) will be abruptly terminated by adenosine. Temporary nodal blockade may also reveal the "sawtooth waves" of atrial flutter that were obscured by the rapid ventricular rate. Adenosine has a short duration of action (15 to 30 seconds), which makes it a useful drug. It also terminates re-entrant tachycardias (AVNRT, WPW). It has no effect on atrial or sinus tachycardia. The initial dose is 6 mg.

AV nodal agents slow conduction through the AV node and are useful in atrial flutter and fibrillation. Drugs in this class include:

▲ beta blockers (propranolol, metoprolol)
▲ calcium channel blockers (verapamil, diltiazem)
▲ digoxin

These drugs are initially given intravenously to slow rapid heart rates associated with atrial tachycardia, flutter, and fibrillation. Verapamil is probably the most effective at slowing the ventricular rate, although it may be associated with hypotension.

Lidocaine is the drug of choice for VT, initially given as a bolus (1 mg/kg), followed by an infusion of 1–4 mg/min. Side effects include confusion and seizures.

Magnesium is given for torsades de pointes, especially drug-induced. Dose is 1 g $MgSO_4$ IV.

▶ TREATMENT

Sinus tachycardia, multifocal atrial tachycardia, and junctional tachycardia are managed long term by correcting the underlying disease. Conditions that may require drug or interventional treatments are listed below.

Atrial Fibrillation

Atrial fibrillation (AF) may be converted to sinus rhythm by electrical cardioversion, type IA or type III agents. Unfortunately, many patients do not remain in sinus rhythm. Increased left atrial size (> 50 mm) and long duration of atrial fibrillation are predictors of relapse. There is also a concern that some antiarrhythmics (like quinidine) may actually increase mortality.

Anticoagulation with warfarin should be considered for all patients with atrial fibrillation to prevent embolic stroke (except patients < 60 years old with no other medical problems). An international normalized ratio of 2 to 3 should be the goal of treatment. The risk of stroke appears to be the same in paroxysmal AF and chronic AF.

Atrial Flutter

Atrial flutter is treated like atrial fibrillation in regards to cardioversion and rate control. However, the risk of embolic stoke appears to be less, and anticoagulation is of uncertain benefit.

Supraventricular Re-entrant Tachycardias

Patients with AVNRT or WPW may be treated with catheter ablation of one arm of the re-entrant loop.

This option may be best for young patients with recurrent symptoms to avoid lifelong drug therapy. Catheter ablation is successful about 90% of the time, although complications such as induced AV block or thromboembolism may occur in rare instances.

Drug treatment to slow AV nodal conduction may be used in AVNRT to prevent recurrence. Drugs used are listed above under AV nodal agents. These drugs, especially digoxin, may **accelerate conduction** in the accessory pathway in patients with WPW and should be avoided or used with caution. Type IA or IC drugs are better choices in these patients.

Ventricular Tachycardia

Ischemic heart disease often is the underlying cause of nonsustained VT (NSVT) and should be appropriately treated. The long-term treatment of NSVT (< 30 seconds of VT) remains controversial, although patients with decreased cardiac ejection fraction and NSVT are at higher risk for sudden death. Beta blockers are often advocated, as well as type III drugs.

Patients with hemodynamic compromise from VT need further evaluation and drug treatment. These patients often undergo electrophysiologic studies, which guide treatment.

▶ KEY POINTS

1. Digitalis toxicity can lead to paroxysmal atrial tachycardia with 2:1 block or nonparoxysmal junctional tachycardia.

2. The WPW syndrome is characterized by a short PR interval, delta wave, and a narrow complex tachycardia.

3. Torsade de pointes is a multifocal ventricular tachycardia, associated with a long QT interval. Treatment is overdrive pacing and magnesium.

4. Adenosine is the drug of choice to treat regular narrow complex tachycardias after vagal maneuvers have been unsuccessful.

5. Patients with long-term atrial fibrillation should be anticoagulated with warfarin.

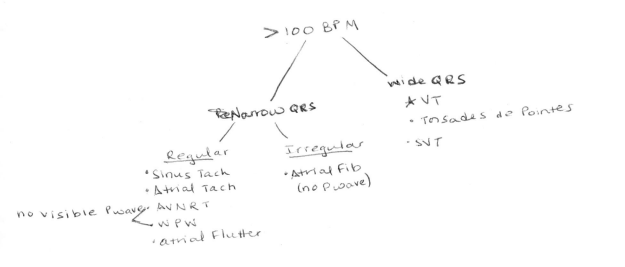

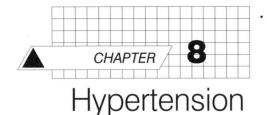

CHAPTER 8

Hypertension

*H*ypertension is a major risk factor for the development of cardiovascular disease, affecting up to 20% of people in developed countries. Uncontrolled hypertension leads to multisystem problems such as stroke, heart disease, renal failure, retinopathy, and peripheral vascular disease.

There is no biologic threshold that separates normal from abnormally elevated blood pressure. The risk of cardiovascular disease increases linearly with increased blood pressure; thus, a number of somewhat arbitrary **definitions of hypertension** have been developed. One common definition uses the cutoff of a diastolic of 90 mmHg and a systolic of 140 mmHg to define the upper limits of normal. Isolated systolic hypertension is defined as a systolic > 160 mmHg with a diastolic < 90 mmHg. Complications of hypertension increase with greater elevation above normal, leading to the **classification of hypertension** into four stages (Table 8-1). These stages correspond to the older classifications of "mild," "moderate," "severe," and "very severe."

▶ EPIDEMIOLOGY AND RISK FACTORS

The prevalence of hypertension in various studies has depended on the definition of hypertension used and the population studied. In the Framingham study, which looked at a white suburban population, nearly half had at least stage I hypertension. A number of **risk factors** for the development of hypertension have been determined:

- ▲ increasing age
- ▲ smoking
- ▲ male sex
- ▲ race (African-American > white)
- ▲ obesity
- ▲ family history
- ▲ sodium intake (applies more to populations than individuals)
- ▲ ethanol intake
- ▲ psychological stress

In the United States, it is estimated that 2 million adults develop hypertension each year. Of individuals with hypertension, about 75% of these have stage 1 disease.

▶ ETIOLOGY AND PATHOPHYSIOLOGY

Greater than 95% of hypertensive individuals have what has been called **essential hypertension**, that is, they do not have an identifiable etiology. Recent research has suggested that most hypertension results from the interplay of a large number of physiologic and environmental factors; thus, essential hypertension is a bit of a misnomer. However, the concept is still useful to distinguish essential hypertension from hypertension where there is a well-defined etiology (i.e., secondary hypertension).

Major **causes of secondary hypertension** include:

- ▲ renovascular disease (atherosclerotic, fibromuscular dysplasia)
- ▲ intrinsic renal disease
- ▲ hyperaldosteronism
- ▲ pheochromocytoma
- ▲ Cushing's disease
- ▲ coarctation of the aorta
- ▲ drugs (especially oral contraceptives)

The suspicion for secondary hypertension should be increased in patients with the following characteristics:

- ▲ age < 35
- ▲ no family history of hypertension
- ▲ severe, rapid onset hypertension
- ▲ hypertension refractory to standard therapy

Uncontrolled or poorly controlled hypertension leads to **complications** in a number of organ systems:

TABLE 8-1		
Staging of hypertension		
	Systolic BP	Diastolic BP
Stage 1	140–159	90–99
Stage 2	160–179	100–109
Stage 3	180–209	110–119
Stage 4	>210	>120

▲ cardiac

▲ cerebrovascular

▲ peripheral vascular

▲ renal

▲ ophthalmologic

▶ CLINICAL MANIFESTATIONS
History

Most newly diagnosed hypertensive patients are **asymptomatic** but may give a positive family history for hypertension. In the new hypertensive, history should focus on **symptoms that may indicate end organ damage** such as:

▲ chest pain

▲ transient ischemic attack symptoms

▲ claudication

▲ peripheral edema

▲ vision changes

Physical Examination

The physical examination should focus on determination of end-organ damage and clues of secondary causes. The major manifestations of **end-organ damage** include:

▲ cardiac (e.g., left ventricular heave, S4, single S2, pulmonary, or peripheral edema)

▲ cerebrovascular (e.g., carotidbruits, neurologic deficit)

▲ peripheral vascular (e.g., loss of one or more major extremity pulses, aneurysms)

▲ renal (e.g., proteinuria, microalbuminuria)

▲ eye (e.g., arterioventricular nicking, hemorrhages, exudates, papilledema)

Clues for secondary causes of hypertension relate to the underlying condition. Examples of this are violaceous striae in Cushing's disease and the presence of renal bruits in renovasular disease.

▶ DIAGNOSTIC EVALUATION

Similar to the physical examination, laboratory studies are focused on defining end-organ damage and looking for secondary causes. A generally accepted panel of studies to be used when evaluating a newly diagnosed hypertensive patient includes:

▲ serum creatinine

▲ urinalysis

▲ potassium

▲ electrocardiogram

This relatively simple and inexpensive panel both defines end-organ damage (renal failure, heart disease) and suggests possible secondary etiologies (hypokalemia in hyperaldosteronism). More specialized tests for other secondary causes should only be undertaken if the history and physical are suggestive.

▶ TREATMENT

Initial management of newly diagnosed hypertension is to look for and correct secondary causes. In patients with essential hypertension or uncorrectable secondary hypertension, the goal of antihypertensive treatment is to reduce the patient's risk of cardiovascular disease by lowering blood pressure to normal. Generally, this goal is aimed for in a graduated step-wise fashion, taking in consideration a variety of specific factors (see below.) The exception to this gradual approach is in the so-called **hypertensive emergency**. Hypertensive encephalopathy, which is the result of cerebral edema from hypertension, and aortic dissection are the two major types of hypertensive emergencies. In these cases, rapid lowering of blood pressure is required, usually in the setting of urgent hospitalization and invasive monitoring.

A number of **nonpharmacologic modalities** may lower blood pressure. Their use is encouraged in all hypertensives and, in some patients with stage 1 disease, may be effective alone:

▲ weight reduction

▲ smoking cessation

▲ sodium restriction

▲ physical exercise

▲ stress reduction

▲ lowering/discontinuing alcohol intake

Antihypertensive medications fall into several major classes:

▲ diuretics

▲ adrenergic blockers (alpha and beta)

▲ angiotensin-converting enzyme inhibitors

▲ calcium channel blockers

▲ vasodilators

There are many considerations in choosing an agent. Diuretics and beta-blockers are preferred initial agents because of a proven reduction in mortality and morbidity. The presence of coexisting medical conditions also influences drug choice. For example, coexisting coronary artery disease may make beta-blockers more attractive because of their mortality benefit in patients who have suffered a myocardial infarction, whereas the presence of severe congestive heart failure may make beta-blockers a less attractive choice.

Once the decision has been made to start antihypertensive drugs, there are a number of recommended strategies:

▲ Maintain lifestyle modifications and initiate therapy with a beta-blocker or diuretic (these are the only drugs that have been shown to have a mortality/morbidity benefit for primary treatment of hypertension).

▲ If there is not an adequate response: a) increase drug dosage *or* b) substitute another drug *or* c) add second agent from a different class (e.g., ACE inhibitor, calcium channel blocker, alpha-blocker).

▲ If there is still not an adequate response add a second or third agent (include a diuretic if one is not already prescribed).

▶ KEY POINTS

1. Blood pressure exists over a range from normal to abnormal, and sequelae of hypertension are related to the absolute elevation of blood pressure over the entire range.

2. The cardiovascular system suffers damage from long-term uncontrolled hypertension.

3. In most (>95%) hypertensives, no single etiology for hypertension can be found.

4. Treatment of hypertension involves coordination of pharmacologic and nonpharmacologic therapies, taking in consideration comorbid conditions and side effects of medications.

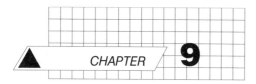

CHAPTER 9

Valvular Heart Disease

$\mathcal{V}$alvular heart disease in the **adult** population is usually due to **acquired valvular defects** as opposed to the situation in the **pediatric** population where **congenital defects** predominate. The **most commonly affected** valves are the **aortic and mitral valves.** The defects generally lead to either **restriction to blood flow (stenotic lesions)** or **incompetency** of the valves and backward flow (**regurgitation/insufficiency**). This chapter focuses on the major clinical entities of aortic stenosis (**AS**), aortic insufficiency (**AI**), mitral stenosis (**MS**), and mitral regurgitation (**MR**).

▶ EPIDEMIOLOGY

With the exception of mitral stenosis, which often presents in the third, fourth, and fifth decades of life, most valvular problems are not clinically manifest until around the seventh decade of life. Traditionally, the most common etiology of valvular heart disease was **rheumatic fever.** With the decreasing incidence of acute rheumatic fever, "wear and tear" degeneration associated with aging is becoming the more common cause of valvular lesions in adults.

▶ ETIOLOGY

Acute rheumatic fever results in **scarring of the valve apparatus and fusion of the valve cusps.** These scarred valves are more prone to **mechanical degeneration** and failure due to the stiffening and thickening of the valve leaflets as well as the resultant turbulent flow. Rheumatic valves are more prone to become involved in **infective endocarditis,** which in turn can result in further valvular damage.

Several valvular entities have particular **etiologic associations** that are common in addition to the association with rheumatic heart disease (RHD):

AS

▲ congenital bicuspid valve,

▲ calcific ("senile") degeneration

AI

▲ infective endocarditis

▲ syphilitic aortitis

▲ connective tissue disease (e.g., Marfan's and Ehlers-Danlos)

MS

▲ mitral annular calcification

MR

▲ mitral valve prolapse

▲ myocardial infarction (papillary muscle dysfunction), mitral annular calcification

▲ infective endocarditis

▶ PATHOGENESIS

In general, **stenotic** valvular lesions lead to **pressure overload** on the upstream cardiac and vascular structures, whereas **regurgitant** lesions cause **volume overload.** Therefore, the following pathogenic **responses** result:

AS

▲ concentric left ventricular (LV) hypertrophy (initial)

▲ left atrial (LA) hypertrophy (secondary to increased role of atrial contraction in diastolic filling of the hypertrophied LV)

▲ decreased LV ejection fraction (late)

AI

▲ LV dilation (early)

▲ LV hypertrophy (secondary)

▲ decreased LV contractility (late)

MS

▲ LA enlargement (early) with subsequent development of atrial fibrillation (AF)

▲ pulmonary venous congestion (early)

▲ pulmonary hypertension (late)

▲ RV hypertrophy (late)

MR

▲ LA enlargement (early, may be massive)

▲ AF (after LA enlargement)

▲ pulmonary congestion

▲ pulmonary hypertension

▲ LV failure (late as LV is no longer able to compensate for regurgitant flow by increased systolic emptying)

It is important to note that the above changes will occur only if the valvular lesions develop slowly over time, as is usually the case in RHD. Initially, these responses are compensatory, but only at the eventual cost of chamber failure. If the valvular lesion occurs rapidly (as in acute AI or MR from infective endocarditis or acute MR in the setting of myocardial infarction), there is no time for compensation and abrupt congestive failure results.

The abnormal valve surfaces are thrombogenic, and this, especially when coupled with associated atrial fibrillation, can result in **embolic phenomena** such as stroke.

▶ CLINICAL MANIFESTATIONS

History

The **symptoms** that are common in each valvular lesion are as follows:

AS

▲ effort-related syncope

▲ exertional angina

▲ dyspnea

▲ congestive failure (late, after LV function declines)

AI

▲ forceful heartbeat/palpitations

▲ exertional dyspnea

▲ angina

▲ congestive failure (late in chronic AI, but early in acute AI)

MS

▲ exertional dyspnea

▲ atrial fibrillation

▲ hemoptysis

▲ congestive failure (early)

MR

▲ fatigue

▲ atrial fibrillation

▲ congestive failure

It is important to elicit a history of RHD in a patient in whom valvular disease is suspected. Known or presumed coronary artery disease may accentuate symptoms (particularly angina) or may even mask symptoms (by limiting exercise before effort-related symptoms are manifest).

Physical Examination

See Table 9-1.

▶ DIFFERENTIAL DIAGNOSIS

Because valvular disease may present with a variety of symptoms ranging from syncope to angina to dyspnea, the differential diagnosis is potentially very large. However, symptoms coupled with physical examination findings of murmurs and peripheral manifestations usually narrow the differential.

▶ DIAGNOSTIC EVALUATION

The principal initial studies are the **electrocardiogram** (ECG), **chest radiograph,** and **echocardiography.** The latter is indicated when the history, physical examination, ECG, and chest film are highly suggestive of the presence of significant valvular disease. **Echocardiography** is useful not only in determining the presence of a stenotic or regurgitant valve but can also **assess the severity of the lesion** and its effect on the myocardium. Along with measuring dimensions of abnormal valves, M-mode, two-dimensional, and Doppler echocardiography can determine magnitude of regurgitant flow and measure the pressure gradients across stenotic valves. Echocardiography can also determine and quantitate **ventricular dysfunction** as well as detect disease in other valves.

If valve replacement surgery is to be undertaken, **cardiac catheterization** allows direct measurement of pressure gradient and intrachamber pressures. It will also detect and quantify concomitant coronary artery disease.

▶ TREATMENT

Once the diagnosis of a significant valvular lesions is made, the main decision is whether to opt for **medical management or surgery.** Of the various lesions, it should be noted that symptomatic AS managed purely medically is associated with the worst prognosis (1-year mortality approaching 50%). In the remainder of the major valvular lesions, medical management is often the initial approach, with surgery being reserved for progression of symptoms. If the valvular lesion arises acutely (see above), surgery may be necessary earlier in the course.

TABLE 9-1
Key Features in Valvular Heart Disease

	Aortic Stenosis	Aortic Insufficiency	Mitral Stenosis	Mitral Regurgitation
Risk factors	Rheumatic heart disease, calcifications ("senile degeneration"), bicuspid valve, male:female 4:1	Rheumatic heart disease, aortic root problems, infective endocarditis	Rheumatic heart disease female:male 2:1	Rheumatic heart disease, mitral annular calcifications, myocardial infarction, mitral valve prolapse, infective endocarditis
Age at presentation (yr)	>65 (calcific)	>65	>20–50	>60
Symptoms	Effort syncope, angina, dyspnea, stroke	Dyspnea on exertion, congestive heart failure	Dyspnea on exertion, paroxysmal nocturnal dyspnea, orthopnea, atrial fibrillation, palpitations	Congestive heart failure
Murmur	"Diamond-shaped" early systolic	Diastolic "blow"	Apical diastolic "rumble"	Late systolic, radiating from apex to axilla
Physical examination	Sustained apical impulse, weak/delayed carotid pulse "Parvus et Tardus"	Increased pulse pressure (Quinke pulses, DeMusse sign, Derosier's sign)	± opening snap, hepatomegaly (pulsatile), lower extremity edema	Hepatomegaly (pulsatile), lower extremity edema
ECG	Left ventricular hypertrophy, left anterior-hemiblock	Left ventricular hypertrophy, no repolarization abnormalities	Left atrial enlargement, right ventricular hypertrophy, atrial fibrillation	Atrioventricular block
Chest film	Poststenotic aortic dilatation, aortic valvular calcifications, "boot-shaped" heart	Congestive heart failure, increased heart size	Left atrial enlargement, congestive heart failure, prominent pulmonary arteries	Congestive heart failure, increased heart size

In some cases, the decision of medical versus surgical management is influenced by the presence of comorbid conditions, particularly coronary artery disease.

Medical management of symptomatic valvular disease is usually similar to the management of **congestive heart failure** (see Chapter 5) with:

▲ digoxin

▲ diuretics

▲ vasodilators

Digoxin is particularly important in the presence of atrial fibrillation. **Anticoagulation** should be considered, especially in the presence of atrial fibrillation but also in mitral stenosis with or without associated AF.

Valve replacement is the most common surgical approach. If valve replacement is to be done, the choice between **bioprostheses** (tissue valves) and **mechanical prostheses** must be made. The decision usually hinges on the need for anticoagulation with its attendant risks when mechanical valves are used and on the durability of the prosthesis. Most of the commonly used tissue valves (e.g., porcine valves) have an expected life expectancy of 10 to 15 years, whereas modern mechanical valves are designed with a durability greater than the normal human lifespan. Generally, unless there are contraindications to anticoagulation, mechanical valves are used in younger patients and tissue valves reserved for the elderly.

Percutaneous balloon valvuloplasty is a newer technique for management of stenotic valvular lesions. Although it is associated with relatively good results in certain cases of MS, balloon valvuloplasty for AS is associated with a high early restenosis rate. However, it may provide symptomatic, if shortlived, relief of symptoms in patients with AS who are not surgical candidates. The procedure carries the risk of subsequent significant valvular regurgitation as well as embolism during the procedure.

If medical management is chosen, patients should be monitored closely for signs and symptoms of clinical decompensation. If this occurs, the patient should be assessed for altered valvular hemodynamics that require adjustment in medicine or consideration of surgery. **Prophylaxis against infective endocarditis** (see Chapter 32) should always be instituted. Patients who receive valve replacement should also receive prophylaxis. The patient should be monitored for prosthetic valvular dysfunction, which may require medical management or repeat valve replacement.

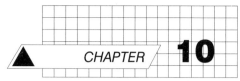

CHAPTER 10

Noncoronary Vascular Disease

𝒱ascular disease is the most common cause of death in the United States. A large part of this is due to disease of the coronary circulation, but diseases of the aorta and the peripheral vasculature are responsible for significant morbidity and mortality. Aortic disease and peripheral vascular disease of the extremities are the focus of this chapter.

▶ EPIDEMIOLOGY

There are approximately 1 million deaths due to vascular disease in the United States each year. About half of these are due to coronary artery disease. Cerebrovascular disease (stroke) is responsible for about 120,000 deaths each year, making it the third leading cause of death.

▶ ETIOLOGY

Damage to vessels can occur via a number of pathogenic mechanisms. Most commonly, **atherosclerotic changes** occur by the formation of atheromatous plaques as outlined in Chapter 3. Progressive atherosclerosis results in increased vascular obstruction and diminished blood flow. Atherosclerotic disease can also lead to the formation of **arterial aneurysms.** Aneurysms of the abdominal aorta are the most common, but aneurysms can form throughout the vascular tree. As an aneurysm grows, it becomes more likely to undergo dissection or rupture.

Acute obstruction of a vessel can occur via **embolization.** An embolus can be thrombotic or atherosclerotic and can originate from a cardiac or proximal vascular source. Cardiac emboli are most common and are generally thrombotic. Thrombi can arise from the **left atrium** (usually in the setting of atrial fibrillation), the valves (in the setting of valvular disease), and the **left ventricle** (most often in the setting of ventricular dysfunction due to coronary artery disease). Cardiac thrombi can also arise in the setting of endocarditis. *In situ* thrombosis, most often at sites of pre-existing atherosclerotic disease, can also be responsible for acute vascular obstruction. A coexisting hypercoagulable state (e.g., due to a neoplasm) can increase the likelihood of *in situ* thrombus formation.

A number of **systemic diseases** can affect the vessels, including:

▲ diabetes mellitus

▲ collagen vascular diseases (see Chapter 58)

▲ hypertension

▲ connective tissue diseases (e.g., Marfan's syndrome)

▶ RISK FACTORS

The same **patient characteristics** that predispose to the development of coronary artery disease are risk factors for the development of vascular disease in general:

▲ hypercholesterolemia (elevated low-density lipoproteins)

▲ low high-density lipoprotein levels

▲ smoking

▲ hypertension

▲ male sex

▲ diabetes mellitus

▲ family history of vascular disease

▶ CLINICAL MANIFESTATIONS
History

The clinical manifestations of vascular disease varies depending on the anatomic location of the vessel affected, but in general, clinical syndromes can be grouped into acute and chronic. In **acute peripheral arterial occlusion,** the cardinal features in an extremity due to arterial occlusion are the "six Ps":

▲ pulselessness

▲ pallor

▲ poikilothermia (temperature of affected extremity varies with the ambient temperature)

▲ pain

▲ paralysis

▲ paresthesia

Acute cerebrovascular arterial occlusion leads to acute ischemic stroke, with clinical neurologic findings dependent on the arterial territory that is affected.

In **acute mesenteric arterial occlusion,** the major clinical feature is of severe abdominal pain. In **chronic arterial occlusive** disease, the most common symptom is **intermittent claudication.** This consists of pain, aching, or numbness that occurs in a muscle during exercise but is relieved by rest. This most commonly occurs in the lower extremities due to the higher incidence of obstructive lesions. Aorto-iliac disease causes claudication in the buttocks and thighs, whereas femoral-popliteal disease results in calf claudication. As the degree of obstruction increases, the pain will progress, requiring less exercise to appear until it occurs at rest. Chronic occlusive disease involving the mesenteric circulation can manifest as **abdominal angina,** a syndrome of abdominal pain that occurs most often after a meal. An **aortic aneurysm** most commonly involves the abdominal aorta (abdominal aorta), and most are asymptomatic. Patients or their physicians may become aware of a pulsatile mass. Rupture or dissection can result in severe pain, often described as tearing (see Chapter 1 for discussion of dissecting aortic aneurym).

Physical Examination

Physical examination findings depend on the anatomic distribution:

▲ Bruits (carotid, renal, femoral) of note; as the degree of obstruction increases, a bruit may diminish and eventually disappear, making bruit intensity a poor indicator of the degree of disease;

▲ Pulselessness, pallor, and poikilothermia as listed above for acute arterial occlusion;

▲ Pulsatile abdominal mass (abdominal aortic aneurysm);

▲ Extremity changes: lack of hair, shiny skin, ulcers, diminished capillary refill/distal pulses (chronic peripheral arterial insufficiency);

▲ Unequal blood pressures/pulses (suggestive of dissecting aortic aneurysm in proper clinical setting).

▶ DIAGNOSTIC EVALUATION

In the setting of possible arterial occlusion (both acute and chronic), the diagnosis can be confirmed by invasive and non invasive tests. **Doppler ultrasound** can attempt to localize flow and obstructions in a noninvasive manner. **Arteriography** has traditionally been the gold standard but is invasive and requires the administration of intravenous contrast. It is generally reserved until the decision for revascularization is made and then used to precisely determine anatomy.

If an occlusion is documented and an embolic event is suspected, **cardiac ultrasound** is generally performed, because most emboli are cardiac in origin.

In addition to ultrasound and arteriography, **contrast CT** and **MRI** can be used to image the aorta to make the diagnosis of aneuryms and dissections. An abdominal aortic aneurysm is usually followed with serial ultrasounds.

The amount of blood flow to an extremity (usually the legs) can be quantitated by means of a **pulse volume recorder.** This device resembles a blood pressure cuff and produces a pressure waveform that can be followed to make serial assessments of blood flow. It can also be used at points along an extremity to localize an obstructive/occlusive lesion.

▶ TREATMENT

An acute arterial occlusion is a medical/surgical emergency, generally requiring referral to a vascular surgeon. Restoration of blood flow is essential to avoid tissue necrosis.

The treatment of chronic arterial occlusive disease is initially medical, with surgical referral for advanced disease no longer responsive to medical therapy. In many instances, the clinical course is not invariably progressive, and surgery may be avoided by a good medical regimen.

The major therapeutic interventions used in the setting of **acute arterial occlusion** include:

▲ surgical thrombectomy

▲ percutaneous catheter thrombectomy

▲ thrombolytic therapy

The decision as to which procedure to perform is based on the immediate danger to the extremity and the location and length of the occlusion. In all cases, **anticoagulation** with **heparin** is started immediately and long-term anticoagulation with **coumadin** continued after intervention.

The treatment of **chronic arterial insufficiency** should begin with a comprehensive **medical regimen:**

▲ cessation of smoking (the vasoconstrictive activity of nicotine increases the limitation to blood flow and smoking is a risk factor for further atherogenesis)

▲ control of hypertension (may decrease incidence of aneurysm/dissection)

▲ meticulous foot care (wear protective properly fitted shoes, keep feet clean and dry, use moisturizing creams)

▲ control of diabetes (can limit further microvascular damage)

▲ control of hypercholesterolemia (can limit progression and may even reverse artheromatous lesions)

▲ regular exercise (to the point of discomfort but not beyond; will improve exercise tolerance)

Pharmacologic measures are of limited benefit. Vasodilators *do not* improve outcome.

▲ Pentoxifylline decreases blood viscosity via an effect on the red cell membrane and only a modest increase is seen in exercise tolerance when compared with placebo;

▲ Aspirin is not shown to increase exercise tolerance but may be of benefit in limiting *in situ* thrombosis at sites of atherosclerosis.

Nonoperative intervention includes:

▲ balloon angioplasty (best results have been with short, segmental stenotic [not occlusive] lesions in the iliac arteries)

▲ atherectomy (using lasers and cutting blades, currently an experimental procedure)

In surgery, the choice of procedure depends on extent of disease and anatomic considerations:

▲ direct bypass (using vein or synthetic material to directly bypass the disease segment, e.g., femoral-popliteal bypass)

▲ extra-anatomic bypass (using a distant artery as the blood source, e.g., axillo-femoral bypass, femoral-femoral bypass)

When considering surgery for peripheral vascular disease, it must be kept in mind that peripheral vascular disease is a marker for coronary artery disease. Therefore, a thorough assessment of the cardiac risk of surgery must be done.

Abdominal aortic aneurysms are generally treated with surgical repair. The risk of rupture and death of an abdominal aorta with a diameter greater than 6 cm is high (about 80% mortality at 2 years). With aneurysms between 4 and 6 cm, the 2-year risk of rupture is between 10 and 30%. Given the average growth rate of about 0.4 cm/yr, early repair in patients is generally recommended for patients who are good surgical candidates.

Acute aortic dissection is also an emergency that requires surgical referral. Proximal thoracic dissections are generally repaired surgically, whereas distal dissections are managed medically (with aggressive blood pressure control and negative ionotropic agents as tolerated). However, overall prognosis in the setting of aortic dissection is poor.

▶ KEY POINTS

1. Disease of the noncoronary circulation is most often atherosclerotic in nature.

2. Acute syndromes involving the vessels includes acute occlusion (embolic and thrombotic), acute dissection, and aneurysmal rupture.

3. Chronic arterial occlusive disease most often manifests as intermittent claudication, which is discomfort that occurs in a muscle during exercise but is relieved by rest.

4. Acute vascular syndromes are generally medical emergencies, often requiring evaluation and treatment by a vascular surgeon.

5. Chronic arterial occlusive disease is initially managed supportively. Revascularization can be accomplished by percutaneous angioplasty or surgical bypass.

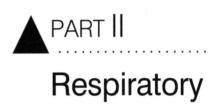

PART II

Respiratory

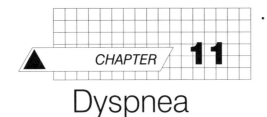

CHAPTER 11

Dyspnea

$\mathcal{D}$yspnea is an **uncomfortable awareness of breathing.** The awareness and control of respiration by the central nervous system (CNS) is influenced by the input of a number of peripheral receptors: central and peripheral chemoreceptors (that measure blood oxygen content, carbon dioxide content, and pH) and mechanical receptors in pulmonary parenchyma, airways, and respiratory muscles. These receptors provide information to the CNS concerning the efficiency of respiration (i.e., gas exchange) as well as the work of breathing. There is a **large subjective component**—the same quantitative respiratory defects in different patients can elicit different degrees of dyspnea.

▶ DIFFERENTIAL DIAGNOSIS

Generally, disorders affecting the cardiopulmonary systems and the blood's oxygen-carrying capacity are the most common causes of dyspnea. It is useful to divide dyspnea into acute and chronic etiologies.

Acute Dyspnea

Pulmonary causes include:

▲ asthma

▲ bronchitis

▲ pneumonia

▲ pneumothorax

▲ pulmonary embolism

▲ large airway obstruction (aspiration of foreign body, epiglottitis)

▲ airway irritants (smoke, aerosols)

Cardiac causes include:

▲ heart failure

▲ tamponade

Other causes include:

▲ hemorrhage

▲ hemolysis

▲ carbon monoxide poisoning

▲ psychogenic (hyperventilation syndrome, panic attack)

Chronic Dyspnea

Pulmonary causes include:

▲ chronic obstructive pulmonary disease

▲ pleural effusions

▲ interstitial lung disease

▲ pulmonary hypertension

▲ neuromuscular disease

▲ severe kyphoscoliosis

Cardiac causes include:

▲ heart failure

▲ restrictive pericarditis

Other causes include:

▲ chronic anemia

▲ severe obesity

Among outpatients, the most commonly encountered causes of dyspnea are chronic obstructive airway disease, asthma, heart failure, and anxiety. Among inpatients, in particular those who are severely ill with another process, the onset of dyspnea may signal an urgent process such as pulmonary embolus or hospital-acquired pneumonia.

▶ CLINICAL MANIFESTATIONS
History

Quickly establish whether the onset of dyspnea was acute or chronic. If acute, check for symptoms of life-threatening conditions such as pulmonary embolus, spontaneous pneumothorax, and pneumonia. Often, the decision regarding hospitalization and empiric treatment will need to be made quickly in cases of acute onset dyspnea.

Historical features in acute dyspnea include:

▲ cough (bronchitis, asthma, pneumonia, airway irritation)

▲ sputum production (bronchitis, pneumonia)

▲ pleuritic chest pain (spontaneous pneumothorax, pulmonary embolus, pneumonia)

▲ visceral chest pain–angina (heart failure)

▲ hemoptysis (pulmonary embolus, bronchitis, pneumonia)

▲ **39**

The evaluation of chronic dyspnea can be more problematic, requiring a stepped diagnostic workup (see below). **Historical features in chronic dyspnea** include:

▲ smoking (chronic obstructive pulmonary disease, bronchitis)

▲ cardiac history (heart failure)

▲ occupational exposures, for example, asbestos, metal dust (interstitial lung disease)

In addition, because chronic dyspnea usually manifests initially as exertional dyspnea, a determination of the **baseline fitness** of an individual is important. Any significant change from baseline indicates possible severe pathology and necessitates further evaluation.

Physical Examination

A directed physical examination is essential in the setting of **acute dyspnea.** Check for:

▲ wheezing (asthma, heart failure)

▲ stridor (upper airway obstruction)

▲ consolidation (pneumonia)

▲ rales, S3, jugular venous distension (heart failure)

▲ tracheal shift from midline

▲ absent unilateral breath sounds (pneumothorax, tension pneumothorax)

In **chronic dyspnea,** check for:

▲ hyperexpansion (chronic obstructive pulmonary disease)

▲ rales (fine rales in interstitial lung disease, more coarse in heart failure)

▲ pulmonary hypertension (fixed split of S2, right ventricular heave, jugular venous distension)

▶ DIAGNOSTIC EVALUATION

In the setting of **acute dyspnea,** a **chest radiograph** is checked for:

▲ pneumothorax (loss of lung markings, pleural reflection)

▲ pneumonia (consolidation)

▲ heart failure (Kerley B lines, effusions)

Measurement of arterial blood gases (see Chapter 19) usually does not suggest a specific etiology, but can help quantitate the degree of respiratory compromise.

The diagnosis of pulmonary embolus is a critical one to make in the setting of acute dyspnea (see Chapter 15). Ventilation perfusion scanning, lower extremity venous ultrasounds, and pulmonary angiography can all be used in the evaluation.

Peak expiratory flow measurements are useful in the evaluation of possible asthma (see Chapter 14).

Evaluation of **chronic dyspnea** should also start with a chest radiograph. Conditions such as chronic obstructive pulmonary disease, interstitial lung disease, and heart failure can have specific radiographic findings (see individual chapters for details). Further imaging with computed tomography can be useful.

A complete blood count to screen for underlying anemia should be performed. If after a routine history physical and these initial tests, more specialized testing, often in consultation with a pulmonary specialist, needs to be done.

Chest radiograph, arterial blood gas measurements, screens for pulmonary embolus, and peak flow measurements generally will yield a diagnosis in **acute dyspnea.** In rare instances, more invasive diagnostic tests such as right-heart catheterization or bronchoscopy will be required.

As mentioned, **chronic dyspnea** can be difficult to diagnose. A common scenario is a patient who presents with chronic progressive exertional dyspnea and who has evidence of both chronic pulmonary disease and coronary artery disease. An ordered evaluation is required to make the diagnosis without unnecessary expensive and invasive tests.

Pulmonary function testing (PFT) is commonly used in the evaluation of chronic dyspnea. This can range from simple **spirometry** that measures expiratory flow rates and volumes (see Chapter 13) to more sophisticated measurement of lung volumes and diffusion capacity. The following parameters can be measured and calculated:

▲ Forced vital capacity (FVC)—the volume of air that can be exhaled going from maximal inhalation to maximal exhalation;

▲ Forced expiratory volume in 1 second (FEV_1)—the volume of air exhaled in 1 second starting at maximal inhalation;

▲ FEV_1/FVC (FEV_1%)—calculated ratio of FEV_1 to FVC;

▲ Total lung capacity (TLC)—the volume of gas contained within the lung after maximal inspiration;

▲ Residual volume (RV)—the volume of gas remaining in the lungs after maximal expiration;

▲ Diffusion capacity of the lung for carbon monoxide (DLCO)—the ability of gas to diffuse across the alveolar-capillary membrane.

Patterns of PFT abnormalities are associated with particular pulmonary diseases (Table 11-1).

Evaluation of the cardiovascular system (see Chapter 5) can reveal a cardiac cause for dyspnea. Generally, an assessment of valvular and ventricular function via an echocardiogram is sufficient. Radionuclide ventriculography can also assess ventricular function and is used during cardiopulmonary exercise testing (see below).

In a patient with chronic exertional dyspnea, if the above pulmonary and cardiac evaluations fail to reveal significant abnormalities, or if the individual abnormalities do not appear to explain the degree of impairment, **cardiopulmonary exercise testing** (CPEx) may be necessary. CPEx involves graded exercise (much as with a cardiac stress test) with cardiopulmonary monitoring. Several parameters can be measured, depending on the clinical setting:

▲ **Vital signs**—continuous heart rate and blood pressure measurement and electrocardiographic monitoring;

▲ **Pulmonary gas** exchange—the patient breathes into a mouthpiece during exercise, with sampling and analysis of the composition (P_{O_2} and P_{CO_2}) of exhaled gas;

▲ **Oxygen delivery and consumption**—oxygenation can be assessed by oxymetry, arterial line. In certain settings measurement of mixed venous oxygen content as well as pulmonary pressure can be measured with a pulmonary artery catheter.

▲ **Cardiac function**—ventricular function during exercise can be assessed by continuous radionuclide ventriculography.

CPEx will determine whether the limitation to exercise is due to a cardiac or pulmonary limit. In normal individuals, pulmonary capacity is greater than cardiac. By determining the function of both the cardiac and pulmonary systems, the relative degree of impairment can be used to guide therapy.

▶ **KEY POINTS**

1. Dyspnea is an uncomfortable awareness of breathing.

2. Dyspnea can arise from abnormalities in the pulmonary, cardiac, hematologic, and musculoskeletal systems.

3. Acute dyspnea can be due to life-threatening conditions such as pulmonary embolism, pneumothorax, and pneumonia.

4. Chronic dyspnea is most commonly due to chronic obstructive pulmonary disease or heart failure.

5. Evaluation of chronic exertional dyspnea requires a careful and orderly assessment of the function of the cardiac and pulmonary systems. Cardiopulmonary exercise testing can determine the physiologic limitations to exercise.

TABLE 11-1

Patterns of PFT Abnormalities

Disease	FVC	FEV$_1$	FEV$_1$ %	TLC	RV	DLCO
Emphysema	↓	↓	↓	↑	↑	↓
Chronic bronchitis	↓	↓	↓	↔	↑	↔
Asthma	↓	↓	↓	↔	↑	↔↑
Interstitial lung disease	↓	↔	↔↑	↓	↓	↓
Extrapulmonary restriction (e.g., kyphosocliosis)	↓	↓	↔	↓	↔↓	↔
Heart failure (early, increased blood flow)	—	—	—	—	—	↑
Heart failure (late, with pulmonary edema)	—	—	—	—	—	↑
Pulmonary embolus	—	—	—	—	—	↑

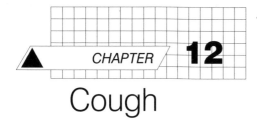

CHAPTER 12

Cough

*C*ough is an important defense mechanism that allows the clearance of secretions and foreign particles. There are three phases to a cough: deep inspiration, glottic closure, and buildup of intrathoracic pressure, and opening of glottis with rapid release of pressure. Cough is triggered by receptors located throughout the upper and lower respiratory tract; therefore, a wide variety of stimuli can trigger the cough reflex, including upper respiratory infection, lower respiratory infection, environmental pollutants, mechanical irritation, chemical irritation, chronic inflammatory states, and drugs.

The final common pathway of most of these causes of cough is mechanical or chemical irritation. It should be noted that cigarette smoking is by far the most common cause of chronic cough. Cough associated with smoking is often dry and worse upon awakening in the morning.

Many irritants that cause cough can also produce bronchospasm in some patients, which may present as wheezing.

▶ DIFFERENTIAL DIAGNOSIS

Causes of cough can be grouped according to the pathogenic stimuli listed above:

▲ Upper respiratory infection—pharyngitis (usually viral), sinusitis (via "postnasal drip"), tracheitis (again, usually viral);

▲ Lower respiratory infection—bronchitis, pneumonia;

▲ Environmental pollutants—dust, pollen, cigarette smoke;

▲ Mechanical irritation (of upper or lower respiratory tract)—tumor, aortic aneurysm, cerumen, pulmonary edema;

▲ Chronic inflammatory states—asthma, chronic aspiration, gastroesophageal reflux disease, sarcoidosis;

▲ Drugs—angiotensin-converting enzyme inhibitors.

▶ CLINICAL MANIFESTATIONS

History

There are a number of important historical features that should be elicited:

▲ Is the cough acute or chronic?

▲ Does the patient smoke and if so is there any history of obstructive airways disease?

▲ Is there sputum production? (If so, what color is it, is there any blood?)

▲ Are there any environmental exposures (e.g., dust, fumes, animal dander)?

▲ Are there any associated constitutional symptoms (e.g., fever, weight loss)?

These historical points can begin to aid in sorting through the differential diagnosis.

Physical Examination

Several elements of the physical examination may provide etiologic clues: **HEENT**, sinus tenderness (sinusitis), conjunctival injection, rhinitis (URI), tympanic membrane erythema (otitis), oropharyngeal "cobblestoning" (chronic sinusitis), and **CHEST**, loose rhonchi (infection, i.e., bronchitis or pneumonia), consolidation (pneumonia), fine crackles (pulmonary edema), focal wheezing (local obstructing lesion, i.e., tumor or foreign body), end expiratory wheezing (obstructive airways disease, i.e., asthma/chronic obstructive pulmonary disease).

The nature of the cough itself can give clues to the etiology, for example, the dry, irritant, nonproductive cough secondary to angiotensin-converting enzyme inhibitors or the loose rattling cough found in chronic bronchitis.

▶ DIAGNOSTIC EVALUATION

Many times the etiology of a cough is suggested by the history and physical. In other cases, if no diagnosis becomes readily apparent, a chest x-ray may be useful. It can reveal an infiltrate, mass, or pulmonary edema. A clear chest x-ray can steer the diagnosis toward tracheobronchitis, asthma, or environmental exposure as the etiology of the cough.

Examination of a Gram stain or Wright stain of **sputum** may also help in diagnosis. Purulent sputum with many white blood cells suggests bronchitis or pneumonia. Eosinophils and mucous casts (so-called Curschmann's spirals) suggests asthma. The presence of red blood cells (with or without frank hemoptysis) may indicate chronic bronchitis, bronchiectasis, tuberculosis, or tumor.

A therapeutic trial such as a course of antibiotics based on the findings of a sputum Gram stain, or the institution of inhaled beta-agonists for a suspected asthmatic, may help establish a diagnosis.

In some instances, usually with chronic cough, the etiology may not be readily apparent, even after trials of therapy. **Pulmonary function testing** (with or without provocative challenge such as methylcholine) may reveal chronic obstruction or reactive airway disease. **Computed tomography** of the chest may reveal anatomic lesions such as extrinsic compression, bronchiectasis, or parenchymal masses. **Bronchoscopy** may be of use, particularly in cases where there are findings on radiography that require biopsy.

▶ TREATMENT

Therapy should be directed at the underlying cause. Because mechanical and/or chemical irritation is the common etiology for most coughs, elimination or avoidance of these irritants is vital. Smoking cessation and avoidance of polluted environments is a major component of management. The use of antibiotic therapy, based on the findings of sputum Gram stain, is indicated when an infectious etiology is suspected.

The use of **antitussives** is often considered. Absolute suppression of the cough reflex is seldom medically necessary or even desired, because the purpose of coughing is to clear foreign particles and secretions. For example, in chronic bronchitis, adequate clearance of secretions is a major component of management. **Reduction** of cough to prevent interference with sleep and improve comfort should be the goal of antitussive therapy rather than full cough suppression.

Antitussives suppress the cough reflex either by anesthetizing the peripheral irritant receptors or increasing the threshold of the central cough center. **Peripheral anesthetics** include benzonatate, phenol preparations, and menthol preparations. Of these agents, benzonatate probably is the most effective. It is chemically related to other local anesthetics such as tetracaine.

Central antitussive agents include **dextromethorphan**, which is the most effective non-narcotic agent, and narcotics such as codeine.

▶ KEY POINTS

1. Cough is usually due to mechanical or chemical irritation of the upper and or lower respiratory tract.

2. A wide variety of agents and conditions can lead to this irritation.

3. History and physical alone can often suggest an etiology for a cough.

4. Chest x-ray is a useful initial test in cases where diagnosis is not readily apparent after history and physical.

5. Further diagnostic testing is usually reserved to rule in or rule out specific diagnoses suggested by history, physical, and chest x-ray.

6. Treatment should be directed at the underlying etiology of the cough, with cough suppression used only to deal with side effects of cough (sleep disturbance, etc.)

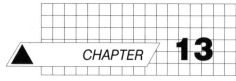

CHAPTER 13

Chronic Obstructive Pulmonary Disease

$\mathscr{C}$hronic obstructive pulmonary disease (COPD) refers to conditions that chronically impair expiratory airflow. Two major entities comprise COPD: **emphysema** and **chronic bronchitis.** Although their pathophysiology differs, both result in airflow obstruction. Chronic bronchitis is defined as excess tracheobronchial mucous production resulting in a productive cough that occurs for at least 3 months a year for more than 2 consecutive years. Emphysema is defined as abnormal dilatation of terminal airspaces with destruction of the alveolar septa. Thus, chronic bronchitis is defined **clinically,** whereas the diagnosis of emphysema is made **pathologically.**

Asthma (see Chapter 14) is another obstructive disease that results in airway obstruction. It differs from COPD in that the obstruction is transient and there is no association with smoking.

▶ EPIDEMIOLOGY

Chronic bronchitis and emphysema are associated with cigarette smoking and are responsible for 80,000 deaths a year, making them two of the most preventable causes of morbidity and mortality. Although cigarette smoking is the most important etiologic factor, occupational and environmental exposures (e.g., air pollution, asbestos, heavy metals) can also have an additive (and independent) effect on risk. In addition, hereditary deficiencies in the protease inhibitor alpha-1-antitrypsin predisposes to a distinct histologic form of emphysema (see below).

In the past, men had a much higher incidence of COPD, but with the increase in the rate of cigarette use by women, there has been a corresponding rise in the incidence of COPD in women.

▶ PATHOLOGY AND PATHOPHYSIOLOGY

In chronic bronchitis, there is distinctive hypertrophy and hyperplasia of the mucus-producing glands that line the airways. In addition, there is chronic mucosal and submucosal inflammation, intraluminal mucous plugging, and smooth muscle hypertrophy. These latter changes are more pronounced in the most distal smaller caliber airways. The loss of ventilation in regions distal to the airway obstruction results in ventilation/perfusion mismatches and hypoxia.

In emphysema, two patterns occur: **centrilobular emphysema,** where the areas most affected are the respiratory bronchioles and the central alveolar ducts, and **panacinar emphysema,** where there is destruction throughout the acinus. Generally, cigarette smoking is associated with centrilobular emphysema and alpha-1-antitrypsin deficiency with the panacinar form. In severe cases, however, it may be difficult to make a definite pathologic distinction as to which pattern is predominant. The destruction of lung parenchyma reduces elastic recoil resulting in increased airway collapsibility and outflow obstruction. The destruction of airspace and blood vessels is equal; therefore, marked ventilation/perfusion mismatch does not occur.

Most patients with COPD have elements of both chronic bronchitis and emphysema, but usually one or the other predominates. When possible, it is important to determine which manifestations are present because it will have impact on the nature of treatment.

The pathophysiologic changes seen in COPD contribute to expiratory obstruction and resultant decrease in maximal expiratory flow. The maximal expiratory flow rate that a person can generate is dependent on a number of variables:

▲ airway diameter

▲ collapsibility of the airways

▲ elastic recoil of the lung parenchyma

Other physiologic changes that result from COPD are:

▲ ventilation/perfusion mismatches (generally shunt, i.e., blood flow to nonventilated areas, resulting in hypoxia)

▲ pulmonary hypertension (in part due to loss of blood vessels from alveolar destruction but more important is vessel constriction due to hypoxia)

▲ abnormal ventilatory responses (blunted response to hypercapnia and a reliance on hypoxic respiratory drive)

▲ right heart failure (due to long-standing pulmonary hypertension, so-called *cor pulmonale*)

The natural history of COPD is generally one of inexorable decline in pulmonary function. Patients with chronic bronchitis have a course that is usually punctuated with multiple exacerbations with episodic increases in sputum production and worsened obstruction. In emphysema, the decline in pulmonary function is generally more continuous and steady.

▶ CLINICAL MANIFESTATIONS

Many patients with COPD will manifest elements of both chronic bronchitis and emphysema. To contrast the clinical presentations, it is useful to consider the presentation of patients who present primarily with one disease or the other.

History

The hallmark of chronic bronchitis is cough with sputum production. Early in the disease, symptoms are much worse during the winter months, but as the disease progresses, they become perennial and increase in frequency and severity. Dyspnea is not a predominant symptom initially, but the onset of exertional dyspnea often triggers medical attention. Weight gain, lethargy, and cyanosis are late findings.

In contrast, patients who present primarily with emphysema have minimal cough that may be productive of scant amounts of thin sputum. The major symptom is that of dyspnea, initially with exertion but then quite significant at rest. Weight loss is common but cyanosis is rare.

Physical Examination

On examination, the chronic bronchitic is generally comfortable at rest. Because of the common obesity and cyanosis, they are often referred to as "blue bloaters." If right-sided heart failure has developed, peripheral edema will contribute to this picture. Lung examination is usually resonant, often with coarse rhonchi and wheezes. Cardiac examination may reveal signs of right ventricular overload (sternal heave, tricuspid regurgitation with neck vein distention, and large v waves). Despite cyanosis, marked clubbing of the digits is rare and, if present, is suggestive of an additional condition, most ominously of lung cancer.

The patient with emphysema reports dyspnea at rest and appears thin without cyanosis. This leads to the description of emphysematous patients as "pink puffers." They will have a markedly prolonged expiratory phase often through pursed lips. Hypertrophy of the accessory muscles of respiration in the neck is common, as is retraction of the intercostal muscles with inspiration. The lung examination is hyperresonant with decrease in breath sounds, an increased antero/posterior chest diameter, and lowered diaphragms. The heart sounds are often distant and signs of right heart overload are absent.

▶ DIAGNOSTIC EVALUATION

Spirometry, the measurement of flow rates and volumes generated during forced expiration, is the primary means of quantifying airway outflow obstruction. The main measurements obtained are:

▲ forced vital capacity (FVC), which is the volume of air that can be exhaled going from maximal inhalation to maximal exhalation

▲ forced expiratory volume in 1 second (FEV_1), which is the volume of air exhaled in 1 second starting at maximal inhalation

▲ FEV_1/FVC (FEV_1%), which is the calculated ratio of FEV_1 to FVC

The calculated FEV_1% (normally 0.75 to 0.8) is usually considered the most accurate and reproducible measure of airway outflow obstruction. With early obstructive disease, the FEV_1% may be normal and the only measurable defect would be a slight decrease in midexpiratory flow rates. But for most patients with symptomatic COPD, the FEV_1% is a very useful assessment of disease.

FEV_1 has been shown to be a predictor of mortality in patients with COPD:

1. > 1.25 L—slight increase in mortality compared to matched controls;
2. 0.75 to 1.25 L—5-year survival 66% of expected;
3. < 0.75 L—5-year survival 33% of expected.

There are other measurements of pulmonary function that can be determined, including measurement of the residual volume (the amount of air that remains in the lungs at the end of maximal expiration), total lung capacity, and diffusing capacity. These require more sophisticated instrumentation than simple spirometry and are generally used for more extensive evaluation, usually in consultation with a pulmonary specialist.

Determination of arterial blood gases at rest is often useful. Patients with emphysema generally have normal $Paco_2$ and only slightly lowered Pao_2, whereas patients with chronic bronchitis often have elevated $Paco_2$ (50 to 60 mmHg) and depressed Pao_2 (45 to 60 mmHg). In addition, patients with chronic bronchitis may have an elevated hematocrit (in the range of 50 to 55%) in response to the hypoxia.

► TREATMENT

The treatment of chronic bronchitis and emphysema differ somewhat because the underlying pathophysiology is not the same. One common aspect of management is **cessation of smoking,** a key intervention. Unfortunately, this does not usually reverse the damage that already exists, but it will usually slow the progression of disease and also limit exacerbations. Other environmental airway irritants should be avoided, including hairsprays, dust, insecticides, and spray deodorants.

Patients with significant airway obstruction (i.e., $FEV_1 < 1.0$ L) require an understanding that a reduced life span is likely. Prospective discussions with such patients concerning endotracheal intubation when there is reduced likelihood of recovery are important. It is much less stressful for the patient and their family if these discussions can take place when the patient is clinically stable rather than during an acute and potentially life-threatening exacerbation.

All patients with COPD should receive yearly influenza vaccines. In addition, they should receive the 23-valent **pneumococcal vaccine.** When patients have acute exacerbations in symptoms, particularly when associated with increase in viscosity, purulence, or volume of sputum, some experts advocate administration of empiric antibiotics. This is not a universally accepted intervention. If administered, antibiotic coverage should encompass pathogens such as *Streptococcus pneumoniae*, *B. catarrhalis*, and *H. influenzae*. Sputum culture and Gram stain can be of assistance.

Bronchodiator therapy can alleviate symptoms significantly in some patients. Agents fall into three classes:

▲ methylxanthines (e.g., theophylline)

▲ beta-adrenergic agonists (e.g., albuterol, metaproternol)

▲ anticholinergics (e.g., ipratropium bromide)

Inhaled **ipratropium bromide** causes bronchodilation through inhibition of vagal stimulation of the airways. It is generally the first choice bronchodilator for use in COPD because tolerance does not develop and systemic side effects are minimal. Inhaled **beta-agonists** can be added to provide additional bronchodilation, but dependence on these agents alone can lead to decreased effectiveness and systemic side effects such as tremulousness and cardiac rhythm disturbances. Oral **theophylline** has moderate bronchodilatory action but may also improve respiratory muscle function and increase respiratory drive. It is useful for the prevention of nocturnal symptoms. Serum levels need to be monitored as nausea, palpitations, and seizures can result from toxic levels.

Corticosteroids can also be of use in certain patients, generally in the setting of acute exacerbations; some patients benefit from long-term steroids. As with bronchodilator therapy, empiric treatment is the only real way to determine which patients will have a beneficial response.

In patients with documented persistent hypoxemia (i.e., $Pao_2 < 55$ mmHg), **continuous supplemental oxygen** is indicated. Patients with signs of cor pulmonale and right heart failure should also receive supplemental oxygen even with less severe hypoxemia. In these patients, oxygen therapy has been shown to increase exercise tolerance, lower pulmonary arterial pressures, and increase life span. Some patients do not require oxygen supplementation during the day but have significant desaturation during sleep and thus benefit from nocturnal oxygen therapy. Patients who do not normally require supplemental oxygen may need supplementation during air travel.

Some patients remain severely incapacitated despite maximal therapy. In selected patients, lung transplantation can restore pulmonary function and relieve symptoms. However, organs are in very limited supply and the selection criteria are generally quite strict, making this a viable option for only a small minority of patients.

In some patients with emphysema who have a small number of large bullae, surgical resection of these bullae can improve symptoms and respiratory function. Again, this is an option only for very selected patients. Consultation with a pulmonologist and a thoracic surgeon is necessary.

► KEY POINTS

1. COPD is a smoking-related disease that results in long-term decrease in maximal expiratory airflow.

2. COPD can be divided into chronic bronchitis, which is characterized by cough and excess sputum production, and emphysema, where destruction of the terminal airspaces is predominant.

3. Spirometry, the measurement of expiratory volumes and flow rates, is the primary means for quantitating the degree of airflow obstruction and can be used to follow the progression of disease.

4. The natural history of COPD is generally one of progressive increase in airflow obstruction. In chronic bronchitis, there are often periodic exacerbations, whereas in emphysema, the decline is more steady.

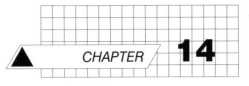

CHAPTER 14

Asthma

Asthma is a disease of the airways that is characterized by abnormally heightened responsiveness of the tracheobronchial tree leading to expiratory airflow obstruction. A key feature of asthma is its episodic nature—acute exacerbations separated by symptom-free periods.

▶ EPIDEMIOLOGY

Asthma affects an estimated 4 to 5% of the population in the United States. Onset is generally among younger patients; about one-half of cases manifest before age 10 and another third before age 40. In childhood, there is a 2:1 male:female preponderance, but by age 30, the sexes are equally affected.

Death related to asthma is infrequent (about 1 for 100,000 population), but there are indications that the mortality rate has been rising over the past 10 to15 years. The precise reason for this rise in asthma-related mortality is not known, but it has been suggested that this is a reflection of improper management of asthma, in particular an overreliance on beta-agonist bronchodilators.

▶ ETIOLOGY AND PATHOGENESIS

Asthmatics have greater degrees of **airway reactivity** (i.e., bronchoconstriction) to inhaled stimuli such as histamine, methylcholine, and cold air than nonasthmatics. Similarly, asthmatics exhibit heightened response to bronchodilators.

The pathophysiology of this airway hypersensitivity is not entirely clear. However, **chronic airway inflammation** appears to have an important role. A number of **stimuli can lead to chronic airway inflammation:**

▲ inhaled allergens

▲ viral and *Mycoplasma* infections,

▲ low-molecular-weight chemicals (including industrial dusts and gases)

Inhaled allergens are the most commonly encountered and important causes of chronic airway inflammation. Patients with so-called **allergic asthma** have increased serum immunoglobulin E (IgE) levels and positive skin-test results to airborne antigens.

In some patients, chronic inflammatory stimuli cannot be identified, yet they still have severe airway inflammation. These patients are referred to as having **intrinsic asthma.**

An **acute asthma attack** is triggered by **stimuli that cause bronchoconstriction,** such as:

▲ cold air

▲ exercise

▲ inhaled irritants (smoke, dust, aerosols, e.g., hairspray)

▲ beta-adrenergic blockers

▲ emotional upset

▲ nonsteroidal anti-inflammatory drugs

▲ food additives (e.g., sulfites)

▲ inhaled allergens

▶ CLINICAL MANIFESTATIONS
History

An acute asthma attack is heralded by **symptoms** of:

▲ dyspnea

▲ wheezing

▲ cough

▲ sputum production (mucorrhea)

▲ sleep disturbance

▲ increased use of bronchodilators

In many patients, these **symptoms develop over days to weeks** after an inciting event. In some patients, however, the onset of an attack can occur acutely, over **hours or even minutes.** This is particularly true if attacks are triggered by nonsteroidal anti-inflammatory agents, beta-adrenergic blockers, or food additives.

Physical Examination

During an acute attack, an asthmatic will be in **respiratory distress** with **tachypnea, wheezing,** and possibly a **cough.** On lung examination, patients will usually have audible **wheezes,** scattered **rhonchi,** and a **prolonged expiratory phase.** The chest will often be **hyperinflated** with an increased anteroposterior diameter.

Vital signs will reveal sinus tachycardia in addition to tachypnea. A **pulsus paradoxus** (an increase in the normal ≤ 10 mmHg fall in systolic blood pressure observed during inspiration) can be seen. Severe paradox (≥25 mmHg) is indicative of a severe attack. It is important to note that as respiratory muscle fatigue develops and the patient can no longer generate increased intrapleural pressure, the paradox can disappear.

Further signs of **respiratory muscle fatigue** are **accessory muscle use** and **paradoxic breathing pattern** (inward movement of the abdominal wall and lower thorax during inspiration).

▶ DIFFERENTIAL DIAGNOSIS

In a patient with known asthma, the diagnosis of an acute attack is relatively straightforward; however, the respiratory signs and symptoms can resemble those seen in:

▲ heart failure (pulmonary edema)

▲ pulmonary embolism

▲ pneumonia/bronchitis

▲ upper airway obstruction

▶ DIAGNOSTIC EVALUATION

The primary test used to determine severity of an acute asthma attack and monitor primary response to therapy is measurement of **peak expiratory flow rates** (PEFR, in L/min). Simple handheld devices are available to measure PEFR that can be used by patients at home and by physicians. Accurate measurements require appropriate patient effort technique. The results are most useful when they can be expressed as a **percentage of normal** or better still, as the percentage of the patient's best obtainable value during an asymptomatic period while on optimal treatment. Most patients present during an **acute attack** with a PEFR in the range of 20 to 30% of predicted. **Symptoms generally resolve** when PEFR returns to about 50% of normal; at about 60 to 70% of normal, **signs** of an attack (e.g., wheezing) disappear. Therefore, signs and symptoms may be absent when the patient still has severe residual disease, making measurement of PEFR important.

Arterial blood gas values are normal early in an attack. As dyspnea and anxiety result in hyperventilation, respiratory alkalosis and hypocapnia result. If respiratory failure develops secondary to respiratory muscle fatigue, an initial **pseudonormalization** of the Pco_2 and eventual hypercapnia with respiratory acidosis develops. Hypoxemia is generally not seen until respiratory acidosis develops. Routine measurement of blood gases during an acute attack is not always nec-

essary. If improvement in the PEFR and symptomatic improvement occurs with initial treatment, blood gas measurement is unnecessary.

Chest radiographs are generally unnecessary but will generally reveal hyperinflation and possibly atelectasis secondary to mucous plugging. Chest radiographs can reveal a pneumonia as well as complications of a severe attack such as pneumothorax and pneumomediastinum and should be considered under such conditions.

▶ TREATMENT

Given the pathophysiology of asthma, prevention of acute attacks depends on **limiting the degree of chronic inflammation,** whereas treatment of an acute attack will involve the **relief of bronchoconstriction.** The use of **anti-inflammatory agents** limits acute attacks and the use of **bronchodilators** provides **symptomatic relief** during exacerabations. Patient education is a key aspect of effective management. Patients need to know the basic pathophysiology of asthma and to understand the difference between the preventative treatment and symptomatic treatment. Patients need to be taught how to recognize exacerbations early and to institute prompt treatment.

Control of the patient's environment is another important aspect of asthma management. It is crucial to avoid sensitizing agents such as inhaled allergens and bronchospastic triggers such as nonsteroidal anti-inflammatory agents.

Corticosteroids are the **most potent anti-inflammatory agents** available. They are generally administered via the inhaled route using a metered dose inhaler (MDI). For stable patients, inhaled steroids can provide benefits equivalent to ingested steroids with fewer systemic effects. Oral steroids are generally reserved for the treatement of acute attacks or for maintenence in the rare patient who is not controlled with inhaled steroids alone.

Sodium chromoglycate and **nedocromil** are two related noncorticosteroid agents that are able to blunt the effect of inflammatory inducers and certain bronchospastic triggers (especially cold air and exercise). They are particularly effective in patients who have a significant **allergic component** to their asthma. The precise mechanism of action of the agents is not yet clear.

Beta$_2$-agonists are the most potent and widely used bronchodilators. Generally administered via MDI to limit systemic side effects (e.g., tachycardia, tremors), they provide prompt symptomatic relief, but because they do not have intrinsic anti-inflammatory action, they do not alter the underlying pathophysiology.

Theophylline and related methylxanthines have moderate bronchodilatory action but may also improve respiratory muscle function and increase respiratory drive. Administered via the oral route (although sometimes used intravenously during an acute attack), they can be useful for the prevention of nocturnal symptoms. Serum levels need to be monitored because nausea, palpitations, and seizures can result from toxic levels. The advent of more potent topical agents has resulted in decreased use of these agents.

Inhaled **ipratropium bromide** causes bronchodilation though inhibition of vagal stimulation of the airways. It has a slower onset and usually a lower peak effect in most asthmatics than beta-agonists. Although ipratropium bromide is the first choice bronchodilator for use in patients with chornic obstructive pulmonary disease (COPD), certain asthmatics, particularly the older patient with intrinsic asthma, benefit from its routine symptomatic use.

Intravenous magnesium sulfate is a mild to moderate bronchodilator that is generally used only in the setting of an acute attack refractory to beta-agonists.

During an acute attack, most asthmatics will benefit from supplemental oxygen. Hypoventilation due to loss of hypoxic drive is extremely rare in asthma as opposed to the case in COPD.

Proper control of asthma involves tailoring an appropriate management strategy to the degree of the patient's disease. For patients who have **infrequent symptoms** (i.e., using a beta-agonist MDI no more than two times a week), only **symptomatic treatment** is required. Once a patient requires beta-agonists more than twice a week, **maintenence therapy with an inhaled corticosteroid** is initiated; titrating dose until symptomatic control is required no more than two times a week. **Exacerbations** and insufficient control

is recognized by an **increased requirement for beta-agonists** and treated by increasing the dose of inhaled steroids. If this is unsuccessful, a short course of ingested steroids followed by a taper is given. For more severe flares that remain unresponsive to more intensive therapy, search for additional conditions such as **pneumonia, sinusitis,** or **gastroesophageal reflux** should be conducted. If a patient is unable to be tapered off ingested steroids, referral to a pulmonary specialist may be indicated.

Key reasons for **failure in asthma control** are patient noncompliance, an overreliance on beta-agonists, improper use of MDIs (requires significant patient education and effort to use properly), and failure to recognize acute exacerbations early and institute proper therapy. It is important to note that failure due to these reasons can be avoided by aggressive patient education.

▶ KEY POINTS

1. Asthma is an episodic disease characterized by abnormally heightened responsiveness of the tracheobronchial tree leading to expiratory airflow obstruction.

2. Chronic airway inflammation appears to be a key pathophysiologic feature of asthma.

3. Acute attacks of asthma are often triggered by stimuli that produce bronchoconstriction in the setting of chronic airway inflammation.

4. Treatment of asthma involves avoiding environmental stimuli that produce inflammation and/or bronchoconstriction, control of chronic inflammation by the use of anti-inflammatory drugs (e.g., inhaled steroids), and the limited symptomatic use of bronchodilators (e.g., beta$_2$-agonists).

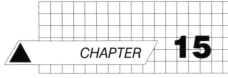
Pulmonary Embolism

► EPIDEMIOLOGY

Pulmonary embolism (PE) is a common but often unrecognized medical disease, with only 10 to 30% of all cases detected antemortem. About 10% of all pulmonary emboli are fatal, accounting for roughly 50,000 deaths per year in the United States.

► ETIOLOGY

Most pulmonary emboli (95%) arise from deep venous thrombosis (DVT) in the lower extremity. The development of thrombosis is increased by three major factors (Virchow's triad):

▲ stasis

▲ alteration in blood vessels

▲ hypercoagulability

High risk conditions may be classified by these factors:

Stasis:

▲ surgery

▲ heart failure

▲ chronic venous stasis

▲ immobility

Alteration in blood vessels:

▲ fractures/surgery of lower extremity

▲ major trauma

Hypercoagulability:

▲ postpartum period

▲ cancer

▲ oral contraceptive pills

▲ deficiencies of protein S, protein C, and antithrombin III

▲ lupus anticoagulant

▲ activated protein C resistance

► CLINICAL MANIFESTATIONS
History

The most prominent symptom in pulmonary embolism is a **sudden onset of unexplained dyspnea** (over 90% of patients). **Pleuritic chest pain** (increased with respiration) occurs in roughly 60%. **Hemoptysis,** although a classic finding, is uncommon and usually indicates pulmonary infarction.

Other presentations include syncope, supraventricular tachycardias, and worsening of underlying heart failure or lung disease.

Physical Examination

Vital sign abnormalities are common in PE. **Tachycardia** is often found and **tachypnea** is almost universal. Low grade fever (< 101°F) is often present.

The pulmonary examination in PE is most often completely normal. Cardiac examination may reveal signs of **right-sided heart strain** if the embolus is extensive. These include:

▲ loud pulmonic component of second heart sound (P2), best heard in left second intercostal space

▲ right-sided S3 (increased with inspiration)

▲ right ventricular heave (palpable lift over left sternal border)

Underlying thrombophlebitis is seen in less than half of all patients.

► DIFFERENTIAL DIAGNOSIS

In the patient who presents with **shortness of breath** and **chest pain,** the differential includes:

▲ pneumothorax

▲ myocardial ischemia

▲ pericarditis

▲ asthma

▲ pneumonia

In the patient with a massive PE who presents with **hypotension** and hemodynamic instability, also consider:

▲ myocardial infarction with shock

▲ cardiac tamponade

▲ tension pneumothorax

▲ aortic dissection

▶ **DIAGNOSTIC EVALUATION**

Arterial blood gas (ABG) classically shows hypoxia, hypocarbia, and a respiratory alkalosis. However, a normal ABG does not conclusively rule out pulmonary embolus. **Chest x-ray** most often shows atelectasis, seen in 60 to 70% of patients. Some classic, but less common, **x-ray findings** include:

▲ increased lung lucency in area of embolus ("Westermark sign")

▲ abrupt cutoff of vessel

▲ wedge-shaped pleural based infiltrate ("Hampton's hump")

▲ pleural effusion, which if tapped is often hemorrhagic

The last two signs occur 12 to 36 hours after symptoms begin and usually indicate pulmonary infarction.

On an **electrocardiogram** (ECG), the classic pattern for PE in the context of **right heart strain** is an S wave in lead I with a Q wave and T wave inversion in lead III ("S1Q3T3 pattern"). Other signs of right heart strain are new right bundle branch block and ST segment changes in V1-V2. However, the most common ECG finding is simply **tachycardia.**

Ventilation/perfusion (V/Q) scan identifies a "mismatch" between areas that are ventilated but not perfused and is the best initial test for PE in patients with a clear chest film. Studies in large numbers of patients evaluated for PE have shown the following:

▲ A **normal** scan basically rules out the diagnosis of PE;

▲ A **high-probability** scan is diagnostic if the clinical suspicion is also high (i.e., a "classic" story for PE in a patient with risk factors);

▲ A **low-probability** scan will rule out the diagnosis only in the low clinical suspicion patient;

▲ An **indeterminate** scan is just that—indeterminate. Chance of PE in these patients ranges from 16 to 66%, depending on the physician's pretest probability.

A **Doppler ultrasound** is a noninvasive test of the lower extremities that accurately detects **proximal deep venous thrombosis** (70 to 80% of all patients with PE have a concomitant proximal DVT). It is **not** useful in asymptomatic post-hip replacement patients (sensitivity < 50%). Some advocate using this test before going to invasive procedures, because a positive result will determine a need for anticoagulation.

A **pulmonary angiogram is the gold standard.** This invasive procedure is generally safe (0.3% mortality) and indicated if the diagnosis remains uncertain after noninvasive testing.

▶ **TREATMENT**

In the high-risk patient for PE, **heparin should be started** while awaiting the diagnostic workup. Delay in therapy will likely increase morbidity, whereas the risk of a brief period of anticoagulation is small. **Contraindications** for anticoagulation include:

▲ active gastrointestinal bleeding

▲ intracranial neoplasm

▲ recent major surgery (relative contraindication)

▲ known bleeding diathesis (relative contraindication)

Patients with **deep venous thrombosis** should also be treated with **heparin.** The treatment of **below-the-knee DVT** is more controversial. These clots have a low risk of embolizing, although 15 to 20% will progress above the knee. Recommendations vary from conservative treatment with elevation of the extremity and nonsteroidal anti-inflammatory drugs to treatment with standard anticoagulation. Others advise follow-up with noninvasive tests every 3 to 4 days over the next 10 to 14 days to detect progression.

In the hypotensive patient with massive pulmonary embolus, **thrombolytic therapy** may be indicated. More stable patients are not believed to benefit from this high-risk therapy.

Heparin should be started with an initial intravenous bolus, equal to 100 U/kg. This is followed by a continuous drip of 15–18 U/hr. Adequate anticoagulation should be achieved within the first 24 hours; if not, the risk of postphlebitic complications and DVT recurrence is increased. The partial thromboplastin time (PTT) should be checked every 4 hours, increasing the heparin dose until the goal of 1.5 to 2.0 times the control value of PTT is obtained.

During heparin therapy, platelet counts should be monitored. **Heparin-induced thrombocytopenia** manifests as a dramatic drop in platelets 1 to 20 days after initiation of therapy and is believed to be an autoimmune destruction mediated through immunoglobulin G. Changing from bovine to porcine heparin or visa versa is not proven to be effective (nor is a change to low-molecular-weight heparin). Discontinuation of heparin is recommended if platelet count is below 75,000.

Once the heparin dose is therapeutic, warfarin therapy may be instituted. A loading dose of warfarin usually consists of 10 mg for 2 to 3 days. This should be adjusted for drug interactions and patient's age. The goal for warfarin therapy is an international normalized ratio (INR) of the prothrombin time of 2 to 3. Heparin should be continued for at least 5 days and overlapped with a therapeutic warfarin dose for 2 to 3 days. Warfarin is then continued for 3 to 6 months in uncomplicated patients.

Recently, low-molecular-weight heparin has begun to replace standard heparin as initial therapy for DVT. Advantages of low-molecular-weight heparin include:

▲ fixed dosages administered subcutaneously (possibly at home)

▲ no need for laboratory monitoring

▲ decreased risk of DVT recurrence in some studies

Some patients are candidates for placement of an inferior vena cava filter. Indications include:

▲ contraindication to anticoagulation (see above)

▲ formation of thrombosis despite adequate anticoagulation

▲ large burden of thrombosis in lower extremities which could be fatal if embolized

Morbidity for pulmonary emboli is best avoided by preventing DVTs in the first place. For patients at risk of DVT, low-dose subcutaneous heparin (5000 U twice a day) or intermittent lower extremity compression is effective. Indications for prophylaxis include:

▲ major surgery

▲ acute myocardial infarction

▲ stroke

▲ prolonged immobility

Special consideration is given to patients at extremely high risk, such as hip fractures or hip/knee replacements. Warfarin to achieve INR of 2 to 3 is indicated in these situations. Low-molecular-weight heparin appears to be effective in these instances as well.

Although cancer is associated with thromboembolism, most cancers are known or obvious at time of PE diagnosis. However, about 10% of patients with idiopathic PE (no known risk factor) will develop cancer over the next few years. Routine cancer screening (stool guaiac, mammograms, etc.) is recommended, but extensive testing is not.

▶ KEY POINTS

1. Patients at risk for DVT/PE are those with an abnormality of blood vessels, stasis, or hypercoagulability. The most common predisposing causes are orthopedic injuries, surgery, and malignancy.

2. Sudden onset of dyspnea and pleuritic pain are classic presentations. A normal chest x-ray and normal arterial blood gas do not rule out the diagnosis but are useful to exclude other causes.

3. Ventilation-perfusion scanning should be performed on all patients suspected of PE. In the high-risk patient, heparin should be initiated if testing is delayed.

4. Given the risks, the need for anticoagulation must be documented by any of the following: angiogram positive for PE, DVT confirmed by ultrasound or venogram, or a high-probability V/Q scan in a patient with a high suspicion of PE.

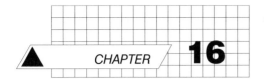

CHAPTER 16

Interstitial Lung Disease

*I*nterstitial lung disease (ILD) refers to a heterogeneous group of disorders that are characterized by inflammation and fibrosis of the alveolar walls and the perialveolar tissue. The spectrum of ILD ranges from idiopathic diseases to diseases resulting from exposure to pharmacologic, environmental, and occupational substances. The **unifying features** of these conditions are the similarity in:

▲ symptoms

▲ alteration in pulmonary physiology

▲ chest radiograph appearance

▲ histologic appearance

▶ ETIOLOGY AND PATHOGENESIS _____

The pathophysiology in ILD centers on chronic inflammation of the alveolar wall and surrounding structures. The inflammatory response can involve polymorphonuclear lymphocytes (PMNs), lymphocytes of B and/or T lineage and macrophages, depending on the specific etiology. Chronic inflammation eventually leads to scarring and fibrosis. Fibrosis leads to the **disturbances in lung function,** such as:

▲ decreased transalveolar gas diffusion

▲ a restrictive respiratory pattern (resulting in decreased lung volumes)

▲ variable obstructive respiratory pattern (depending on the underlyin getiology)

There are close to 200 described causes of ILD. However, most of them can be grouped into four **major divisions:**

▲ the pneumoconioses

▲ hypersensitivity pneumonitis

▲ drug-induced disease

▲ idiopathic

Pneumoconioses _____

These are a group of disorders characterized by pulmonary exposure to inorganic and organic **dusts** (e.g., asbestos, coal dust, rock dust [talc, silica, cement], metals [beryllium, antimony, tin, silver, iron], graphite, cotton dust, and grain dust) and **gases** (e.g., acid fumes, chlorine, nitrogen dioxide, and phosgene). Chronic inflammation develops, characterized by mucous hypersecretion, scarring, and fibrosis. As compared with other causes of ILD, the mucous hypersecretion can result in a prominent obstructive picture.

Hypersensitivity Pneumonitis (HP) _____

These are conditions in which the inflammation is immunologically mediated. Deposition of antigen (again usually in the form of dusts) in the alveoli results in the formation of antigen-antibody complexes. There is early infiltration by PMNs and later mononuclear cells and mast cells. Granuloma formation, in a classic delayed-type hypersensitivity reaction, can result.

Exposure to a variety of antigens can result in the development of HP. These antigens can be from various microorganisms (fungi and bacteria), plants, or animals:

▲ themophilic **actinomycetes** (farmer's lung, bagassosis or sugar cane worker's lung, potato riddler's lung)

▲ *Aspergillus* spp. (malt worker's lung, tobacco worker's lung, compost lung, allergic bronchopulmonary aspergillosis)

▲ *Botrytis cinerea* (wine grower's lung)

▲ bird proteins (e.g., feathers, droppings; bird fancier's/bird breeder's lung)

▲ animal fur dust (furrier's lung)

▲ wood dust (woodworker's lung)

▲ *Bacillus subtilis* enzymes (detergent worker's lung)

The **appearance of HP** is influenced by the degree and length of antigen exposure, the specific antigen, and host factors.

Drugs _____

A large number of drugs can cause diffuse pulmonary injury:

Cytotoxic drugs

▲ bleomycin

▲ vinblastine

▲ alkylating agents (cyclophosphamide, melphalan)

▲ antimetabolites (methotrexate, azathioprine, cytosine arabinoside)

Noncytotoxic drugs

▲ antibiotics (nitrofurantoin, amphotericin, penicillins, sulfas)

▲ nonsteroidal anti-inflammatory agents

▲ beta-blocking agents

▲ antiarrhythmic agents (lidocaine, amiodarone)

For cytotoxic agents, the pathophysiology is believed to be direct pulmonary toxicity. For noncytotoxic drugs, a combination of direct pulmonary toxicity and immunologic injury may be involved.

Idiopathic

ILD can develop in the setting of a number of **collagen vascular disorders**:

▲ systemic lupus erythematosis (ILD less common than pleural disease and acute pneumonitis)

▲ rheumatoid arthritis

▲ ankylosing spondylitis (upper lobe fibrosis)

▲ progressive systemic sclerosis

▲ polymyositis

▲ Goodpasture's syndrome (pulmonary hemorrhage and glomerulonephritis due to anti-basement membrane antibodies)

▲ Wegener's granulomatosis

Sarcoidosis and the group of diseases referred to as **histiocytosis X** can also result in **idiopathic pulmonary fibrosis** (IPF), a well-defined disease in which there is typical immunologic damage to the lung without identification of a causative antigen as in HP. The disease is characterized by an alveolar infiltrate composed of PMNs and activated macrophages. Fibrosis results, but without granuloma formation (which can distinguish it from some forms of HP).

▶ CLINICAL MANIFESTATIONS
History

The typical history in ILD is one of months or years of gradually **progressive dypsnea** (particularly on exertion) and a **nonproductive cough.** Some patients can have a more acute onset as in HP, where it occurs several hours after allergen exposure. If no further allergen exposure occurs, symptoms will diminish over several days. Patients with occupational HP may give a history of relatively symptom-free weekends, with an increase in symptoms associated with return to work on Monday.

A detailed history of possible environmental and occupational exposures, both past and present, must be obtained when evaluating possible ILD.

Physical Examination

Initially, the physical examination in patients with ILD may be unremarkable, but as the disease progresses, the classic finding of **fine expiratory crackles** appears. With progressive fibrosis and resultant pulmonary hypertension, signs of right heart overload and failure develop (accentuated pulmonary component of the second heart sound, right-sided heave, hepatic congestion, lower extremity edema).

If ILD is associated with a systemic illness such as lupus, physical finding of these diseases may be present.

▶ DIFFERENTIAL DIAGNOSIS

The major differential diagnosis is among the illnesses that compromise ILD, but the pulmonary symptoms of dyspnea and cough can also be seen in:

▲ heart failure (congestive)

▲ asthma

▲ chronic obstructive pulmonary disease

▶ DIAGNOSTIC EVALUATION

The initial diagnostic test in suspected ILD is the chest radiograph. The typical **chest radiograph** findings in ILD are **reticular** or **reticulonodular infiltrates** with diminished lung volumes. A variety of abnormalities, including alveolar infiltrates, hilar and mediastinal adenopathy, pleural disease, and honeycombing, can also be seen. Larger nodules are more common in granulomatous diseases such as sarcoidosis and Wegener's as well as in silicosis and asbestosis.

The **anatomic location of the infiltrates** can suggest different etiologies:

Upper lung zones

▲ sarcoidosis

▲ silicosis

▲ berylliosis

▲ hypersensitivity pneumonitis

Lower lung zones

▲ idiopathic pulmonary fibrosis

▲ collagen vascular disease-associated ILD

▲ asbestosis

It is important to note that up to 10% of patients with biopsy proven ILD will have a normal or near normal chest radiograph. **High resolution computed**

► CLINICAL MANIFESTATIONS
History

Symptoms in setting of a pleural effusion can reflect the underlying causes:

▲ pleuritic chest pain (bacterial pneumonia, pulmonary embolism, viral infection, tumor)

▲ cough (pneumonia, tumor)

▲ sputum production (pneumonia)

▲ hemoptysis (pulmonary embolism)

▲ shortness of breath (heart failure, pneumonia)

Symptoms directly related to the effusion itself can be minimal, but if the effusion becomes large enough, dyspnea can result. This is often seen in the large pleural effusions associated with malignancy.

Physical Examination

A large pleural effusion can result in:

▲ decreased tactile fremitus

▲ dullness to percussion

▲ absent or diminished breath sounds

▲ shift of trachea and heart away from affected side

In addition, findings related to the underlying etiology may be present:

▲ adenopathy (malignancy, tuberculosis)

▲ elevated neck veins, peripheral edema (heart failure)

▲ ascites (cirrhosis)

► DIAGNOSTIC EVALUATION

Large pleural effusions are readily seen on routine **chest radiographs.** Smaller effusions can be seen by obtaining bilateral lateral **decubitus films** in addition to the routine upright films. **Chest computed tomography** is useful in detecting small pleural effusions and is also more sensitive in detecting parenchymal masses and enlarged lymph nodes in cases of suspected malignant pleural effusion.

Once a pleural effusion is detected by examination and radiographic studies, a sample should be obtained by **diagnostic thoracentesis** to determine whether it is an exudate or transudate. For large free-flowing effusions, this can be done blindly with guidance based on physical examination (via percussion to determine the extent of the effusion). Smaller effusion and loculated effusions may need to be sampled under ultrasound guidance.

A number of criteria have been proposed to differentiate transudates from exudates, but the most common **criteria** was proposed by Light and colleagues:

▲ pleural fluid to serum protein (albumin) ratio > 0.5

▲ pleural fluid lactate dehydrogenase (LDH) > 200 IU

▲ pleural fluid to serum LDH ratio > 0.6

If **any one** of the critical values is exceeded, the effusion is judged to be an exudate.

An effusion occurring in the setting of a bacterial pneumonia or lung abscess (so-called *parapneumonic effusion*) needs further evaluation. The diagnosis of a **complicated parapneumonic effusion** is made if any of the following conditions are found:

▲ gross pus is present in the pleural space

▲ organisms are visible on Gram stain of the pleural fluid (defines an *empyema*)

▲ the pleural fluid glucose is less than 50 mg/dL

▲ the pleural fluid pH is below 7.00 (with an arterial pH greater than 7.15)

Culture of a suspected empy ma should be done as well as Gram stain.

If a **malignant pleural effusion** is suspected, the pleural fluid should be sent for **cytology.** If this is negative, a needle biopsy of the pleura should be performed. If this is also negative, thoracoscopic or open biopsy of the pleural may be needed. These latter procedures are often needed to make the diagnosis of **malignant mesothelioma.**

► TREATMENT

The treatment of pleural effusions varies between transudates and exudates. **Transudative effusions** are managed simply by correcting the underlying problem. Because the pleural membranes are intact, restoring the normal Starling forces will permit reabsorption of the excess fluid. Management of an **exudate** may require local control of the effusion (drainage or sclerosis) as well as correction of the underlying disorder.

For **transudates, diuretic treatment** is the mainstay of therapy, reducing the intravascular hydrostatic pressure. In rare cases, a therapeutic thorac entesis is required to relieve dyspnea until the Starling forces are in proper balance and further accumulation stops.

A **complicated parapneumonic effusion** requires drainage with **tube thoracostomy.** This is to prevent loculation of the effusion and also because antibiotics penetrate and perform poorly in such effusions. If loculation has already occurred, multiple tubes may be required. Alternately, streptokinase or urokinase can be instilled via the chest tube in an attempt to dissolve the loculations. In severe cases, **surgical decortication** may be required.

The treatment of **malignant pleural effusions** is often problematic. Treatment of the underlying malignancy is generally not possible. Malignant effusions are often quite large and reaccumulate after therapeutic needle thoracentesis. Alternatives include:

▲ instillation of sclerosing agents such as bleomycin or minocycline via a chest tube

▲ application of talc or direct abrasion via thoracoscopy

▲ insertion of a pleuroperitoneal shunt

▶ KEY POINTS

1. A pleural effusion is the accumulation of excess fluid between the parietal and visceral pleura.

2. Pleural fluid can form because of excess production due to a disturbance in the Starling forces across the pleural membrane (transudates) or due to damage to the pleural membrane and/or the draining lymphatics (exudates).

3. Transudates can be distinguished from exudates by measuring the protein and LDH measurements in the pleural fluid and comparing them to serum values.

4. Treatment of a transudate involves restoration of the normal Starling forces by correction of the underlying condition.

5. Treatment of a transudate often requires drainage and, in severe cases, pleural sclerosis in addition to correction of the underlying condition.

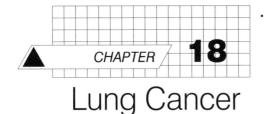

CHAPTER 18

Lung Cancer

*L*ung cancer is the leading cause of cancer death in the United States. Because most of these cancers are due to **cigarette smoking,** many of these deaths are preventable.

▶ EPIDEMIOLOGY

There are approximately 170,000 new cases of lung cancer diagnosed each year in the United States, with about 150,000 deaths occurring each year. Formerly, most of these cases occurred among men, but with the increased rate of cigarette use among women over the past 50 years, there has been a corresponding increase in the incidence of lung cancer among women.

Eighty to 90% of all lung cancers occur among **smokers.** There is a 10% mortality from lung cancer among smokers, whereas the mortality among non-smokers is less than 1%. The major determinants of risk among smokers is the number of cigarettes smoked per day and the total number of years smoked (usually expressed as **pack years,** i.e., the number of packs smoked per day multiplied by the number of years a patient has smoked).

If a person quits smoking risk declines, and by 10 years the lung cancer risk is only slightly above that of someone who had never smoked. The risk never returns to baseline.

There are **other exposures** that increase a person's risk of developing lung cancer, generally in a cocarcinogenic manner along with smoking:

▲ radon gas (a naturally occurring radioactive gas)

▲ asbestos

▲ environmental pollutants (automobile exhaust)

These other carcinogens may be responsible for some nonsmoking-related lung cancers that are encountered.

▶ PATHOPHYSIOLOGY

There are four major pathologic types of lung cancers that can be grouped into **two major groups** based on clinical grounds:

▲ small cell (100% of which are associated with smoking)

▲ non–small cell (further divided into squamous cell, large cell, and adenocarcinoma)

These cancers account for about 95% of all lung cancers. Other **rarer types of lung neoplasms** include:

▲ carcinoid tumors

▲ bronchoalveolar cancers (usually encountered in nonsmokers)

▲ mesotheliomas

The grouping of lung cancers into small cell and non–small cell cancers is based on clinical characteristics. **Non–small cell lung cancers** arise as a discrete mass within the lung parenchyma that can spread to regional lymph nodes and then metastasize to distant sites. As such, they are staged with the tumor-node-metastasis system used to stage many solid tumors. For patients with limited tumors, surgical resection can result in cure. Unfortunately, these tumors are not very responsive to chemotherapy, limiting treatment options in disseminated disease.

In contrast, **small cell lung cancers** metastasize rapidly to regional lymph nodes and distant sites. As such, the staging of small cell lung cancers is either as **limited disease** (overt disease confined to one hemithorax and the regional lymph nodes) and **extensive disease** where there is further spread. Only about 30% of patients present with limited disease. Because of the early spread of small cell lung cancer, surgery is generally reserved to relief of symptoms due the mass effect of the tumor. Unlike non–small cell cancer, small cell cancers are generally **quite responsive to chemotherapy.** About half of all patients with limited stage disease and about a third of those with extensive disease will have a complete remission, and 90% will have at least a partial response. Unfortunately, recurrence is common, leading to overall survival of about 5%. Patients with limited disease appear to have about a three- to fivefold better long-term survival rate than those with extensive disease.

Lung cancers are somewhat unique among neoplasms in that they are relatively more likely to produce active substances that result in a variety of **paraneoplasmic syndromes** (see also Chapters 48 and 69):

▲ hypercalcemia (due to PTH-like substance)

▲ syndrome of inappropriate antidiuretic hormone release (SIADH)

▲ ectopic corticotropin secretion (with resultant Cushing's syndrome)

▲ Eaton-Lambert syndrome (a myasthenia-like disorder seen in the setting of small cell cancer)

▲ hypercoagulable state (including migratory venous thrombophlebitis, Trousseau's syndrome)

▶ CLINICAL MANIFESTATIONS
History

The symptoms of lung cancer can arise from the local mass effect and systemic effects (e.g., constitutional symptoms) of the tumor itself, effect of metastatic disease (local or distant), and effect of products produced by the tumor (paraneoplasmic syndromes).

Because most lung cancers arise in patients with a long smoking history, the symptoms of **cough** and **dyspnea** are relatively nonspecific. However, an acute change in previously stable symptoms can be a clue of an underlying malignancy. Other symptoms related to the tumor can be **chest pain** and **hemoptysis.** Hemoptysis is generally not massive and can also be seen in patients with chronic obstructive pulmonary disease (COPD). Patients may present with the nonspecific constitutional symptoms of **anorexia, weight loss,** and **fevers/night sweats.**

Symptoms attributable to tumor **mass effect** include:

▲ cough (due to irritation of nerves including the phrenic nerve)

▲ hoarseness (with tumor compression of the recurrent laryngeal nerve)

▲ facial and/or upper extremity swelling (see SVC syndrome below)

Lung neoplasms commonly metastasize to the pleura, bone, brain, liver, and adrenal glands, where they can also produce symptoms. Patients may present with symptoms that are due to a paraneoplastic process.

Physical Examination

The physical examination generally provides few clues to the presence of an underlying lung cancer. However, typical physical findings associated with lung cancers are:

▲ Horner's syndrome (sympathetic ganglion dysfunction with ptosis, miosis, and anhydrosis)

▲ a supraclavicular mass due to a Pancoast tumor (apical tumor involving C8 and T1–2 nerve roots causing shoulder pain radiating down the arm)

▲ SVC syndrome (upper extremity ± facial swelling due to vascular obstruction)

In addition, clubbing and adenopathy (axillary or supraclavicular) are suggestive (but not pathognomonic) of an underlying malignancy.

▶ DIFFERENTIAL DIAGNOSIS

Lung cancer figures prominently in the differential diagnosis of lung masses and the so-called *solitary pulmonary nodule* (defined as a < 4-cm mass that appears on chest x-ray). The differential diagnosis of lung masses includes:

▲ tuberculosis

▲ fungal infection (histoplasmosis, coccidiomycosis, cryptococcus)

▲ metastatic cancer to the lung

▲ other granulomatous diseases (e.g., sarcoid)

The significance of the solitary pulmonary nodule is that about half are proven to be malignancies. If a solitary nodule is found to be malignant, it is associated with a 40% 5-year survival rate, significantly better than all lung cancer patients as a group.

▶ DIAGNOSTIC EVALUATION

The diagnosis of a lung cancer is first suggested on routine **chest x-ray,** which can reveal a mass as well as hilar adenopathy. The ability of chest radiograph to detect lung cancers has led to attempts to use the test as a screening method for smokers. However, it was shown that detection of asymptomatic masses on yearly chest x-ray **did not** lower mortality, presumably due to the rapid growth rates of the tumors and the relatively advanced stage of disease once a mass is visible on chest film.

If a potential mass is found on chest x-ray, further imaging with **computed tomography** (CT) can define the mass and better detect nodal disease. Magnetic resonance imaging has also been used but is less well studied.

Tissue diagnosis can be obtained in a number of ways. **Sputum cytology** can yield a diagnosis of malignancy. Generally, first morning sputums give the highest yield. **Bronchoscopy** (with bronchial washings, brushings, and/or biopsy) can also yield tissue. The location of a lesion determines accessibility. The flexible bronchoscope can only be inserted as far as secondary branches of the bronchial tree. Peripheral masses can be sampled with CT-guided **transthoracic needle biopsy.** Pneumothorax occurs in about a third of patients undergoing the procedure, but usually less than half of these require a chest tube.

Sampling of potentially involved nodes can be performed via:

▲ transbronchial biopsy via flexible bronchoscopy

▲ mediastinoscopy, where an incision is made in the suprasternal notch and a biopsy is taken via a mediastinoscope

▲ mediastinotomy, where an incision is made along the lower sternal border, allowing access to paratracheal nodes not accessible to mediastinoscopy

However, mediastinotomy is associated with a higher risk of complications.

Thoracoscopy can allow sampling of nodes and provide tissue samples of peripheral masses. It requires general anesthesia and the insertion of a chest tube.

▶ TREATMENT

Once a lung cancer has been diagnosed, studies must be done to determine the histologic type and stage of disease. Once this has been determined, therapeutic options can be discussed, generally in consultation with an oncologist.

As mentioned above, surgery with removal of the mass can be curative in some patients with non–small cell lung cancer. In patients with parenchymal tumors with either no nodal disease or involvement of only ipsilateral peribronchial or hilar nodes (stage I or II disease), surgery can be curative in 30 to 50% of patients. Once disease has progressed past this, a few selected patients can be cured surgically, but the proportion is much smaller.

Before surgery, the ability of the patient to survive the procedure needs to be assessed. Because many patients with lung cancer have underlying COPD, assessment of predicted postsurgical residual lung function must be done, usually with spirometry and/or nuclear perfusion studies.

Radiotherapy is generally not as effective as surgery but can be curative in some patients with limited disease who are unable to tolerate surgery or in some cases of more advanced disease. More often, radiation is used in a palliative manner (see below).

Chemotherapy in non–small cell lung cancer is still experimental. After referral to an oncologist, some patients can be candidates for clinical trials.

Small cell lung cancer is considered to be clinically or subclinically metastatic at time of diagnosis, and therefore surgery is unlikely to be curative. Combination chemotherapy is the standard treatment. In some cases, cranial and/or thoracic irradiation is added. As mentioned previously, most patients have a good initial response but most will relapse, giving an overall 5-year survival rate of about 5 to 10%, depending on the protocol used.

Patients with non–small cell cancer who have undergone surgery with the intent of cure need to be monitored for local recurrence and the appearance of metastatic disease. The same applies to patients with small cell cancers who have undergone chemotherapy. (The toxicity of cancer therapy is discussed in Chapter 68.)

Patients who have advanced disease and/or severe mechanical problems due to their cancer (e.g., airway obstruction, SVC syndrome, tracheal compression) are candidates for palliative therapy involving:

▲ radiation therapy (generally in lower doses and for shorter duration than curative radiation)

▲ laser surgery (for endobronchial obstructing lesions)

▲ brachytherapy (local application of radioactive material, generally via an endobronchial catheter)

In palliative care, the main goal is the relief of symptoms for the patient. Use of pain medications and hospice care are generally considered.

▶ KEY POINTS

1. Most lung cancer is associated with cigarette use and is the leading cause of cancer death in the United States.

2. Clinically, lung cancers can be divided into small cell lung cancers, which metastasize early, are very responsive to chemotherapy, but frequently recur, and non–small cell cancers, which in some cases of limited disease can be cured with surgery but are not very responsive to chemotherapy.

3. Lung cancers are associated with a number of paraneoplasmic syndromes, which in a number of cases is the presenting finding of the cancer.

4. In the case of a solitary pulmonary nodule (a <4-cm mass found on x-ray), about half of these will turn out to be malignant, and among those that are malignant, 40% will have a 5-year survival rate.

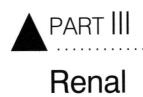

PART III

Renal

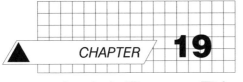

CHAPTER 19

Acid-Base Disturbances

▶ PRODUCTION AND ELIMINATION OF ACID

Acids are continually produced as a by-product of metabolism. Despite this addition of acid, the pH of the extracellular fluids is normally maintained between 7.35 and 7.45. Acid is produced in two forms: carbonic acid (H_2CO_3), also known as volatile acid, principally produced by metabolism in the form of carbon dioxide, and nonvolatile acids, such as sulfuric acid from sulfur-containing amino acids; organic acids from the partial metabolism of carbohydrates and fats; uric acid from nucleic acid metabolism; and inorganic phosphates and protons from the metabolism of organic phosphorus compounds.

Most of the daily acid load is carbonic acid (about 15,000 to 20,000 mmol/day), with nonvolatile acids being produced at the rate of about 80 mmol/day. Although nonvolatile acids are produced in a much lower amount on a molar basis, they can have a profound effect on the acid-base balance because of the differential elimination of carbonic acid and nonvolatile acids (see below).

The primary organs that deal with the removal of this acid load are the lungs and kidneys. The lungs rapidly eliminate carbon dioxide, maintaining a concentration of CO_2 in the body fluids of 1.2 mmol/L (Pco_2 of 40 mmHg). The protons produced by nonvolatile acids are removed by buffering with bicarbonate, converting it to water and carbon dioxide, which is then excreted by the lungs. In the process, the bicarbonate buffer is destroyed. The respiratory response to changes in extracellular pH is rapid, with acidosis stimulating ventilation and alkalosis depressing it.

The kidneys function to maintain the bicarbonate buffer system. They do this by retaining existing bicarbonate and generating new bicarbonate to replace that destroyed by the buffering of nonvolatile acids. Preservation of bicarbonate is accomplished by tubular reabsorption. New bicarbonate is generated by secretion of protons into urinary buffers (phosphate and ammonia) that are then eliminated. Proton secretion is stimulated by acidosis and aldosterone secretion. Bicarbonate reabsorption is stimulated by hypercapnia, extracellular volume contraction, and severe potassium depletion. The renal response to changes in extracellular pH is slower than the respiratory response, generally requiring 24 to 48 hours for a maximal response.

▶ DISTURBANCES IN THE HANDLING OF ACID

Acidosis is any abnormality that results in addition of acid or removal of alkali from the body fluids, whereas alkalosis is any abnormality that removes acid or adds base. If the primary disturbance is in the concentration of bicarbonate, it is referred to as metabolic. Conversely, if the primary disturbance is in the concentration of carbon dioxide, it is referred to as respiratory. Mixed disturbances are possible (e.g., a mixed metabolic acidosis and respiratory alkalosis). The term acidemia refers to a decrease in blood pH from normal, whereas alkalemia refers to an abnormal increase in blood pH. These terms are particularly useful when referring to mixed acid-base disturbances, when the direction of pH change can be the opposite from what is expected (e.g., a mild respiratory alkalosis in the setting of a severe metabolic acidosis will manifest as an acidemia).

Metabolic acidosis can arise via:

▲ increased production of nonvolatile acids

▲ decreased acid excretion by the kidney

▲ loss of alkali (generally from the gastrointestinal tract)

The first mechanism leads to a so-called *increased anion gap* acidosis. The serum anion gap (calculated as $[Na] - [HCO_3] + [Cl]$) is normally 8 to 12 and is due to unmeasured anions such as serum proteins. Nonvolatile acids will contribute to these unmeasured anions and increase the calculated gap. Decreased acid excretion by the kidney and loss of alkali do not increase the anion gap.

Metabolic alkalosis arises by increased loss of acid (generally from the stomach or kidney). Excess intake of base generally does not cause alkalosis unless large amounts are given continuously or in the setting of renal insufficiency.

Primary respiratory abnormalities can either be failure of respiration, leading to accumulation of carbon dioxide and acidosis, or hyperventilation, leading to a reduction in carbon dioxide and alkalosis.

An important aspect of acid-base balance is that the lungs and kidneys attempt to **compensate** for any abnormality that arises. A change in the plasma bicarbonate induces a compensatory change in ventilation that tries to counteract the effect of the bicarbonate change on the extracellular pH. Conversely, a primary change in carbon dioxide will result in a renal alteration in bicarbonate handling to offset this. The magnitude of an **appropriate** compensatory response has been determined from empiric observation of the responses in humans and experimental animals.

The following are the **expected compensations** for a primary acid-base disturbance:

▲ metabolic acidosis, 1.0 to 1.5 mmHg fall in Pa_{CO_2} for each 1 mEq/L decrease in HCO_3 (maximal decrease is to Pa_{CO_2} 12 to 15 mmHg)

▲ metabolic alkalosis, 0.25 to 1.0 mmHg rise in Pa_{CO_2} for each 1 mEq/L rise in HCO_3

▲ respiratory acidosis, acute, 0.1 mEq/L rise in HCO_3 for each 1 mmHg of Pa_{CO_2} rise over 40 mmHg, and chronic, 0.3 mEq/L rise in HCO_3 for each 1 mmHg of Pa_{CO_2} rise over 40 mmHg

▲ respiratory alkalosis, acute, 0.1 to 0.3 mEq/L fall in HCO_3 for each 1 mmHg of Pa_{CO_2} decrease below 40 mmHg, and chronic, 0.2 to 0.5 mEq/L fall in HCO_3 for each 1 mmHg of Pa_{CO_2} decrease below 40 mmHg.

▶ DIFFERENTIAL DIAGNOSIS

It is useful to divide the differential of acid-base disorders based on the primary abnormality.

Causes of Metabolic Acidosis

With increased anion gap include:

▲ lactic acidosis (from inadequate tissue oxygenation, hepatic failure, neoplasms)

▲ ketoacidosis (from diabetes, starvation, alcoholism)

▲ poisons/drugs (salicylates, methanol, ethylene glycol)

▲ renal failure (chronic, end-stage disease)

With normal anion gap include:

▲ renal tubular disorders (renal tubular acidosis, potassium sparring diuretics, hypoaldosteronism)

▲ loss of base (diarrhea, carbonic anhydrase inhibitors, ureterosigmoidoscopy, pancreatic fistula)

▲ excess acid intake (ammonium chloride, cationic amino acids)

Causes of Metabolic Alkalosis

Disorders include:

▲ volume loss with chloride depletion (vomiting, gastric drainage, diuretics, villous adenoma)

▲ hypermineralocorticoid states (exogenous steroid treatment, primary aldosteronism, Cushing's syndrome, renovascular disease)

▲ severe potassium deficiency

▲ excess alkali intake (milk-alkali syndrome, bicarbonate administration)

Causes of Respiratory Acidosis

Disorders include:

▲ acute respiratory failure (drug intoxication, cardiopulmonary arrest)

▲ chronic respiratory failure (chronic obstructive pulmonary disease, neuromuscular disorders, obesity)

Causes of Respiratory Alkalosis

Disorders include:

▲ hypoxia stimulating hyperventilation (asthma, pulmonary edema, pulmonary fibrosis, high altitude, congenital heart disease)

▲ increased respiratory drive (pulmonary disease, anxiety, salicylate intoxication, cerebral disease, fever)

▲ cirrhosis, pregnancy

▲ excessive mechanical ventilation

▶ CLINICAL MANIFESTATIONS
History and Physical Examination

There are few specific clinical findings for most acid-base disorders. Diagnosis depends on recognition of the appropriate clinical setting as described above and appropriate laboratory studies (see below). Given their role in maintaining acid-base balance, disease of the pulmonary and renal systems increases the likelihood of developing acid-base abnormalities.

Nonspecific signs such as fatigue and mental status changes can be seen along with findings related to the underlying etiologies. Some **signs and symptoms** that can be suggestive are:

▲ profound hyperventilation in the setting of acute metabolic acidosis (Kussmaul respiration)

▲ papilledema with severe, acute hypercapnia in the setting of acute respiratory acidosis

▲ neurologic symptoms in acute respiratory alkalosis (paresthesias, numbness, lightheadedness)

▶ DIAGNOSTIC EVALUATION

The diagnosis of acid-base disorders is made by measurement of **serum electrolytes** and obtaining **arterial blood gases.** Measurement of the **urine pH** and **plasma creatinine** can be useful in assessing renal function.

Arterial blood gas measurement is useful, but it should be noted that several technical aspects can affect the accuracy of the results:

▲ delay in processing sample or not keeping sample on ice

▲ contamination of the sample with excess heparin

▲ failure to purge air from the syringe

▲ a difficult arterial puncture leading to a respiratory alkalosis due to pain and anxiety

▲ sampling of venous blood instead of arterial blood can cause severe errors (usually decreased pH and Po_2 and increased Pco_2). This is particularly true in disease states that impair peripheral oxygen delivery and/or increase peripheral metabolism.

▶ TREATMENT

The treatment of acid-base disorders should proceed through a series of logical steps:

▲ Determine the magnitude and direction (i.e., acidemia versus alkalemia) of the acid-base disturbance through measurement of arterial blood gases;

▲ Determine the primary abnormality (in terms of acidosis versus alkalosis and metabolic versus respiratory);

▲ Determine whether there is an appropriate compensatory response;

▲ If the compensatory response is not appropriate, determine whether there is a secondary abnormality;

▲ Find and correct the underlying abnormality(ies).

Generally, if the underlying disturbance is corrected, the kidneys and lungs will restore acid-base balance.

Several conditions may require specific therapeutic interventions: metabolic acidosis in the setting of chronic renal failure (administration of oral bicarbonate), severe uncorrectable metabolic acidosis in the setting of acute renal failure (temporary hemodialysis), and metabolic alkalosis from volume and chloride loss (fluid replacement with saline solution). The administration of bicarbonate in the setting of severe anion-gap acidosis (e.g., lactic acidosis) is controversial. There is some evidence that this can actually increase cerebrospinal fluid acidosis.

▶ KEY POINTS

1. Metabolic acid can be in the form of carbonic acid (i.e., eliminated as exhaled CO_2) or nonvolatile acids (that are buffered by the blood bicarbonate system).

2. The lungs serve to eliminate CO_2 and the kidneys are responsible for maintenance of the bicarbonate buffer system.

3. Disturbance in the acid-base balance can be classified as acidosis (addition of acid or loss of base) or alkalosis (loss of acid or addition of base). If the primary abnormality is bicarbonate, the disturbance is said to be metabolic. If the primary abnormality is CO_2, the disturbance is said to be respiratory.

4. For each primary acid-base disturbance, there is an appropriate compensatory response that attempts to counteract the primary change.

5. Correction of the underlying abnormality is the mainstay of treatment for acid-base disturbances.

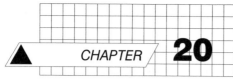

CHAPTER 20

Fluid and Electrolytes

*W*ater constitutes about 50 to 60% of the body weight. About two thirds of total body water (TBW) is intracellular fluid (ICF) and the remainder is extracellular (ECF). The plasma volume constitutes about 25% of the ECF, and the remaining 75% is interstitial fluid.

All principal electrolytes in the body are asymmetrically distributed across cell membranes. **Sodium** is the **principal extracellular cation**, with **chloride** and **bicarbonate** the main extracellular anions. **Potassium, calcium, magnesium,** and **organic anions** (e.g., proteins) the main intracellular electrolytes.

The asymmetric distribution of electrolytes is maintained by a variety of energy-requiring electrolyte "pumps" that move the electrolytes against their electrochemical gradients. The action of these pumps results in the vast majority (>95%) of sodium staying in the ECF and a similar majority of potassium staying intracellularly.

Because sodium salts account for >90% of the osmolality of the ECF, the plasma sodium concentration generally reflects the osmolality of the ECFs. Because water rapidly moves across membranes to dissipate osmotic gradients, the plasma sodium concentration not only reflects the osmolality of the ECF but is a marker for the relationship between total body solute and TBW.

▶ REGULATION OF SODIUM AND WATER

The **kidneys** tightly **regulate** the total body **sodium** content. Sodium depletion triggers decreased excretion, whereas sodium overload results in increased excretion. Peripheral receptors in the atria, central arteries, and juxtaglomerular apparatus sense the effective blood volume. These receptors regulate renal sodium handling via the **renin-angiotensin** system and a number of **natriuretic hormones.**

Plasma osmolality is regulated via the action of antidiuretic hormone (ADH). ADH is produced by the hypothalamus in response to increased plasma osmolality. ADH acts upon the kidney to reduce urine volume and increase urine osmolality, thus conserving water. Similarly, in the absence of ADH, the kidneys produce very dilute urine, allowing water diuresis at rates up to 20 L/day.

▶ DISTURBANCES IN SODIUM AND WATER BALANCE

Disturbances in sodium and water balance can reflect an excess or deficit in either or a combination of abnormalities. Pure sodium or water deficits are uncommon compared with combined deficits. Pure or disproportionate **water excess** leads to **hyponatremia,** whereas absolute or disproportionate **water deficit** leads to **hypernatremia.** A **pure excess of sodium** results in **edema** as seen in heart failure, cirrhosis, and the nephrotic syndrome.

Volume Depletion

ECF can be lost via renal or extrarenal routes:

Renal loss includes:

▲ excess diuretics

▲ osmotic diuresis (diabetic glycosuria)

▲ renal disease (end-stage renal disease, diuretic phase of acute renal failure)

▲ adrenal disease (mineralocorticoid deficiency)

Extrarenal loss includes:

▲ gastrointestinal losses (vomiting, nasogastric suction, diarrhea)

▲ abdominal sequestration (ascites, pancreatitis, ileus, peritonitis)

▲ skin (sweating, burns)

Clinical Manifestations

The clinical manifestations of volume loss depend on the magnitude and on the plasma osmolality (see hyponatremia and hypernatremia below):

▲ fatigue, weakness

▲ orthostatic lightheadedness and syncope

▲ orthostatic hypotension/tachycardia

▲ decreased skin turgor, lack of axillary sweat, sunken eyes, dry mucous membranes

▲ oliguria

Treatment

Volume depletion requires replacement of the lost fluid and electrolytes. In mild cases, this can be accomplished orally, but in severe cases, intravenous fluids are provided. Monitoring of serum electrolytes and avoidance of fluid overload are necessary.

Hyponatremia

Hyponatremia is the result of an **excess of water relative to total solute.** Because this results in a dilution of body fluids and hypoosmolality, there is usually a defect in production of dilute urine, which is the normal response to hypoosmolar states:

- ▲ volume depletion with sodium loss in excess of water loss (by mechanisms listed above for volume depletion)
- ▲ edematous states (cirrhosis, heart failure)
- ▲ euvolemic hypoosmolar states (renal failure, syndrome of inappropriate antidiuretic hormone, water intoxication, glucocorticoid deficiency)
- ▲ normoosmolar states (hyperglycemia, hyperlipidemia, hyperproteinemia)

Clinical Manifestations

Symptoms of hyponatremia are generally neurologic as water moves into brain cells, resulting in swelling. Symptoms include:

- ▲ lethargy
- ▲ confusion
- ▲ coma
- ▲ hyperexcitability, muscular twitching, and seizures (usually occur only with rapid onset hyponatremia)

  These symptoms are related to the degree of hyponatremia and the rapidity with which it develops.

Treatment

Treatment of hyponatremia generally involves correction of the underlying etiology. When there is severe volume depletion, then intravenous fluid replacement may be needed. Edematous states generally require free water restriction. Care must be taken not to raise the plasma sodium too rapidly because it can cause neurologic damage (central pontine myelinolysis).

Hypernatremia

Hypernatremia results from a deficit in water relative to solute. Hypernatremia invariably results in hyperosmolarity. This in turn normally results in ADH secretion that stimulates renal water conservation and thirst. Therefore, sustained hypernatremia will usually only occur in patients who are unable to respond to thirst by drinking (young children and mentally and/or physically limited adults).

Etiology

The **causes of hypernatremia** can be divided into:

- ▲ pure water deficits (insensible losses via skin and lungs, diabetes insipidus)
- ▲ water loss in excess of sodium loss (sweating, osmotic diuresis)
- ▲ sodium overload (administration of hypertonic oral or intravenous solutions)

Clinical Manifestations

As with hyponatremia, the **clinical features** of hypernatremia are due to central nervous system dysfunction and can manifest as lethargy, confusion, neuromuscular hyperexcitability, and coma.

Treatment

Correction of hypernatremia involves oral or intravenous replacement of water as well as sodium replacement if required. The **free water deficit** can be calculated as desired TBW (TBW) − current TBW, where current TBW = $0.6 \times$ body weight (kg) and desired TBW = $[Na]_{serum} \div 140 \times$ current TBW. As a rule of thumb, **only half of the free water deficit should be replaced in the first 24 hours** and the remainder of the deficit over the next 24 to 48 hours.

▶ DISORDERS OF POTASSIUM BALANCE

Potassium is the main intracellular anion. The **ratio of intracellular to extracellular potassium is the principal determinant of membrane excitability** in nerve and muscle cells. Because the extracellular potassium is low, small absolute changes in concentration can influence this ratio greatly. Similarly, small changes in the plasma potassium level may reflect large changes in the total body potassium level.

Excess potassium is mainly **eliminated by the kidneys.** Aldosterone stimulates renal potassium excretion. Additionally, the balance between intracellular and extracellular potassium is influenced by acid-base balance, with acidosis favoring a shift of potassium out of cells. Hormones also influence this balance. Insulin and beta-adrenergic catecholamines promote the movement of potassium into cells.

Hypokalemia

Potassium depletion results from insufficient dietary potassium intake or increased loss. **Potassium loss** can occur via:

▲ gastrointestinal loss (diarrhea, vomiting, villous adenoma, ureterosigmoidostomy)

▲ diuretic use

▲ metabolic alkalosis (renal wasting due to bicarbonate excess)

▲ mineralocorticoid excess

▲ licorice intoxication (due to a compound with mineralocorticoid-like activity)

▲ glucocorticoid excess

▲ renal tubular disease (renal tubular acidosis, certain antibiotics)

In addition, shift of potassium into the intracellular compartment (from insulin effect, alkalosis) can result in hypokalemia without an actual total body potassium deficit.

Hypokalemia manifests as disturbances in the function of excitable tissues:

▲ skeletal muscle (weakness, particularly of the lower extremities, rhabdomyolysis)

▲ smooth muscle (gastrointestinal ileus)

▲ cardiac muscle (prominent U-waves on electrocardiogram, cardiac arrest—with rapid reduction of serum potassium, enhanced digitalis toxicity)

▲ peripheral nerves (decreased or absent tendon reflexes)

Potassium replacement is generally done via oral supplementation, with potassium chloride the usual form. Severe hypokalemia or hyperkalemia in patients who cannot absorb oral supplements can be treated with intravenous supplementation. However, potassium solutions should normally contain at most 60 mEq/L and should be administered no faster than 20 mEq/hr to avoid cardiac toxicity from transient hyperkalemia.

Hyperkalemia

Hyperkalemia can occur via a number of mechanisms:

▲ inadequate renal excretion (acute renal failure, end-stage renal failure, tubular disorders)

▲ adrenal insufficiency

▲ administration of "potassium-sparing" diuretics (spironolactone, amiloride)

▲ tissue damage with release of intracellular potassium (muscle crush injury, hemolysis, internal hemorrhage)

▲ shift of potassium from the intracellular compartment (acidosis, insulin deficiency, digitalis poisoning, beta-adrenergic antagonists)

▲ excess potassium intake (usually in the setting of underlying renal insufficiency)

The **major toxicity of hyperkalemia is the development of cardiac arrhythmias.** Electrocardiographic manifestations of hyperkalemia include:

▲ peaking of T-waves (earliest sign)

▲ PR prolongation

▲ complete heart block

▲ atrial asystole

▲ QRS widening

▲ ventricular fibrillation/standstill

Severe hyperkalemia is a medical emergency, requiring immediate treatment. Therapies can be divided into those that immediately lower the serum potassium concentration (by causing shift of potassium from the extracellular compartment to the intracellular compartment) and those that eliminate excess potassium from the body. **Emergency management includes:**

▲ insulin (with concomitant glucose administration to avoid hypoglycemia)

▲ intravenous bicarbonate

▲ calcium administration (does not lower plasma potassium levels but counteracts the effect of hyperkalemia on excitable membranes—transient effect)

Elimination of excess potassium can be done by:

▲ using oral potassium-binding resins

▲ dialysis (hemodialysis and peritoneal dialysis)

▲ diuretics and saline infusion

[Handwritten notes:]

C BIG K

pseudohyponatr.
• ↑glycemia
• ↑Lipidemia
• ↑ Protienemia

Hyponatremia

↑Volume Normo ↓Volume

↑Volume
*Edema
1. cirrohsis
2. CHF
3. Nephrosis

Normo
• SIADH
• Water Introx
• Renal Fail.

↓Volume
*Volume Depletion
① Renal
 • Diuretics
 • DZ
② Extrarenal
 GI (Diarrhea, vomit)
 Abdomen (ascites, pancreatitis)
 Skin

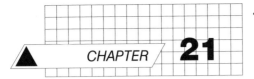

Acute Renal Disease

*7*he kidneys normally serve a number of important functions, such as:

▲ maintenance of water and electrolyte balance

▲ removal of metabolic wastes

▲ vitamin D metabolism

▲ blood pressure regulation (via secretion of renin and prostaglandins)

Acute renal failure (ARF) is that which arises over hours to weeks. Often arising in patients with comorbid conditions, ARF needs to be quickly recognized and the underlying etiology determined.

▶ ETIOLOGY AND PATHOPHYSIOLOGY

The etiologies of ARF can be divided into three major groups based on the anatomic nature of lesion. **Prerenal** refers to conditions that lead to an overall decrease in the normal renal perfusion, including:

▲ hypovolemia

▲ decreased cardiac output

▲ renovascular disease

▲ systemic vasodilation

▲ renal vasoconstriction

▲ impairment of renal autoregulation of blood flow (often due to drugs such as angiotensin-converting enzyme inhibitors or nonsteroidal anti-inflammatory drugs).

Intrinsic renal refers to conditions affecting the renal parenchyma itself, such as:

▲ glomerulonephritis

▲ acute tubular necrosis (can be due to an ischemic insult or nephrotoxic drugs such as aminoglycoside antibiotics)

▲ interstitial nephritis (often an allergic type reaction to various drugs)

▲ tubular obstruction

Postrenal refers to conditions that lead to impairment in the flow of urine from the kidneys:

▲ ureteral obstruction

▲ bladder neck obstruction

▲ urethral obstruction (e.g., secondary to an enlarged prostate)

Given the normal functions of the kidney listed above, **complications of ARF** commonly seen are:

▲ intravascular volume overload

▲ metabolic acidosis

▲ anemia

▲ hyperkalemia

▲ uremic syndrome (see below)

▶ RISK FACTORS

ARF occurs in both the hospital and ambulatory setting. Among ambulatory patients, it is more frequently seen in patients with comorbid conditions and a debilitated state. ARF is generally more frequent in the hospital setting (occurring in up to 5% of all hospitalized patients) where it is associated with:

▲ surgery

▲ trauma (hemorrhage, muscle injury)

▲ administration of nephrotoxic drugs (aminoglycoside antibiotics, contrast agents)

▲ bladder catheterization

▲ sepsis

▲ shock (low cardiac output states)

▶ CLINICAL MANIFESTATIONS
History

Symptoms of acute renal failure are usually not present until the glomerular filtration rate falls to about 10 to 15% of normal. Most symptoms (e.g., fatigue, nausea, vomiting, puritus, and mental status changes) are due to the accumulation of toxic metabolites. Oliguria or even anuria is frequent but not invariably seen. Fluid overload can result in **dyspnea** and **orthopnea** that can be quite severe.

Because symptoms are generally present only with greater degrees of renal impairment, the diagnosis of ARF is often made by routine laboratory assessment. History can give clues as to the etiology. A drug history is important, as is a history of recent surgery, trauma, or infection.

Physical Examination

The physical examination of a patient with ARF can give an assessment of the degree of renal failure and provide clues to the underlying etiology. The patient's fluid balance can be assessed by orthostatic vital signs, assessment of skin turgor, and examination of jugular veins. Signs of fluid depletion can indicate a prerenal condition, whereas fluid overload can indicate the degree of renal dysfunction. The presence of abdominal bruits suggests renovascular disease. A pelvic or rectal examination can reveal causes of urinary outflow obstruction such as an enlarged prostate or a pelvic mass. The kidneys can be palpable in cases of hydronephrosis or polycystic kidney disease (which generally causes chronic renal failure).

The **uremic syndrome** is a constellation of symptoms (described above) and physical findings that are due to the accumulation of toxin normally handled by the kidney:

▲ pericarditis (manifested by a cardiac rub)

▲ uremic frost (crystals of urea that collect on the skin)

▲ asterixis

▲ uremic fetor (a urine-like odor to the breath)

▶ DIFFERENTIAL DIAGNOSIS

Generally, in acute renal failure the main diagnostic challenge is to determine the underlying cause. However, the fluid and electrolyte abnormalities can cause a symptom complex that can mimic a number of other conditions, such as congestive heart failure, dehydration, and intoxication.

▶ DIAGNOSTIC EVALUATION

The diagnosis of ARF is often made by the finding of an elevated blood urea nitrogen and creatinine. Once the diagnosis of renal failure is made, measurement of serum electrolytes (sodium, potassium, chloride, bicarbonate, calcium, and phosphate) is important for monitoring the patient because life-threatening abnormalities can develop.

Analysis of urine sediment can provide important information. The presence of red blood cells, either alone or in casts, suggests a glomerular or vascular lesions. White cells and white cell casts are seen in interstitial nephritis. Granular casts (in particular, "muddy-brown" casts) are often seen in acute tubular necrosis but are generally less specific than the other types of casts.

Assessment of the degree of proteinuria by a 24-hour urine collection can give clues to the etiology. Generally, nephrotic range proteinuria (i.e., > 3 g/24 hours) indicates a glomerular lesion. Lesser amounts are usually seen in interstitial disorders.

Calculation of the fractional excretion of sodium (FENA), which is defined as:

$$100 \times (\text{urine Na/serum Na} \div \text{urine Cr/serum Cr})$$

can distinguish prerenal azotemia from other etiologies. In prerenal conditions, the FENA is generally < 1 as the kidneys try to preserve intravascular volume by maximally conserving sodium.

If a glomerular process is suspected from the clinical context, immune-mediated disease can be screened for by measurement of antinuclear antibodies, antineutrophil cytoplasmic antibodies (ANCA; seen in Wegener's granulomatosis), antiglomerular basement membrane (anti-GBM) antibodies, complement levels, and cryoglobulins.

Renal imaging can determine the etiology of ARF. **Renal ultrasound** is commonly used, because it can allow assessment of kidney size and can detect hydronephrosis. It has largely replaced the intravenous pyelogram for screening for hydronephrosis because it avoids the risk of radiocontrast nephrotoxicity. If hydronephrosis indicative of obstruction is found, a urologist should be consulted and a search for the precise location of the obstruction can be undertaken with further tests such as computed tomography, retrograde pyelography, and cystoscopy.

The nuclear medicine **renal scan** can detect unilateral renal artery stenosis but is less sensitive in detecting bilateral renal artery disease.

The use of the **renal biopsy** has decreased in recent years. Traditionally used in the diagnosis of glomerulopathies, the development of serologic tests such as ANCA and anti-GBM has allowed many diagnoses to be made without biopsy. However, in cases where the diagnosis is uncertain, consultation of a nephrologist with possible biopsy can be useful in making a diagnosis or in giving prognostic information.

▶ TREATMENT

Treatment of acute renal failure involves correction of fluid and electrolyte abnormalities and attempting to find and correct the underlying cause. The search for an etiology is important because it will influence the long-term management.

The presence of prerenal azotemia dictates restoration of intravascular volume. In many cases of acute tubular necrosis, which is often due to nephrotoxic agents, once the offending agent is removed, renal function will eventually return and supportive measures are all that is necessary. Other disease(s) such as glomerulonephritis in Wegener's granulomatosis require treatment (immunosuppression with prednisone and cyclophosmamide) to prevent irreversible renal damage (see Chapter 23). The management of postrenal azotemia involves prompt determination of the level and then relief of the obstruction to urinary flow.

In prerenal and intrinsic renal azotemia, fluid and electrolytes should be managed using the general principles outlined in Chapter 20. In prerenal azotemia that is secondary to absolute hypovolemia, replacement of fluid depends on the mechanism of loss. Fluid deficit due to hemorrhage should be corrected with both saline and red cells. Gastrointestinal fluid loss is generally hypotonic and should be replaced accordingly.

Hyperkalemia in ARF can be life threatening, and emergent management is required in patients with extreme elevation (>6.5 mmol/L) or in any patient with electrocardiogram abnormalities (see Chapter 20).

For patients with urinary outflow obstruction, once the level of obstruction is determined, relief of obstruction (with urologic consultation if needed) will result in reversal of the azotemia. For urethral obstruction, bladder catheterization or placement of a suprapubic tube (if catheterization is not possible) will be sufficient. If the obstruction is higher (at the vesicoureteral junction or in the ureter or renal pelvis), percutaneous nephrotomy or ureteral stent placement by a urologist will be needed.

In intrinsic renal failure, supportive methods are generally sufficient while waiting for reversal of the underlying problem. In more severe cases, temporary dialysis (see Chapter 22) may become necessary.

Once therapy for ARF has begun, continued monitoring for both complication of renal failure and return of renal function is maintained. One important consideration is dose adjustment of renally excreted drugs, both to avoid systemic drug toxicity and to direct renal toxicity. The need for dialysis can arise later in the course if recovery is delayed or not forthcoming. In some cases (glomerulonephritis in particular), renal function may not return to a sufficient degree and long-term dialysis is required.

▶ KEY POINTS

1. ARF can be divided into prerenal (due to decreased renal perfusion), intrinsic renal (due to defects in the renal parenchyma), and postrenal (due to obstruction of the flow of urine).

2. ARF leads to complications due to the malregulation of fluid and electrolyte balance and the accumulation of toxic waste products.

3. Signs and symptoms of ARF generally do not appear until renal function falls to about 10% of normal.

4. Treatment of ARF involves determining the underlying etiology, correction of the etiology, and supportive management of fluids and electrolytes.

5. In more severe cases of ARF, temporary or permanent dialysis may be necessary.

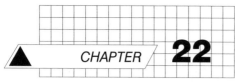

CHAPTER 22

Chronic Renal Disease

*C*hronic renal failure (CRF) can develop in the setting of acute renal failure (ARF; see Chapter 21) but more often arises as a complication of a chronic systemic illness such as diabetes and hypertension. CRF is characterized by progressive loss of functioning nephrons, eventually leading to a condition known as end-stage renal disease (ESRD). In ESRD, signs and symptoms of renal failure appear as the functional reserve of the kidneys is lost.

▶ EPIDEMIOLOGY AND ETIOLOGY

There are approximately 160,000 patients who are on chronic dialysis in the United States. The incidence of patients who require dialysis is 150/million/year (i.e., about 42,000 new dialysis patients a year). The incidence of ESRD that requires dialysis is about 1.3 to 1.4 times higher among men than women. The peak age is between 65 and 75 years.

The major underlying **conditions leading to end-stage renal disease** include:

▲ diabetes (33%)

▲ primary hypertension (29%)

▲ glomerulonephritis (15%)

▲ interstitial nephritis (4%)

▲ polycystic kidney disease (4%)

▲ other (15%)

It is important to note that the two leading causes of ESRD, diabetes and hypertension, can be controlled and that adequate control of these conditions can prevent or at least delay the development of ESRD.

▶ PATHOPHYSIOLOGY

Uremia refers to the syndrome that results from the failure of the kidneys to perform their normal excretory, metabolic, and endocrine functions. Uremia is a complex syndrome that includes a variety of physiologic and clinical abnormalities:

▲ **fluid and electrolyte abnormalities**, such as fluid overload, metabolic acidosis, sodium imbalances, hyperkalemia, hyperphosphatemia, hypocalcemia

▲ **endocrine/metabolic abnormalities**, such as hypertriglyceridemia, vitamin D deficiency, second-ary hyperparathyroidism, osteomalacia, hyperuricemia, impotence

▲ **cardiovascular disorders**, such as hypertension, heart failure, pericarditis, accelerated atherosclerosis

▲ **gastrointestinal disturbances**, such as anorexia, nausea/vomiting, peritonitis, ascites

▲ **dermatologic abnormalities**, such as pruritus, uremic frost, hyperpigmentation

▲ **hematologic/immunologic abnormalities**, such as anemia (generally normochromic, normocytic), impaired platelet function, leukopenia, T-cell dysfunction (leading to increased risk of infection)

▲ **neurologic/neuromuscular abnormalities**, such as fatigue, asterixis, headache, myoclonus, seizures, peripheral neuropathy, altered mentation, coma

Some abnormalities are due to accumulation of toxic metabolites, and others are due to underproduction (e.g., vitamin D, erythropoietin) or overproduction (e.g., renin) of substances produced by the kidney. For other abnormalities, the exact pathophysiology is unclear.

Because of the significant functional reserve of the kidneys, symptoms generally do not appear until renal function (as measured by glomerular filtration rate [GFR]) declines to 10 to 15% of normal. At about 30 to 40% of normal GFR, biochemical evidence of renal failure can be seen, but patients are generally asymptomatic.

▶ CLINICAL MANIFESTATIONS
History and Physical Examination

The history and physical examination findings in a patient with chronic renal failure are manifestations of the abnormalities associated with uremia:

▲ fatigue, shortness of breath, pruritus, headache

▲ peripheral edema, ascites

▲ asucultatory rales, pericardial rub

▲ bruising, uremic frost, hyperpigmentation

▲ asterixis, peripheral neuropathy, and altered mental status

▶ DIAGNOSTIC EVALUATION

In a patient with a condition known to predispose to the development of chronic renal failure, biochemical monitoring is usually performed to detect renal failure before it becomes clinically overt. As with acute renal failure, monitoring of the **serum creatinine** can track the progression of CRF. Given the functional reserve of the kidneys, the GFR (normally about 125 mL/min) can fall to 40 to 50% of normal with only modest change in creatinine.

GRF can be estimated in a number of ways. A 24-hour urine collection can provide an estimate of GFR using the equation:

$$(U_{Cr} \times V/P_{Cr}) \div 1440$$

where U_{Cr} is the urine creatinine concentration (mg/dL), P_{Cr} is the plasma creatinine (mg/dL), V is the 24-hour urine volume (mL), and 1440 is the number of minutes in 24 hours. It can be difficult to accurately obtain a 24-hour urine collection, especially from an ambulatory patient. Alternately, the GFR can be estimated using the formula:

$$[(140 - age) \times bodyweight\ (kg)] \div [72 \times P_{cr}]$$

This formula is more convenient, because it does not require a 24-hour urine collection.

Routine monitoring of the complete blood count can detect anemia secondary to erythropoietin deficiency. Monitoring of urinalysis can detect increasing proteinuria. When renal function declines further, closer monitoring of routine laboratory tests to detect dangerous electrolyte imbalances (e.g., hyperkalemia) and acidosis is required.

▶ TREATMENT

The treatment of chronic renal failure is based on:

▲ determination and control of the underlying etiology

▲ monitoring changes in renal function

▲ conservative treatment of effects of CRF

▲ instituting more aggressive treatment (dialysis and/or renal transplantation) when appropriate

Aggressive control of diabetes, hypertension, and acute glomerulonephritis can delay or even prevent the development of CRF. In patients who present with CRF, control of these underlying etiologies can delay progression.

Diet modification is a key element in the conservative treatment of CRF. **Restriction of fluid and sodium** can diminish secondary hypertension. In some cases, diuretics may be required. At the same time, **dehydration must be avoided** to prevent prerenal azotemia. As renal function declines further, restriction of dietary phosphate and potassium becomes necessary. **Protein reduction** can relieve uremic symptoms and delay progression of renal failure. Dietary protein intake of 0.55 to 0.6 g/kg/day is sufficient to prevent negative nitrogen balance while relieving uremia.

The progression of CRF is initially monitored by following the blood urea nitrogen, creatinine, and creatinine clearance. As disease progresses to the more advanced stages, conservative management begins to fail and the patient has problems with fluid balance and may experience repeated episodes of hyperkalemia, hypertension, acidosis, and severe uremia. At this stage (generally when GFR falls below 10 mL/min), the decision for **advanced therapy** may need to be made. Options include hemodialysis, peritoneal dialysis, and renal transplantation.

Hemodialysis involves circulating the patient's blood through a machine that uses diffusion across a semipermeable membrane to remove unwanted substances while adding other desirable materials. The composition of the dialysate (i.e., the solution the blood is equilibrated against) can be altered to increase the amount of solute that is removed or added. A prerequisite for hemodialysis is vascular access. For emergent (e.g., in severe ARF) hemodialysis, a catheter can be placed, but for long-term dialysis, permanent access is required. This can be a surgically constructed arteriovenous fistula, usually involving the radial artery of the nondominant arm. If the patient's vessels are inadequate, synthetic graft material can be placed, but these tend to be more prone to clotting and infection. An arteriovenous fistula generally needs to mature for 1 to 2 months before it can be used, making it important to place it before dialysis is imminent or to use temporary access while it matures.

Chronic hemodialysis is generally performed three times a week. Each session lasts about 3 to 4 hours, during which time the patient remains attached to the dialysis machine.

Peritoneal dialysis is a procedure in which the dialysate is placed via a specialized permanent catheter directly into the peritoneal cavity of the patient. In this case, fluid and toxic solutes are transferred across the mesenteric capillary bed into the dialysis fluid. The fluid is then removed via the catheter. The most common method, **continuous ambulatory peritoneal dialysis (CAPD)**, involves having the patient continually carry about 2 L of dialysis fluid in the peritoneal cavity. The fluid is then exchanged four times a day. Because exchange is accomplished by gravity flow, no machinery is required and dialysis can be performed virtually anywhere.

In **renal transplantation**, kidneys for transplantation are either **cadaveric** or from **living-related donors**. The best success rates involve organs from living-related donors who are HLA identical. Close to 100,000 renal transplants have been performed in the United States, with about 9000 new transplants performed each year. The best candidates for renal transplants are younger patients who have minimal comorbid disease. Referral to a center where transplants are commonly performed is generally required.

The decision to move to dialysis and/or transplantation is usually made in consultation with a nephrologist. Patient characteristics often determine which modality would be appropriate. Hemodialysis requires several periods a week of being hooked up to the dialysis machine, which can make travel and scheduling problematic, but in between dialysis, patients have only to continue their conservative treatment measures. CAPD allows more lifestyle freedom but requires a much greater degree of patient responsibility to manage the dialysate changes and to maintain the dialysis catheter. Transplantation offers the best treatment option for relieving the various manifestations of renal failure, but patients must be able to adhere to and tolerate their immunosuppressive regimen. As with all organ transplants, organ supply is limited.

Patients who are on hemodialysis generally tolerate the procedure well. Hypotension during the procedure is a common complication but is generally easily managed by adjusting the flow rates and dialysate. Psychiatric problems related to the loss of independence and altered self-image can arise. Long-term hemodialysis has been associated with a dementia that may be related to aluminum contamination of dialysate water. Failure of the vascular access can occur.

The major complication of peritoneal dialysis is the development of peritonitis. A patient on CAPD who develops fever, abdominal pain, and notices a change in the clarity of the dialysate should be evaluated for possible peritonitis. Treatment of peritonitis generally involves administration of antibiotics, which can be given as an outpatient in a patient who is not systemically ill. CAPD can usually be continued during treatment. In severe cases, catheter removal and temporary hemodialysis is required.

Patients who undergo a successful renal transplant usually have normalization of most abnormalities associated with renal failure. The major complications are either due to the immunosuppression required or rejection of the transplanted organ.

▶ KEY POINTS

1. Chronic renal failure most often occurs as a complication of a chronic systemic illness. In the United States, the leading conditions are diabetes and hypertension.

2. Chronic renal failure can lead to the syndrome of uremia, which is manifested as signs and symptoms related to the loss of the excretory, metabolic, and endocrine functions normally performed by the kidneys.

3. When conservative treatment (fluid/electrolyte management, dietary modification) fails, patients will require more aggressive treatment.

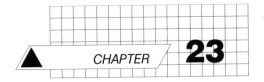

CHAPTER 23

Glomerular Disease

*T*he glomerulopathies are a heterogeneous group of disorders that are characterized by direct injury to the glomerulus. The etiologies of glomerular injury are varied and give rise to a number of distinct clinical syndromes. A particular etiology can give rise to more than one clinical syndrome, making classification of the glomerulopathies difficult.

▶ PATHOGENESIS

Glomerular injury can be divided into two major categories based on pathology:

- ▲ **nephritis,** which is characterized by glomerular inflammation and/or necrosis
- ▲ **nephrosis,** which is characterized by abnormal permeability of the glomerular membrane, allowing macromolecules such as albumin to pass.

These two forms of injury are not mutually exclusive and a single etiology can produce both forms of injury.

The immunologic injury that characterizes **glomerulonephritis** can be subdivided into:

- ▲ **antiglomerular basement membrane disease (anti-GBM disease),** which is due to direct glomerular damage occurring as a result of inflammation triggered by antibodies directed against components of the glomerular basement membrane. **Linear** deposits of immunoglobulin are seen by immunofluorescence microscopy (IF) of renal tissue.

- ▲ **Immune complex disease** is another subdivision, which is glomerular deposition of immune complexes, composed of antibody bound to a variety of circulating antigens, that results in an inflammatory response. IF reveals **granular** immunoglobulin deposits.

- ▲ Finally, **pauci-immune (anti-neutrophil cytoplasmic antibody) disease** is a group of disorders characterized by the presence of serum antibodies against the neutrophil cytoplasm (ANCA) that are associated with multisystem disease. Minimal or no immunoglobulin is seen by IF, hence the name "pauci-immune." Despite this name, the glomerular injury is still believed to be immunologic in nature.

In **nephrosis,** the hallmark is a marked increase in the permeability of the glomerular capillary wall to macromolecules including serum proteins. Inflammatory changes are generally not seen (but can be present). In classic forms, the nephrotic syndrome (see below) develops, but various degrees of proteinuria can be seen. In about two thirds of adults, and most children, nephrotic syndrome is idiopathic. In the remainder, nephrosis is a result of a systemic disease. In adults, this is usually diabetes, lupus, or amyloidosis.

▶ CLINICAL MANIFESTATIONS

Glomerular disease can manifest as a number of clinical syndromes:

- ▲ acute glomerulonephritis (AGN)
- ▲ rapidly progressive glomerulonephritis (RPGN)
- ▲ nephrotic syndrome (NS)
- ▲ chronic glomerulonephritis

AGN (also known as the acute nephritic syndrome) is characterized by the abrupt onset of **hematuria, proteinuria,** and **acute renal failure.** The latter can lead to salt and water retention, hypertension, and edema. The renal failure is generally associated with transient **oliguria** but is usually followed by a spontaneous diuresis and return of normal renal function.

RPGN refers to glomerulonephritis that advances to end-stage renal disease in days to weeks. It most commonly occurs in the setting of AGN, but drug-induced and idiopathic forms exist. Of patients with AGN who progress to RPGN, about 20% have anti-GBM disease and the remainder are evenly divided between immune-complex and pauci-immune (ANCA) disease. The key pathologic finding in RPGN is extensive formation of extracapillary **crescents** in over half of glomeruli, giving rise to the synonym crescentic glomerulonephritis.

NS is defined as proteinuria in excess of 3.5 g/day. Secondary findings due to this extreme proteinuria are hypoalbuminemia, **edema,** and **hyperlipidemia**. Unlike AGN, the onset of NS can be insidious. Gross hematuria is rare, and patients may present without azotemia.

Chronic glomerulonephritis refers to slowly progressive glomerular disease that leads to end-stage renal disease over a period of months to years. Any acute glomerular disease can lead to chronic glomerulonephritis. The most important cause of chronic glomerulonephritis in the United States is diabetes mellitus.

▶ HISTORY AND PHYSICAL EXAMINATION

Patients with glomerular disease can present with a variety of signs and symptoms. These can be related to the underlying etiology or due to the development of renal dysfunction.

▶ DIAGNOSTIC EVALUATION

Workup of a patient with possible glomerular disease should start with:

▲ measurement of electrolytes and creatinine to detect and quantify renal insufficiency and associated electrolyte abnormalities

▲ urinalysis to detect proteinuria and hematuria. In addition, microscopic examination of the urine sediment can reveal the presence of **dysmorphic** red blood cells and **red blood cell casts** that are highly suggestive of glomerular disease.

In patients who present with AGN or RPGN, **serology** has become an important part of the workup. Screens for **anti-GBM antibodies** and **ANCA** are readily available in many hospitals and can diagnose Goodpasture's syndrome, Wegener's granulomatosis, and microscopic polyarteritis. Immune complex disease is often accompanied with low **serum complement levels**. Several anti-streptococcal antigen antibodies can develop in poststreptococcal AGN.

Renal biopsy with examination by light microscopy, immunofluorescence, and electron microscopy is often useful for establishing a diagnosis in the setting of AGN, RPGN, and NS. It is usually reserved for those patients who have negative serology and an unclear clinical diagnosis. Done in consultation with a nephrologist, it is a relatively safe procedure.

▶ TREATMENT

For most glomerular disease, supportive care with fluid and electrolyte management (as outlined in

Chapters 20 and 21) is the initial intervention. For diseases that are usually self-limited (e.g., poststreptococcal AGN), this supportive care is sufficient.

Treatment with **immunosuppressive agents** (e.g., steroids, cyclophosphamide, chlorambucil) is usually recommended in diseases such as Goodpasture's, Wegener's, and polyarteritis. In addition, it can limit disease in idiopathic nephrotic syndrome, lupus nephritis, and idiopathic RPGN. Immunosuppression is controversial in other diseases such as immunoglobulin (Ig)A nephropathy and amyloidosis. In other diseases such as poststreptococcal AGN and AGN in the setting of infections such as endocarditis, the use of immunosuppression has not been shown to be useful.

The management of diabetic nephropathy is outlined in Chapter 47.

Prognosis in the glomerular diseases varies. In general, for a given disease, patients who develop RPGN have a poorer chance of preservation of renal function than those who manifest with AGN. For idiopathic NS, prognosis varies on histologic subtype, with about 95% of patients with minimal change disease maintaining baseline renal function compared with only about 50% with the membranoproliferative form.

Once fluid and electrolyte balance is achieved and any specific treatment initiated, close monitoring is maintained, awaiting return of normal renal function.

Patients who develop chronic renal failure from glomerular disease are managed as outlined in Chapter 22. Patients who develop end-stage renal failure may be candidates for long-term dialysis or renal transplantation.

▶ KEY POINTS

1. Causes of glomerular injury can be divided into those that cause inflammation and those that alter the permeability of the glomerular membrane.

2. There are four major clinical syndromes of glomerular disease: acute glomerulonephritis, rapidly progressive glomerulonephritis, nephrotic syndrome, and chronic glomerulonephritis.

3. A given etiology of glomerular disease can manifest as one or more clinical syndromes.

4. In addition to maintenance of fluid and electrolyte balance, immunosuppression is a part of treatment of specific glomerular diseases.

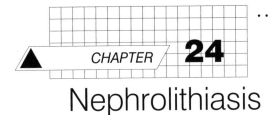

CHAPTER 24

Nephrolithiasis

*C*alcium and oxalate are normally present in the urine in amounts exceeding their solubility (supersaturated solution). However, most people do not form kidney stones, in part due to the kidney's natural inhibitors such as citrate or kidney proteins (Tamm-Horsfall mucoprotein and nephrocalcin).

This balance can be disturbed either by increased excretion of solutes or a change in urine volume. When this occurs, calcium and oxalate may precipitate on their own (homogeneous nucleation) or, more commonly, crystallize on another source such as urate crystals, epithelial cells, or urinary casts (heterogeneous nucleation).

► EPIDEMIOLOGY

Most kidney stones occur in men, with a peak incidence between the ages of 20 and 30. The exception is struvite stones, which are more common in women.

► ETIOLOGY

Nephrolithiasis may be grouped into four categories on the basis of stone composition. First, **calcium** constitutes 75 to 85% of all stones. Calcium oxalate predominates but stones may occur as calcium phosphate. The following abnormalities lead to calcium stones. **Hypercalciuria** is the most common urinary abnormality (>50% of patients). It is important to exclude secondary causes, such as malignancy, hyperparathyroidism, sarcoidosis, or Cushing's syndrome, but most patients have idiopathic hypercalciuria (caused by increased intestinal absorption, renal leak of calcium, or both). **Hypocitruria** is a deficiency of this natural inhibitor found in about 30% of patients. It is usually idiopathic but may be due to distal renal tubular acidosis (type 1) or chronic diarrhea, both of which create a nonanion gap acidosis. **Hyperoxaluria** is found in 8% of stone formers. This is caused by high dietary oxalate, malabsorption, or ileal disease. The latter two increase oxalate absorption by two mechanisms: malabsorbed fat binds calcium leaving oxalate free for absorption and colonic mucosa injured from bile acids absorbs more oxalate. **Hyperuricosuria** may serve as nucleating agent for calcium.

The second category of stones, **uric acid**, occurs as a predominate crystal in 5 to 10% of stones. Patients often have gout (50%), myeloproliferative disease, or a family history of nephrolithiasis. **Struvite**, the third category, comprises 10 to 20% of all stones, composed of magnesium ammonium phosphate crystals. This type is associated with urease-producing bacteria (e.g., Proteus) and may grow quite large. Finally, **cystine**, which is an uncommon cause (1%) of stones, occurs only in patients with cystinuria, an inherited defect of amino acid transport.

► CLINICAL MANIFESTATIONS
History

Flank pain is the hallmark symptom. It begins gradually and then escalates to a severe pain in 20 to 60 minutes. Pain radiating to the groin or testicle (labia in women) indicates migration of the stone into the lower third of the ureter. There can be associated nausea and vomiting. The patient with hematuria may describe pink or grossly bloody urine.

Physical Examination

The physical is often unrevealing. There can be tenderness to palpation or costovertebral tenderness. If there are peritoneal signs, consider another diagnosis. Fever is also not typical and indicates a complicating infection.

► DIFFERENTIAL DIAGNOSIS

In the clinical presentation of **abdominal pain**, the following diseases may have similar pain and radiation:

▲ aortic dissection

▲ lumbar disc disease

▲ renal infarct

If **gross hematuria** predominates the picture, the following diagnoses should be considered as well:

▲ renal malignancy or tuberculosis

▲ infection

▲ glomerulonephritis

▲ trauma

TABLE 24-1

Clinical Features of Kidney Stones

Type of Stone	Urine pH (nl 5.5–6.0)	X-ray findings
Calcium	Increased	Radioopaque
Uric acid	Decreased	Radiolucent
Struvite	Increased	Radioopaque
Cystine	Decreased	Radioopaque

Adapted from N Engl J Med 327:1142;1992.

▶ DIAGNOSTIC EVALUATION

The urinalysis is the key to diagnosis, with hematuria as the predominant feature. The urine should also be examined for crystals and tested for pH. Typical findings for each stone are listed in Table 24-1. A plain film of the abdomen should be obtained in all patients to look for radiopaque stones (90% of all stones).

An intravenous pyelogram should be obtained to confirm the diagnosis or detect radiopaque stones. A nonfunctioning kidney, partially obstructed solitary kidney, or extravasation of dye are indications for immediate urologic referral.

A recent National Institutes of Health consensus panel recommended a minimal workup for first-time stone formers consisting of serum electrolytes, creatinine, calcium , phosphorus, and urinalysis. Only hypercalcemic patients should be tested for hyperparathyroidism.

▶ TREATMENT

The initial treatment should focus on adequate hydration, pain relief, and evaluation for possible urologic procedure. Patients often require narcotic analgesia, but those patients who can maintain adequate fluid intake may be discharged home on oral medication.

Stone retrieval is an essential feature because further workup and treatment are dictated by type of stone. Patients should be instructed to strain urine at home or in the hospital.

Recurrence of a kidney stone occurs in most patients within a decade (14% at 1 year, 35% at 5 years, 50 to 60% at 10 years). Patients with an inherited defect, such as cystinuria, may have a malignant course, leading to renal failure.

All physicians agree that patients who have had a kidney stone should ensure an adequate daily urine volume (>2 L) by increasing fluid intake (6 to 8 glasses a day). However, because the advent of extracorporeal shockwave lithotripsy (see below) has de-

creased the morbidity of nephrolithiasis, there is continued debate over what workup (if any) a patient should receive after the first stone.

▶ THERAPEUTICS

All hospitalized patients should receive intravenous fluids and adequate analgesia. Stones that are < 5 mm usually pass on their own. Larger stones may require one of the following procedures. Extracorporeal shock wave lithotripsy (ESWL) has greatly diminished the need for invasive procedures. Shock waves fragment the stone into smaller pieces that can then pass. Referral for this procedure should be considered:

▲ when stone fails to progress

▲ infection, severe bleeding, or intractable pain is present

▲ stone is >0.5 and <2 cm

Stents may be used to assist passing the stone.

In percutaneous nephrolithotomy, stones are manually extracted under fluoroscopy by a percutaneous approach. It is most useful in stones not well treated by ESWL (such as those >2 cm).

Struvite stones often grow quite large and may require percutaneous or even open nephrolithotomy for removal. Removal is essential because these stones are often infected and will recur unless adequately removed.

More extensive workup, involving 24-hour urine collection, is indicated in recurrent stone formers. Some advocate this workup in first-time stone formers given the high rate of recurrence. Almost all patients (97%) will have some detectable abnormality on the urine test, and most will have more than one.

Urine should be sent for calcium, uric acid, citrate, and oxalate. Cystinuria, a rare cause of kidney stones, may be screened for with the nitroprusside test. This sensitive test may also detect a symptomatic heterozygotes; therefore, a positive test should be followed up with a quantitative cystine analysis.

Long-term follow-up is aimed at preventing recurrent stones. Although medications may be effective in changing the results of urine tests, the results on stone recurrence are mixed. Risks and benefits must be weighed for each individual patient.

Alkalinization of urine with potassium citrate may be useful for stones that form in an acid urine. These include uric acid stones, cystine stones, and those calcium stones associated with hypocitraturia.

For **calcium stones,** sodium restriction and thiazide diuretics, both of which decrease calcium excretion, are used for hypercalciuria. Calcium wasting may continue to occur with a calcium restricted diet, so this is not recommended. In **hyperoxaluria,** decreased dietary oxalate, calcium supplements to bind oxalate (not with concurrent hypercalciuria), or cholestyramine to bind fatty acids, bile salts, and oxalate are used.

Treatment for **uric acid stones** includes dietary restriction (avoid meats, fish) and allopurinol in refractory cases.

Struvite stones often need to be surgically removed followed by a course of antibiotics effective against the offending organism.

For **cystine stones,** penicillamine forms a soluble complex with cystine to prevent stones, but its toxic side effects limit its use.

▶ KEY POINTS

1. Calcium stones, specifically calcium oxalate, are the most common type of kidney stone.

2. The clinical picture of nephrolithiasis consists of flank pain, often radiating to the groin, and hematuria. An abdominal plain film will show kidney stones (except for radiolucent uric acid stones), and diagnosis is confirmed with an intravenous pyelogram.

3. Treatment is hydration and pain control, with lithotripsy used for more complicated cases.

4. Systemic conditions often predispose to nephrolithiasis. Calcium stones may be caused by hyperparathyroidism, sarcoidosis, or Cushing's syndrome. Uric acid stones are associated with myeloproliferative disorders, chemotherapy (tumor lysis syndrome), or gout. Patients with intestinal malabsorption and ileal disease usually have calcium oxalate stones.

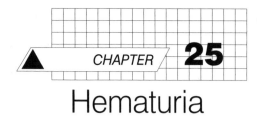

CHAPTER 25

Hematuria

*H*ematuria (the presence of blood in the urine) is a very common disorder and can be classified as **gross** or **microscopic** depending on whether or not blood is visible to the naked eye. Normal individuals excrete up to 2 million red blood cells (RBCs) into the urine each day; more than this is considered to be abnormal hematuria. Gross and microscopic hematuria share a common differential diagnosis.

In many instances, hematuria is asymptomatic and patients have no evidence of renal or systemic disease. In other cases, hematuria may be a manifestation of a systemic disease such as a vasculitis. Determination of the cause of hematuria is important because up to 10% of patients with hematuria are found to have an underlying malignancy.

Differential Diagnosis

The **causes of hematuria** can be divided based on the anatomic site of the blood source (asterisk indicates most common causes):

Kidney

▲ *Infection (pyelonephritis, tuberculosis, parasites)

▲ *Nephrolithiasis

▲ Malignancy (renal cell carcinoma)

▲ Trauma

▲ Glomerular disease (vasculitis, idiopathic)

▲ Cysts (single and polycystic disease)

▲ Allergic interstitial nephritis (drug induced)

▲ Ischemia (embolism, thrombosis, papillary necrosis)

Ureters

▲ *Nephrolithiasis

▲ Tumor

▲ Endometriosis

Bladder

▲ *Infection (bacterial cystitis, parasites)

▲ *Calculus

▲ Tumor

▲ Vascular malformations (hemangiomas, telangiectasias)

▲ Endometriosis

▲ Drugs (e.g., hemorrhagic cystitis from cyclophosphamide)

Prostate/male reproductive tract

▲ *Infection (prostatitis, epididymitis)

▲ Benign prostatic hypertrophy (BPH)

▲ Tumor

Urethra

▲ *Urethritis (gonococcal, nongonococcal)

▲ Stricture

▲ Calculus

▲ Trauma

Systemic illnesses/other

▲ *Intense exercise

▲ Coagulopathy

▲ Thrombocytopenia

▲ Hemoglobinopathy

▶ CLINICAL MANIFESTATIONS
History

Although many times hematuria is diagnosed in asymptomatic patients, certain **symptoms** can suggest particular etiologies:

▲ flank pain (pyelonephritis, nephrolithiasis, neoplasms, ischemia, glomerulonephritis)

▲ dysuria (cystitis, pyelonephritis, prostatitis, BPH, urethritis)

▲ urethral discharge (urethritis)

▲ weight loss

▲ fever (pyelonephritis, neoplasms, tuberculosis)

▲ nocturia (cystitis, BPH, pyelonephritis)

In women, the **menstrual history** is important. Hematuria can be caused by urologic endometriosis, but more commonly, blood in a clinical urine specimen is vaginal in origin.

Other historical findings are associated with specific causes of hematuria and should be sought:

▲ recent streptococcal infection (poststreptococcal glomerulonephritis)

▲ gross painless hematuria (bladder cancer)

▲ recent heavy exercise (exertional hematuria)

▲ history of nephrolithiasis

▲ medication history (allergic interstitial nephritis, hemorrhagic cystitis)

▲ family history (polycystic kidney disease, benign familial hematuria)

▲ travel (parasitic infections)

Physical Examination

The physical examination can provide important clues regarding the origin of hematuria:

▲ skin lesions, for example, ecchymoses, petechiae (coagulopathy, vasculitis)

▲ costovertebral angle tenderness (pyelonephritis, tumor, glomerulonephritis)

▲ abdominal mass (polycystic kidneys, renal cell cancer)

▲ urethral discharge (urethritis)

▲ suprapubic tenderness (cystitis)

▲ enlarged prostate (BPH)

▲ tender prostate (prostatitis)

▲ prostatic nodule (prostate cancer)

▶ DIAGNOSTIC EVALUATION

The **initial diagnosis** of microscopic hematuria is commonly made with either a urine dipstick or microscopic examination of spun urine sediment. The **urine dipstick** detects the presence of hemoglobin and can detect free hemoglobin or hemoglobin contained in red blood cells. The **microscopic examination** will only detect intact RBCs but provides additional information. Normally performed on a spun urine sediment (obtained by centrifuging about 10 mL of fresh urine), it can detect the presence of 1.2×10^6 RBCs per 100 mL. This corresponds to the presence of two to three RBCs per high-powered field (hpf). Most nephrologists will accept up to two to three RBC/hpf as normal in a routine urinalysis. Microscopic examination can also reveal the presence of **bacteria** in the setting of urinary tract infections. The presence of **red blood cell casts** indicates a renal origin for the hematuria.

Examination of the **morphology** of RBCs present in the urine using **phase-contrast microscopy** can provide clues as the etiology of hematuria. RBCs originating from **glomerular disease** are often **dysmorphic,** whereas nonglomerular disease is associated with normomorphic RBCs. It is important to examine a fresh urine sample because changes in morphology can occur if the urine is allowed to sit.

Routine chemistries, such as complete blood count, platelet count, and blood urea nitrogen and creatinine, should be performed in the initial evaluation of hematuria.

In many cases, an asymptomatic patient is found to have hematuria on a routine screening urinalysis and no clear source is found by history and physical. Such patients are said to have **isolated asymptomatic hematuria.** The challenge for the clinician is to determine the cause for the hematuria with a minimum of invasive testing while detecting potentially malignant causes.

The initial test for isolated asymptomatic hematuria should be **urine culture.** If positive, appropriate treatment should be instituted and then culture and urinalysis repeated. If hematuria is still present, further evaluation is necessary.

Patients with isolated asymptomatic hematuria who are over the age of 40 should be evaluated extensively because the incidence of urologic tumors is much higher in this group. In patients under the age of 40, a 3-month period of "watchful waiting" with repeat urinalyses performed **at least** monthly is acceptable. If hematuria is still present after this time, evaluation should be continued as with patients over the age of 40.

The next step in evaluation is **structural examination of the kidney.** An **intravenous pyelogram** is generally the initial test, provided the patient has adequate renal function. This can detect the presence of stones, soft tissue masses, hydronephrosis, and cysts. **Ultrasonography** can be used to further evaluate possible cystic lesions and also as the initial study in the case of a patient where the use of contrast is contraindicated. **Computed tomography** is the preferred follow-up test if a possible solid renal mass is found.

At the same time that structural evaluation is undertaken, additional tests can be performed, including:

▲ prothrombin time, partial thromboplastin time

▲ purified protein derivative (PPD) followed by urine acid-fast bacilli stains and cultures if positive

▲ erythrocyte sedimentation rate

▲ antinuclear antibody test

▲ complement levels

▲ antistreptococcal enzyme titers (anti-ASO, anti-DNase B)

▲ cryoglobulin screen

▲ urine cytology

The choice of test should be based on the clinical picture. For example, evidence of glomerular disease (heavy proteinuria, dysmorphic RBCs) should be followed up with complement levels, sedimentation rate, and appropriate serology (see Chapter 23). **Urine cytology** is performed on three consecutive first-voided urines. Sensitivity is only about 30%.

If the source of bleeding is still not apparent, referral to a urologist for **cystoscopy** is indicated. In addition, cystoscopy is often performed as part of the initial evaluation of **gross hematuria.** At this point, if the etiology is still elusive, further evaluation can involve computed tomography or magnetic resonance imaging (if not already performed) or angiography to detect small structural abnormalities. Renal biopsy can be considered.

If, after exhaustive evaluation, no etiology is found, long-term follow-up at 6-month intervals should occur. This consists of repeat history and physical, urinalysis, complete blood count, and blood urea nitrogen and creatinine. In the patients over age 40, repeat cytology should be done. Imaging (radiologic and cystoscopic) should be performed or repeated as indicated by results of follow-up testing.

▶ KEY POINTS

1. Hematuria is detected by the presence of hemoglobin on a urine dipstick or finding greater than two to three RBCs per hpf on examination of a spun urine sediment.

2. Up to 10% of patients with hematuria have an underlying malignancy.

3. Determining the source of hematuria involves a stepped approach using a variety of laboratory and imaging techniques.

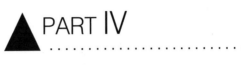

PART IV

Infectious Diseases

CHAPTER 26

Fever and Rash

A patient who presents with fever and rash poses a diagnostic challenge to the clinician. The causes of this combination form a broad differential that includes a wide variety of infectious and noninfectious conditions. Some conditions are trivial, whereas others can be life threatening.

Rashes can be classified according to their appearance:

▲ Maculopapular—a **macule** is a spot with a change in normal skin color without elevation or depression or the surrounding skin. A **papule** is a raised area of skin (i.e., a "bump"). Therefore, a maculopapular rash is an outbreak of pigmented bumps.

▲ Petechial—**petechiae** are small red or brown spots that are formed by extravasation of blood into the skin. When pressure is applied with a glass slide (diascopy), the lesions **do not** blanche.

▲ **Vesicles** and **bullae** are small and large blisters. If the fluid within a vesicle is cloudy (purulent), it is referred to as a **pustule.**

▲ Erythematous—diffuse erythema can be a manifestation of a number of systemic illnesses. Generally, diascopy will result in blanching because extravasation of red blood cells is not occurring.

▲ Urticarial—urticaria (wheals) are rounded or flat-topped raised areas. They may have slight pale-red discoloration or may have normal coloration. They are characteristically evanescent and disappear within several hours.

▶ DIFFERENTIAL DIAGNOSIS

The differential diagnoses are listed in Table 26-1.

▶ CLINICAL MANIFESTATIONS

When a patient presents with fever and rash, the clinician must determine whether empiric treatment needs to be started along with diagnostic tests. As a rule of thumb, patients who present with a petechial rash and fever, particularly if there are other systemic signs of illness, are most likely to have a potentially life-threatening illness. Among the potential fatal **"do-not-miss" diagnoses** that present with fever and rash are:

▲ meningococcemia

▲ bacterial sepsis (e.g., Staphylococcal sepsis)

▲ endocarditis

▲ Rocky Mountain spotted fever

▲ gonococcemia

▲ typhoid fever

If any of these life-threatening illnesses are suspected, proper diagnosis and immediate treatment (see below) should be initiated.

History

A number of **important historical features** should be sought:

▲ food and water history

▲ drug ingestions

▲ recent travel

▲ animal exposure

▲ insect bites/exposure

▲ ill contacts

▲ sexual history

▲ prior rashes/illnesses

The presence of a prodrome (fatigue, malaise, myalgias) before the appearance of rash is often suggestive of an infectious illness (viral, Rocky Mountain spotted fever, bacterial). The pattern of appearance and spread of the rash also have diagnostic significance (Table 26-1).

Physical Examination

On physical examination, the extent and morphology of the rash needs to be determined carefully. Mucosal surfaces, genitalia, scalp, palms, and soles all need to be examined. Patients may not be aware of the full extent of the lesions and a careful examination is important. Examination of the fundi can reveal embolic phenomena indicative of an intravascular bacterial infection (e.g., endocarditis).

Signs of severe systemic illness (e.g., hypotension, meningismus) suggest potentially a life-threatening condition (meningococcemia, toxic shock, endocarditis, Rocky Mountain spotted fever, Kawasaki disease).

TABLE 26-1

Conditions Presenting with Fever and Rash

Disease	Type of Rash	Epidemiology	Clinical Findings
Infectious			
Endocarditis	P	Abnormal heart valves, intravenous drug use (IVDU)	Cardiac murmur, mucosal lesions, retinal findings
Meningococcemia	P,MP,VB	Outbreak of *Neisseria meningitidis*	± meningitis, septic shock (hypotension, oliguria), pustules may be present—organisms visible on Gram stain
Gonococcemia	P,VB	Sexual activity, esp. with prostitutes or multiple partners	± urethritis, joint pain/effusions
Typhoid fever	MP ("rose spots")	Poor sanitation (fecal/oral spread), contact with asymptomatic carriers	Prolonged, persistent fever, constipation relative bradycardia during febrile episodes
Staphylococcal sepsis	VB	IVDU, poor skin hygiene	Evidence of dermatologic Staphylococcal infection
Vibrio vulnificus	VB	Ingestion of raw seafood, exposure to seawater	Patients with cirrhosis are most susceptible to septic shock, lesions are on extremities, legs > arms
Folliculitis	MP, VB	Hot tubs (*Pseudomonas*), freshwater exposure (swimmer's itch from avian schistosomes)	Diffuse rash, marked pruritus in swimmer's itch
Streptococcal infection	E	Outbreaks of scarlet fever	Diffuse erythematous rash with "sandpaper" texture, well circumscribed cellulitis (erysipelas)
Staphylococcal infection	MP, VB, E	Tampon use (toxic shock), poor skin hygiene	Shock, with diffuse erythema and later palmar desquamation (toxic shock), folliculitis, pustules (Staphbacteremia)
Ehrlichiosis	E	Endemic area in summer, tick bite, outdoor exposure	Headache, leukopenia, LFT abnormalities
Rocky Mountain spotted fever	P	Endemic area in summer, tick bite, outdoor exposure	Severe headache, rash starts in extremities and spreads centripetally
Secondary syphilis	MP	Sexual activity, esp. with prostitutes or multiple partners	Involves palms and soles
Mycoplasma	MP,U	Younger patients	Bullous myringitis, pneumonia
Lyme disease	MP	Endemic area in summer, tick bite, outdoor exposure	Erythema migrans rash, joint effusions, headache
Enteroviral infection	P,MP,VB,E,U	Winter months	Myalgia, diarrhea, headache, meningitis
Rubella	P,MP	No history of immunization	Viral prodrome, rash starts on forehead and spreads downward to feet, adenopathy
Rubeola	MP	No history of immunization	Viral prodrome with conjunctivitis, small, irregular mucosal lesions (Koplik's spots), rash starts on forehead and spreads downward to feet
Adenovirus	MP,U	Year-round occurrence, but greatest in winter months	Upper respiratory illness, conjunctivitis, adenopathy
Primary HIV infection	MP	Sexual activity, esp. with prostitutes or multiple partners, IVDU	Viral syndrome with fever, malaise, headaches, and myalgia
HIV	VB,U	Sexual activity, esp. with prostitutes or multiple partners, IVDU	Often with no other symptoms
Varicella-zoster	VB	No history of disease (primary infection)	Reactivation in dermatomal distribution
Herpes simplex virus	VB	Multiple sexual partners, other STD	HSV-1 typically oral HSV-2 typically genital

TABLE 26-1

Conditions Presenting with Fever and Rash (Continued)

Disease	Type of Rash	Epidemiology	Clinical Findings
Infectious (cont.)			
EBV	U,MP	Outbreaks occur among college students and military recruits	Mononucleosis (fever, adenopathy, pharyngitis, malaise, splenomegaly) 5% incidence of rash in mononucleosis, almost 100% if ampicillin is administered
Hepatitis	U	IVDU, multiple sexual partners	Urticaria may occur during acute hepatitis, but also during chronic disease
Noninfectious			
Allergy	P,MP,VB, E,U	Exposure to various drugs, foods, animals	Manifestations vary greatly
Thrombocytopenia	P	Previous viral syndrome, known idiopathic thrombocytopenia	Easy bruising as well as spontaneous petechiae
Henoch-Schonlein purpura	P	Mostly in children	Abdominal pain, arthralgias, glomerulonephritis, IgA deposits in skin and kidneys
Hypersensitivity vasculitis	P	Antigen exposure (infectious agent, drug)	Biopsy reveals leukocytoclastic vasculitis with antigen/antibody immune complex deposition
Vasculitis (e.g., SLE, polyarteritis nodosum, dermatomyositis)	P,MP	Known history of vasculitis	Manifestations vary as to type of vasculitis
Erythema multiforme	MP	Drug exposure	Characteristic "target" lesions, can have mucosal involvement (Stevens-Johnson syndrome)
Plant dermatitis (poison ivy, poison oak)	VB	Known exposure to plants	Weepy, vesicular-bullous lesions in areas of contact, pruritus
Vasodilatation	E	Shock, vigorous exercise	Blanching, bright erythema
Psoriasis	E	Known history	Silvery scale present over diffuse erythema, pustular variant seen
Lymphoma	E	Middle-aged men (cutaneous T-cell lymphoma)	Diffuse erythema can occur in all lymphomas, T-cell lymphoma of skin (mycosis fungoides and Sezary syndrome)
Kawasaki disease	E	Generally children	Resembles scarlet fever, but without evidence of Streptococcal infection

P, petechial; MP, maculopapular; VB, vesicular/bullous; E, erythematous; U, urticarial.

Other important physical examination findings are listed in Table 26-1.

▶ DIAGNOSTIC EVALUATION

When history and physical examination narrows the differential to a group of relatively benign illnesses, extensive diagnostic testing is unnecessary. In cases where the diagnosis is unclear, **routine laboratory tests** (complete blood count, creatinine, liver function tests, urinalysis, chest radiographs) can provide useful information.

The overall diagnostic test strategy is to limit the differential diagnosis based on history and physical examination and then use selected tests to confirm potential diagnoses. Certain test results (e.g., serology and pathology) can take days to become available and thus are used only to confirm a diagnosis and not to guide therapy.

If the patient is systemically ill, **blood cultures** should be obtained. Pustules can be sampled and the material subjected to **Gram stain and culture.** Vesicles can be unroofed and material sent for **Tzanck prep,** direct **antibody stain,** and **viral culture** to identify varicella-zoster and herpes viruses.

Patients with meningeal signs should have a **lumbar puncture** with Gram stain and culture and cell count performed on the fluid.

Serology can be useful to identify diseases such as syphilis, Rocky Mountain spotted fever, Lyme disease, and Ehrlichiosis. Paired acute and convalescent serology is often more helpful.

In patients with severe systemic illness, **empiric antibiotic therapy** is often initiated to cover meningococcemia, Rocky Mountain spotted fever, and typhoid fever. A third-generation cephalosporin such as ceftriaxone and a tetracycline provides broad empiric coverage pending culture results.

Skin biopsy and culture may be necessary. Special stains for certain organisms and for vasculitis (e.g., immunoglobulin [Ig]A in Henoch-Schonlein purpura) can be done.

Skin testing for possible allergic reactions can be useful in selected cases.

▶ KEY POINTS

1. The combination of fever and rash can indicate a variety of benign and life-threatening diseases.

2. The nature of the rash coupled with the history and physical play a key role in narrowing the differential diagnosis.

3. In cases of severe systemic illness, empiric antibiotic treatment is initiated at the same time as the diagnostic workup.

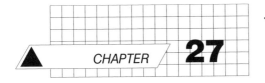

CHAPTER 27

Pneumonia

*P*neumonia can occur among otherwise healthy (from an immunologic standpoint) individuals, so-called community acquired pneumonia. Organisms, management, and outcome vary between patients based on host characteristics. The physician must be able to identify pneumonia and, based on host characteristics and a variety of physical and laboratory findings, start empiric antimicrobial therapy when indicated.

▶ EPIDEMIOLOGY

Pneumonia is the sixth leading cause of death in the United States, and among infectious causes of death, it ranks number one. It is estimated that there are approximately 4 million cases of community-acquired pneumonia occurring each year in the United States. About 20% of these cases will require hospitalization, and among these patients, mortality approaches 25%, compared with only 1 to 5% of patients who can be managed as an outpatient.

▶ ETIOLOGY

The microbial agents responsible for pneumonia range from bacteria to viruses. Specific etiologic agents of pneumonia occur with different frequencies and depend on specific host factors:

▲ age

▲ socioeconomic status

▲ prior antibiotic use

▲ alcohol abuse

▲ chronic obstructive pulmonary disease (COPD) or other respiratory illness

▲ diabetes mellitus

▲ chronic liver disease

▲ chronic renal insufficiency

▲ congestive heart failure

These host factors not only influence the etiology of pneumonias in patients, they also impact on the prognosis.

▶ CLINICAL MANIFESTATIONS
History

Patients presenting with pneumonia may present with pulmonary or extrapulmonary symptoms such as:

▲ fever, chills, rigors

▲ cough

▲ sputum production

▲ chest pain

▲ shortness of breath

Other important historical points are the presence of underlying disease (see list above), history of recent travel, and exposure (sick individuals, animals, environmental irritants).

Physical Examination

The physical examination is geared to establish the diagnosis and extent of a possible pneumonia and to assess the severity of disease. Classically, pneumonias present with signs of consolidation, including:

▲ bronchial breath sounds

▲ egophony ("e" to "a" changes)

▲ dullness to percussion

▲ increased tactile fremitus

Even if evidence of frank consolidation is not present, most patients with pneumonia will have crackles on lung examination. The presence of a pleural effusion is usually manifested as dullness to percussion with decreased tactile fremitus and decreased breath sounds.

Physical findings in patients with community-acquired pneumonia that are associated with increased morbidity and mortality include:

▲ tachypnea (respiratory rate >30)

▲ fever (>38.3°C)

▲ hypotension (diastolic < 60, systolic < 90)

▲ extrapulmonary disease (meningitis, septic arthritis)

▲ confusion or altered mental status

▶ DIFFERENTIAL DIAGNOSIS

Upper respiratory illness, sinusitis, pharyngitis, and bronchitis are infectious illnesses that can present with respiratory findings seen in patients with pneumonia. **Noninfectious conditions** that can mimic pneumonia include pulmonary embolus, congestive heart failure, obstructing bronchogenic carcinoma, and inflammatory lung disease (e.g., Wegener's granulomatosis, eosinophilic pneumonia).

▶ DIAGNOSTIC EVALUATION

A number of tests can be useful in detecting the presence and extent of pneumonia. A **standard PA and lateral chest radiograph** can differentiate pneumonia from conditions such as bronchitis (which is associated with a normal chest radiograph) and detect other conditions such as lung abscesses, pleural effusions, and masses. Differences in the radiographic findings in pneumonia (lobar versus diffuse) are not specific enough to allow diagnosis of a specific etiology of a pneumonia but can be suggestive.

Gram stain and culture of sputum can help define the etiologic cause of a pneumonia. The exact utility of the Gram stain has been debated, but overall it generally adds information helpful in determining empiric antibiotic therapy, pending results of culture.

In addition to sputum cultures, blood cultures (both anaerobic and aerobic) should be collected from those patients who require hospitalization. Although positive in only some cases (in particular, in cases of pneumococcal pneumonia), they can provide useful information about the etiologic agent and, if positive, are also predictive of a more severe clinical course.

In a manner similar to certain physical findings (see above), certain laboratory results are predictive of **higher morbidity** and **mortality:**

▲ total white blood cell count $< 4 \times 10^3/mL > 30 \times 10^3/mL$ or absolute neutrophil count less than $1 \times 10^3/mL$

▲ $Pao_2 < 60$ or $PaCo_2 > 50$ mmHg (Fio_2 0.21)

▲ hematocrit $< 30\%$ or hemoglobin < 9 g/dL

▲ serum creatinine > 1.2 mg/dL or blood urea nitrogen > 20 mg/dL

▶ TREATMENT

Once the diagnosis of a pneumonia has been established, the two main management questions are does the patient require admission to the hospital? and what is appropriate initial antibiotic therapy? There are some guidelines for determining which patients with community-acquired pneumonia require admission. Overall, the severity of the illness and social factors (homelessness, support services, etc.) all play a role in determining the need for hospitalization. In general, if multiple risk factors coexist, hospitalization should strongly be considered, at least long enough to monitor clinical status and determine response to therapy.

A number of classic clinical pictures based on patient characteristics, chest radiograph, and sputum findings have been recognized (Table 27-1).

TABLE 27-1

"Classic" Pneumonia Syndromes

Organism	Host Factors	Chest Radiograph	Sputum	Gram Stain
Klebsiella pneumoniae	Alcoholics	Lobar	Dark red, mucoid "currant jelly"	PMNs encapsulated GNR
Streptococcus pneumoniae	All ages, generally older	Lobar	Purulent with blood "rusty"	PMNs Gram-positive diplococci "lancet-shaped"
Haemophilus influenzae	Smokers, COPD	Lobar	Purulent	PMNs pleiomorphic GNR
Mycoplasma	Younger patients	Interstitial infiltrate	Scant, may be purulent	PMNs but no organisms
Aspiration	Alcoholic, altered mental status	Multilobar, often lower	Foul smelling	PMNs mixed morphologies
Staphylococcus aureus	Previous influenza infection	Lobar, may be cavitary	Bloody	PMNs Gram-positive cocci in clusters

COPD—chronic obstructive pulmonary disease; PMN—polymorphonuclear lymphocyte; GNR—gram-negative rod.

Attempts have been made to guide initial antimicrobial therapy in community-acquired pneumonia based on patient characteristics. The **American Thoracic Society** has broken patients into four groups (Table 27-2). For each group, the major pathogens encountered and appropriate empiric therapies based on these pathogens are delineated (Table 27-2). Gram stain can be used to further narrow the choice if a predominant organism is seen.

The presence of a pleural effusion on chest radiograph may indicate a possible empyema. See Chapter 17, Pleural Effusions. Consideration should be given to sampling of pleural fluid to determine whether it is infected and if so, placement of a chest tube is indicated.

Once empiric antimicrobial therapy is initiated, the patient's response needs to be carefully monitored. Generally, therapy should not be altered in the first 72 hours. **Early change in therapy** is indicated if:

▲ initial diagnostic studies identify a pathogen not covered by original empiric therapy (e.g., tuberculosis)

▲ a resistant organism is isolated from blood or other sterile site (e.g., pleural fluid)

▲ there is marked clinical deterioration

When determining clinical response, it is important to note that signs and symptoms can persist even if appropriate therapy is being given. Fever may last for several days, although the magnitude should decrease each day. Leukocytosis may also persist for 2 to 4 days. Physical findings (e.g., crackles, egophony) can persist beyond a week, and chest radiograph changes can be present for several weeks.

If a patient does not improve or worsens on empiric therapy, consideration must be given to several causes:

▲ inadequate antimicrobial selection (e.g., due to resistance, presence of a viral pathogen)

▲ undrained infection (i.e., pulmonary abscess or empyema)

TABLE 27-2

Etiologies and Empiric Treatment of Pneumonia

Group I: Outpatient, Age ≤ 60, No Coexisting Disease	Group II: Outpatient, > 60 or with Coexisting Disease	Group III: Inpatient, Not Requiring ICU Admission	Group IV: Inpatient, Severe, Requiring ICU Admission
Major pathogens			
S. pneumoniae	S. pneumoniae	S. pneumoniae	S. pneumoniae
M. pneumoniae	Respiratory viruses	H. influenzae	Legionella spp.
Respiratory viruses	H. influenzae	Polymicrobial (including anaerobes)	Gram-negative bacilli
C. pneumoniae	Gram-negative bacilli	Gram-negative bacilli	M. pneumoniae
H. influenzae	S. aureus	Legionella spp.	Respiratory viruses
		S. aureus	
		C. pneumoniae	
		Respiratory viruses	
Miscellaneous pathogens			
Legionella spp.	M. catarrhalis	M. pneumoniae	H. influenzae
S. aureus	Legionella spp.	M. catarrhalis	M. tuberculosis
M. tuberculosis	M. tuberculosis	M. tuberculosis	Endemic fungi
Endemic fungi	Endemic fungi	Endemic fungi	
Gram-negative bacilli			
Empiric therapy			
Macrolide	Second-generation cephalosporin	Second- or third-generation cephalosporin	Macrolide
or	or	or	plus
Tetracycline	TMP/SMZ	Beta-lactam/beta-lactamase inhibitor ± macrolide	Antipseudomonal third-generation cephalosporin
	or		or
	Beta-lactam/beta-lactamase inhibitor ± macrolide		Other antipseudomonal agent (e.g., quinolone, imipenem/cliastatin)

TMP/SMZ—trimethropin/sulfamethoxazole.

▲ unusual pathogens (e.g., fungal pneumonias, psittacosis)

▲ noninfectious illness

If a patient is failing initial therapy, consideration should be given to **further diagnostic testing,** including:

▲ bronchoscopy with sampling of respiratory secretions

▲ computed tomography

▲ pulmonary arteriogram (if pulmonary embolism is suspected)

▲ serology (not usually useful in the acute setting)

▶ **KEY POINTS**

1. Pneumonia is the leading infectious cause of death in the United States.

2. Etiologic agents differ depending on various host factors including age and coexisting illness.

3. Empiric therapy for pneumonia should be based on patient characteristics and data from sputum Gram stain.

4. Failure of initial therapy may be due to resistant organisms, unusual organisms, or a noninfectious cause and may warrant further diagnostic testing, including bronchoscopy.

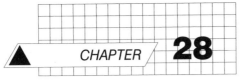
Sexually Transmitted Diseases

► EPIDEMIOLOGY

Sexually transmitted diseases (STDs) are among the most common infections. In the United States, there are an estimated 8 to 12 million cases of STDs each year. Accurate estimation is made difficult by the fact that not all STDs are reported because social stigma leads to underreporting. The rates of many STDs are influenced by:

▲ socioeconomic class

▲ drug use

▲ sexual practices (number of partners, rate of partner change, prostitution, oral-fecal exposure)

In the United States, STDs are most prevalent among young individuals of low socioeconomic class. The notable exception is infection with *Chlamydia trachomatis*, which is more evenly distributed across the population. Human immunodeficiency virus (HIV) infection, an important STD, is discussed separately in Chapters 34 and 35.

► ETIOLOGY AND PATHOGENESIS

A variety of organisms can be transmitted by sexual contact including bacteria, viruses, and arthropods. Annually, the most common STD agents encountered in the United States are *C. trachomatis* (4 to 5 million cases), *Neisseria gonorrhoeae* (620,000 cases), *Treponema pallidum* (35,000 cases), human papilloma virus (HPV; ~500,000 new cases, 40 million chronic cases), herpes simplex virus type 2 (HSV-2; ~400,000 new cases, 30 million chronic cases), hepatitis B virus (~250,000 cases), and HIV infection (~50,000 new cases and 1.5 million chronic infections).

Most nonviral STDs can induce acute inflammation when the organisms colonize the mucosa. This inflammation leads to the symptoms associated with infection (see below). In addition, infection of the upper female reproductive tract (endometrium, fallopian tubes, and pelvic peritoneum), also known as pelvic inflammatory disease (PID), can lead to a variety of sequelae, including ectopic pregnancy, tubal infertility, and chronic pelvic pain. Infection can be completely asymptomatic. This is important in maintaining a reservoir of infection.

Infection with HPV and HSV is lifelong. Recurrences (which may be asymptomatic) are common and are responsible for continued spread of the viruses. In addition, chronic infection with certain types of HPV (e.g., type 16 and 18) is associated with the development of a premalignant lesion (cervical intraepithelial neoplasia) and frank cervical cancer.

► CLINICAL MANIFESTATIONS

Urethritis (men and women), epididymitis (men), vulvovaginitis/cervicitis (women), acute pelvic inflammatory disease (women), genital ulcers (men and women), genital warts, and hepatitis are distinct clinical syndromes that can arise from STDs (Table 28-1). Although the specific clinical syndromes manifest with typical symptoms and physical findings, STDs can be clinically silent, particularly in women.

History

Most patients who seek medical attention for a possible STD do so because of symptoms such as:

▲ dysuria

▲ discharge

▲ genital lesions (ulcers, warts)

▲ abdominal pain

▲ fever

Other patients may seek attention because of a high-risk sexual exposure (e.g., prostitutes) or because they were notified by a sexual partner of possible infection. A thorough sexual history can provide clues as to which infections may be likely. Sexual history should include:

▲ number of sexual partners (both lifetime and recent)

▲ details of sexual practices (anal-oral, oral-genital, anal receptive, vaginal)

▲ condom use (specifically frequency of use)

▲ high-risk sexual contacts (prostitutes, intravenous drug users)

▲ past history of STDs

▲ history of abnormal Pap smears

TABLE 28-1

Clinical Syndromes Seen in STDs

Clinical Syndrome	Common Etiologies	Clinical Findings	Laboratory Findings	Treatment
Urethritis (male)	*N. gonorrhoeae, C. trachomatis, Ureaplasma urealyticum*	Dysuria, urethral discharge, fever, arthritis, Reiter's syndrome	Gram-negative diplococci inside PMNs (*N. gonorrhoeae*), PMNs without organisms (NGU)	Third-generation cephalosporin *or* quinoline (*N. gonorrhoeae*), doxycycline *or* azithromycin *or* quinolone (NGU)*
Urethritis (female)	*N. gonorrhoeae, C. trachomatis, E. coli*	Dysuria (without frequency and urgency), ± cervicitis	Pyuria	Third-generation cephalosporin *or* quinoline (*N. gonorrhoeae*), doxycycline *or* azithromycin *or* quinoline (NGU)*
Epididymitis	*C. trachomatis, N. gonorrhoeae,* Enterobacteriaceae	Testicular pain and tenderness (usually unilateral)	None specific	Doxycycline (*C. trachomatis*), third-generation cephalosporin (*N. gonorrhoeae*), quinoline (Enterobacteriaceae)
Vulvovaginitis	*Trichomonas vaginalis, Candida albicans*	Vulvar itching, "cottage cheese" discharge (candidiasis), vulvar itching, purulent, malodorous discharge, mucosa visibly inflamed (*T. vaginalis*)	PMNs, budding yeast on KOH prep or Gram stain (candidiasis), PMNs with motile organisms seen (trichomoniasis)	Intravaginal azoles e.g., clotrimazole, miconazole (candidiasis), metronidazole (trichomoniasis)
Bacterial vaginosis	*Gardnerella vaginalis, Mycoplasma hominis,* anaerobic bacteria	Malodorous, thin discharge (clear to white)	"Clue cells" on wet prep, replacement of *Lactobacilli* with mixed organisms of Gram stain, few PMNs	Metronidazole (either orally or intravaginally)
PID	*C. trachomatis, N. gonorrhoeae*	Abdominal pain, purulent vaginal discharge, cervicitis (purulent), nausea/ vomiting, fever, cervical motion tenderness	Elevated WBC, PMNs in vaginal discharge, Gram-negative diplococci seen within PMNs (*N. gonorrhoeae*)	Inpatient: third-generation cephalosporin *or* clindamycin and gentamicin *or* ampicillin/sulbactam Outpatient: third-generation cephalosporin × 1 *plus* doxycycline *or* quinoline *plus* metronidazole*
Genital ulcers	Herpes simplex virus (HSV), *Treponema pallidum* (syphilis), *Haemophilus ducreyi* (chancroid)	Painful ulcers (HSV, chancroid), painless ulcers (syphilis), painful ulcers, and inguinal adenopathy with overlying erythema (chancroid)	Multinucleated giant cells/positive DFA/viral culture (HSV), spiro-chetes seen on dark field microscopy (syphilis), isolation of *H. ducreyi* from lesion or lymph node aspirate	Acyclovir (HSV), penicillin G (syphilis)—single IM dose for early disease, benzathine penicillin, three doses for late disease (not neurosyphilis) doxycycline for penicillin allergy, ceftriaxone or erythromycin (chancroid)
Genital warts	Human papilloma virus	Visible papillomas, associated with the development of epithelial cancers	Molecular typing is available but not usually needed to make the diagnosis	Local wart removal (cryosurgery, laser surgery, podophyllin)
Hepatitis	Hepatitis B virus, possibly hepatitis C virus, hepatitis A (fecal-oral contact)	Fever, hepatomegaly, abdominal pain (see Chapter 40)	Elevated liver transaminase, serologic testing available	None available

*When treating presumed *Neisseria gonorrhoeae*, empiric treatment for *Chlamydia trachomatis* is also added.
PMN, polymorphonuclear lymphocyte; NGU, nongonococcal urethritis.

Physical Examination

When evaluating a patient with a possible STD, the physical examination should include a close examination of the genitalia (including a speculum and bimanual examination for women and testicular and prostate examination for men) and other mucosal surfaces (conjunctiva, oral cavity, rectum). Lymphadenopathy should be sought as well as skin lesions such as rashes and ulcers. Certain findings are suggestive of specific etiologies (Table 28-1).

▶ DIFFERENTIAL DIAGNOSIS

Certain conditions can mimic STD syndromes; urethritis (e.g., urinary tract infection, prostatitis), PID (e.g., ectopic pregnancy, appendicitis, pyelonephritis, cystitis), and vulvovaginitis/cervicitis (e.g., normal cyclical changes in vaginal secretions during menstrual cycle, dysfunctional uterine bleeding).

▶ DIAGNOSTIC EVALUATION

Diagnosis of specific STDs can be made by culture and various nonculture methods, including:

▲ direct microscopy

▲ immunofluorescence

▲ serology

▲ DNA diagnosis (e.g., polymerase chain reaction)

Nonculture methods have been proven to be useful for organisms that cannot be cultured (e.g., *T. pallidum*) or are difficult and/or expensive to culture (HSV, HPV, *Chlamydia*). Nonculture methods are sometimes much more rapid than culture.

Evaluation of specific STDs varies with the particular clinical entity encountered. In a male, the presence of urethritis should be confirmed by examination for discharge, which may require milking the urethra after the patient has not voided for several hours. If no discharge is found, an endourethral sample should be obtained by inserting a small urethral swab about 2 to 3 cm into the urethra. The sample should be examined by Gram stain, looking for the presence of polymorphonuclear lymphocytes (PMNs) and/or organisms. Further workup and treatment can then be based on the findings listed in Table 28-2. For women with presumed urethritis, the workup is similar. However, it is important to rule out cystitis, pyelonephritis, and vulvovaginitis first.

For vulvovaginitis/bacterial vaginosis, in a woman who presents with abnormal vaginal discharge ($\pm$ malodor) and/or vaginal discomfort (pruritus, burn-ing, dyspareunia, with or without dysuria), it is again important to rule out urinary tract infection. In addition, vaginal discharge can be a sign of infection higher in the reproductive tract (cervicitis or PID). A careful pelvic examination is thus indicated with collection of samples for microscopic examination and culture (Table 28-2).

For cervicitis/pelvic inflammatory disease, because of the severe sequelae that can result from PID, particularly when not treated in a timely fashion, prompt evaluation and empiric treatment are necessary when evaluating a woman who presents with cervical discharge and/or abdominal pain and fever. As mentioned above, the important distinction is between PID and surgical emergencies such as appendicitis and ectopic pregnancy. Gram stain and culture should be performed, and empiric treatment for chlamydia and gonorrhea should be instituted.

▶ TREATMENT

The treatment of most STDs is accomplished on an outpatient basis. Specific and/or empiric therapy can be initiated based on clinical findings while awaiting the results of specific laboratory diagnosis. In certain populations (e.g., young individuals of low socioeconomic status), empiric treatment is important because of the likelihood of poor follow-up. Similarly, simple (preferably single-dose) drug treatment is preferable.

In cases of suspected PID, consideration should be given to hospitalization in cases when the diagnosis is uncertain, surgical emergencies must be ruled out, severe systemic illness is present (severe emesis, high fever, hypotension), close outpatient follow-up cannot be arranged or the patient is judged to be unable to complete or tolerate outpatient management, or the patient has failed outpatient management.

TABLE 28-2

Evolution of Suspected PID/Urethritis

< 5PMNs per high-powered field and no organisms	Culture for *N. gonorrhoeae,* repeat urethral sampling. If both are negative, assess for prostatitis, cystitis
PMNs with intracellular Gram-negative diplococci	Culture molecular probe for *N. gonorrhoeae,* treat for gonorrhea
PMNs with atypical Gram-negative diplococci (extracellular or abnormal morphology)	Culture/probe for *N. gonorrhoeae* and *C. trachomatis,* treat for gonorrhea and *Chlamydia* infections
PMNs and no Gram-negative diplococci	Culture/probe for *N. gonorrhoeae,* treat for presumed Chlamydia infection

For nonviral STDs, antimicrobial therapy is the mainstay of therapy (Table 28-1). Generally, empiric therapy based on clinical picture and preliminary diagnostic tests is started pending definitive diagnosis by culture or other nonculture methods.

Acyclovir and other similar antiviral agents (e.g., famciclovir) is used for the treatment of HSV. Even though HSV infection cannot be cleared, acyclovir can shorten the course of outbreaks, shorten viral shedding time, and shorten healing time. Patients who have frequent outbreaks may be candidates for chronic acyclovir suppression.

From the public health standpoint, the screening and treatment of sexual partners of patients diagnosed with an STD is a critical part of management. Practices vary widely, from supplying medication for partner treatment to requiring the partner to appear in person for assessment. The risks of treating partners without the opportunity to assess for possible drug allergies and provide education needs to be balanced against the public health risk of not treating a partner at all.

Primary prevention, mainly through latex condom use and avoiding high-risk contacts, should be encouraged in all sexually active patients, particularly those who have had a previous diagnosis of STD.

▶ SYPHILIS

Infection with *T. pallidum* deserves separate attention because of its varied clinical manifestations, serious late complications, and diagnostic difficulties. Syphilis is characterized by stages of active clinical disease separated by periods of asymptomatic latent infection. The duration of each stage may vary, the stages may overlap, and a given patient may not progress through each stage. All patients, however, manifest the initial or primary stage, which is a painless indurated ulcer (known as a chancre) at the inoculation site. If untreated, about half of the patients will progress to a disseminated (hematogenous) stage, and the rest will go directly to a stage of latent disease. In the disseminated (also known as secondary) stage, the organisms are widely dispersed throughout the body. Physical findings in secondary syphilis commonly include:

▲ generalized maculopapular rash (characteristically involves palms and soles)

▲ mucous patches (silver-gray erosions with an erythematous periphery that are generally painless)

▲ condyloma lata (wart-like enlarged papules that are moist and pink to gray-white; these lesions are highly infectious)

▲ generalized nontender lymphadenopathy

About 15% of cases will still have the primary chancre. Patients with secondary syphilis can also have a variety of nonspecific constitutional symptoms (fever, sore throat, malaise, headache). Syphilis has been called the "great imitator" because there is a wide variety of less common manifestations, including:

▲ hepatitis

▲ nephropathy

▲ arthritis

▲ iridocyclitis

▲ nephrotic syndrome

▲ gastritis

▲ ulcerative colitis

Patients in the latent stage, which is divided into early latent in the first year after infection and late latent thereafter, will have serologic evidence of infection (see below) but no clinical manifestations. This stage can last for the patient's lifetime or end with spontaneous clearance of infection or progression to late syphilis. Late syphilis is marked by end-organ damage involving the nervous system (general paresis, tabes dorsalis, paresthesias, loss of position, pain, and temperature sensation), the cardiovascular system (syphilitic aortitis), and gumma formation (granulomas with central necrosis most commonly involving the skin, skeletal system, mouth, larynx, liver, and stomach, but all organs have been reported to be involved).

The laboratory diagnosis of syphilis can be performed by dark field microscopy of lesions (to demonstrate the presence of spirochetes), direct immunofluorescence microscopy, and serology (both nontreponemal tests such as RPR and VDRL, which are used for screening, and treponemal tests such as immunofluorescence and hemagglutination to detect antibodies specific for *T. pallidum*).

The nontreponemal tests are also used to monitor response to therapy, using the guideline as a fourfold decline in titer within 6 to 12 months after treatment indicative of cure.

▶ KEY POINTS

1. Sexually transmitted diseases are among the most common infections, with an estimated 8 to 12 million new cases a year in the United States.

2. A number of viruses and bacteria are responsible for the most commonly encountered STDs.

3. STDs can manifest a number of clinical syndromes, including urethritis, genital ulcers/warts, and upper reproductive tract disease in women (PID).

4. PID can result in a number of serious sequelae, including tubal infertility, ectopic pregnancy, and chronic pelvic pain.

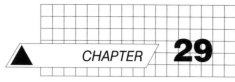

CHAPTER 29

Urinary Tract Infections

*U*rinary tract infections (UTIs) are often divided into lower tract infections involving the urinary bladder (cystitis) and upper tract infections involving the kidneys and collecting system (pyelonephritis). In practice, the precise determination of upper tract involvement in a UTI is difficult but is not always necessary for successful treatment.

▶ EPIDEMIOLOGY AND PATHOGENESIS

UTIs are much more prevalent among women than among men presumably due to a shorter urethra. Among hospitalized patients, the presence of an indwelling urinary catheter is a major risk for the development of a UTI.

Most (>90%) UTIs are caused by **aerobic Gram-negative bacteria.** About 80% of community-acquired and 50% of nosocomial UTIs are caused by *Escherichia coli,* with most of the remainder caused by Gram-negative bacteria such as *Enterobacter, Klebsiella, Proteus,* and *Pseudomonas.* Gram positives only cause about 10% of UTIs, most notably *Staphylococcus saprophiticus* among young sexually active women and Enterococci among men and women with indwelling urinary catheters. Another etiologic agent in catheterized patients is yeast (most often *Candida* spp.).

Some organisms that commonly cause UTIs have particular **virulence factors** that allow them to successfully colonize the urinary tract:

▲ pili/fimbriae (hairlike bacterial appendages that allow adherence to urinary tract epithelial cells)

▲ hemolysins (often with strains that produce pyelonephritis)

▲ aerobactin (an iron scavenging molecule)

▶ RISK FACTORS

As mentioned above, most community UTIs occur among women. **Risk factors** that increase the incidence of UTIs **among women** are:

▲ history of recent UTI

▲ increased sexual activity

▲ use of diaphragm and/or spermicide

▲ failure to void after intercourse

Among men, the presence of an anatomically abnormal urinary tract is the major factor that predisposes to UTIs.

▶ CLINICAL MANIFESTATIONS
History

Lower tract infection usually presents with **symptoms** of **bladder irritation,** such as:

▲ frequency

▲ urgency

▲ dysuria

Gross hematuria may sometimes be present but is not a common feature. **Upper tract infections** also present with **symptoms** of bladder irritation, but features that tend to distinguish them from lower tract infections are:

▲ fever

▲ flank pain

▲ abdominal symptoms of pain, nausea, and vomiting

It is important to note that there can be much overlap in symptoms between upper and lower disease.

Physical Examination

In a patient presenting with classic symptoms of a UTI, the physical examination often does not add much. Other than the finding of a fever and flank tenderness that raises suspicion of upper tract disease, diagnosis is usually suggested by the history.

▶ DIFFERENTIAL DIAGNOSIS

A number of **other conditions** may produce signs and symptoms that can mimic a bacterial UTI, including:

▲ vulvovaginitis

▲ gonococcal and nongonococcal urethritis

▲ bladder calculi

▲ bladder tumor

▲ chemical- or drug-induced cystitis

▲ prostatitis

A pelvic examination in women (with vaginal or cervical cultures) and a prostate examination in older men may help distinguish a UTI from other conditions that can produce symptoms suggestive of a UTI.

▶ DIAGNOSTIC EVALUATION

Urinalysis and **urine culture** are the most important laboratory tests used in diagnosis and guiding treatment. If examination of a cover-slipped slide of unspun urine under 40× power reveals one organism per field, this correlates with an organism count of 10^6/mL. The presence of white blood cell (WBC) casts is suggestive of pyelonephritis.

In practice, it is often not feasible or practical to examine all urines under a microscope. However, the presence of both WBC and nitrites on a urine "dipstick" correlates with the presence of a UTI in about 90% of cases.

Urine culture with susceptibility testing is important to determine whether empiric antibiotic therapy is appropriate for the isolated organism. The initial empiric therapy may need to be altered to match the sensitivities of the isolated organism.

▶ TREATMENT

In most cases of community-acquired UTIs, including those with upper tract involvement, treatment as an outpatient with oral antibiotics is adequate. Factors that could lead toward inpatient (i.e., intravenous antibiotics) treatment include severe nausea and vomiting (which could interfere with oral administration of antibiotics) and signs of sepsis (including high fever and signs of hemodynamic compromise).

In the setting of catheter-related UTI, removal of the urinary catheter, if possible, is the most important consideration. If removal is not possible, directed antibiotic therapy for an isolated organism may be effective, but reinfection with different organisms is common.

Uncomplicated UTIs can be treated with an empiric **3-day course of antibiotics.** This length of treatment can give cure rates equivalent to more traditional 7-day courses and is more effective than one-dose therapy. If upper tract disease is suspected, the length of therapy should be extended to 7 to 14 days, reflecting the increased difficulty in clearing upper tract infections.

Standard oral drugs to treat UTIs include:

▲ beta-lactams such as ampicillin and amoxicillin

▲ trimethoprim-sulfamethoxazole

▲ quinolones

▲ tetracyclines

These drugs have good activity against most Gram negative bacteria, although resistance to beta-lactams has been rising among community isolates. Therefore, initial empiric therapy with trimethoprim-sulfamethoxazole is usually recommended. However, beta-lactams remain important with pregnant patients where other drugs carry the risk of fetal injury. Along with antibiotics, symptomatic relief can be given with a short course of the bladder analgesic phenazopyridine.

The standard 3-day regimen of oral antibiotics is usually effective in most cases of UTI. The most common **causes of treatment failure** are lack of patient compliance and infection with a resistant microorganism. It is important in patients who fail to respond to empiric therapy to obtain culture and sensitivity results so that therapy can be altered based on microbial resistance.

Other complications of UTIs that must be watched for are the development of perinephric abscesses, formation of renal calculi (particularly with recurrent infections with **Proteus,**) and the development of sepsis by bloodstream seeding.

Frequent recurrent UTIs in a woman may signal the presence of anatomic abnormalities that can be worked up with an intravenous pyelogram. If the urinary tract is found to be structurally normal, there are a number of **preventative measures** that can be tried, including:

▲ voiding after intercourse

▲ alternative contraception other than diaphragm

▲ high fluid intake early after symptoms occur

▲ prophylactic antimicrobials (often trimethoprim-sulfamethoxazole, nitrofurantoin, or cephalexin) at bedtime or after sexual intercourse if other methods fail

The latter treatment is usually used for limited time periods (3 to 6 months) before discontinuing and observing but may need to be extended if frequent UTIs recur after prophylaxis is stopped.

▶ KEY POINTS

1. Urinary tract infections most often present with symptoms of bladder irritation: frequency, urgency, and dysuria.

2. Most are caused by Gram-negative bacteria.

3. Urinalysis (dip stick and or microscopic) and culture are the most important laboratory tests.

4. Empiric 3-day courses of antibiotics for lower tract disease and 7- to 14-day courses for upper tract infections are usually sufficient.

5. Treatment failure may suggest antimicrobial resistance and recurrent UTIs may be an indication to check for anatomic abnormalities of the urinary tract.

6. Chronic use of antimicrobials may be needed to prevent recurrent UTIs.

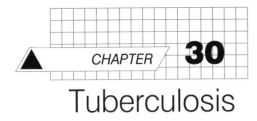

Tuberculosis

Tuberculosis (TB) is the chronic infection with the organism *Mycobacterium tuberculosis*. The characteristic pathology of *M. tuberculosis* infection is the formation of granulomas via cell-mediated immunity. Although TB can affect a wide number of organ systems, pulmonary tuberculosis remains the most important.

▶ PATHOGENESIS

M. tuberculosis is usually spread via inhalation of droplets, setting up the initial site of infection in the lungs and then spreading via lymphatics to regional (i.e., mediastinal) lymph nodes. About 90 to 95% of immunocompetent individuals control the initial infection via a cellular immune response involving *M. tuberculosis* ingestion by macrophages, both in the lung and the lymph node. Granuloma formation results with eventual control of the infection. This effective cellular response takes about 3 to 9 weeks to develop, at which time the tuberculin skin-test will become positive. In some patients, the early immune response is so robust that severe necrosis occurs, leading to cavity formation or local extension of disease. In still others, dissemination occurs very early in the course with systemic spread to **extrapulmonary sites** including the pericardium, extrapulmonary lymph nodes (scrofula), kidneys, epiphyses of long bones, vertebral bodies, and meninges.

In most cases the initial infection is walled off by granuloma formation, but viable organisms may persist within the granuloma. With waning cellular immunity (e.g., with age, advancing human immunodeficiency virus [HIV] disease, malignancy, or corticosteroid administration), these organisms may escape from the granuloma, resulting in **reactivation tuberculosis.**

▶ EPIDEMIOLOGY

After falling since the early part of the century, the incidence of TB in the United States has been rising since 1985. A number of factors (see below) have led to this increase, including the human immunodeficiency virus epidemic and the appearance of multidrug-resistant *M. tuberculosis.*

M. tuberculosis is spread from person to person mainly by the **respiratory route** via droplets formed by coughing. Most people with tuberculosis shed relatively few bacteria, with the exception of those with endobronchial or cavitary disease. Therefore, transmission usually requires several months of close (i.e., household) contact.

▶ RISK FACTORS

In the United States, important **risk factors** for the development of TB include:

▲ older age (thought to be reactivation)

▲ lower socioeconomic status (via crowding, homelessness, poor nutrition, etc.)

▲ minority status

▲ HIV seropositivity

▶ CLINICAL MANIFESTATIONS

History

Early pulmonary TB is usually asymptomatic and often discovered by chance on routine chest x-ray. When symptoms do develop later in the disease, they are usually nonspecific and constitutional:

▲ fevers

▲ chills

▲ night sweats

▲ anorexia

▲ weight loss

▲ fatigue

▲ cough

Development of **hemoptysis** denotes advanced disease.

Because the symptoms outlined above are nonspecific, clinical suspicion for TB must be raised in patients with the appropriate risk factors who present with these features.

Physical Examination

Physical examination findings are dependent on the nature of disease present and in general may underestimate its severity. Pulmonary findings of **dullness with decreased fremitus** may be present with pleural effusions or pleural thickening. Signs of consolidation may be present. A cavity may produce distant hollow breath sounds that suggest the sound of blowing across the mouth of a jar (**amphora**).

Extrapulmonary TB is manifest by signs of the particular organ system involved, for example, spine pain and tenderness with skeletal TB and cervical adenopathy (**scrofula**) in tuberculous adenitis.

▶ DIFFERENTIAL DIAGNOSIS

A number of different diseases may present with the clinical findings found in TB, including fungal diseases (histoplasmosis, coccidioidomycosis), sarcoidosis, and malignancy.

▶ DIAGNOSTIC EVALUATION

The chest x-ray is important in determining the presence and extent of pulmonary disease in TB. Important radiographic patterns that can be seen in pulmonary TB include:

▲ calcified primary parenchymal lesion and calcified mediastinal node (Ghon complex)

▲ apical pleural scarring

▲ cavitary disease

▲ diffuse (miliary) disease

▲ lobar consolidation

It is important to note that in early disease, the chest radiograph may be completely normal.

Evaluation of sputum, when present, may be useful. *M. tuberculosis* stains positive in an acid-fast stain. Acid-fast positivity requires a heavy organism burden in the patient, and early disease may be missed. Culture is more sensitive but time consuming due to the slow growth of *M. tuberculosis*.

Skin testing is important for the diagnosis of TB. The administration of the intermediate (5TU) skin test has been shown to be useful in documenting exposure and infection with *M. tuberculosis*. Population studies have determined levels of skin test reactivity that help identify infected individuals with sufficient sensitivity and specificity:

▲ >15 mm in a normal host from a low-risk group

▲ >10 mm in a high-risk individual

▲ >5 mm in an HIV-infected individual

Other laboratory findings (anemia, liver function test abnormalities) may be found in TB, particularly with extrapulmonary disease, but are not specific.

▶ TREATMENT

Management of TB is closely tied to the diagnosis of the disease. Distinction has to be made between active disease (i.e., with symptoms and positive physical findings and/or chest x-ray) and early asymptomatic disease (characterized by a newly reactive skin test). Immunologically normal patients with only a newly reactive skin test have an approximate 3% chance of going on to symptomatic disease within the first year after conversion. New skin test converters are treated with chemoprophylaxis. Patients with active disease require more intensive therapy.

Active TB requires various combinations of the so-called **first-line TB drugs** such as:

▲ isoniazid (INH)

▲ rifampin (RMP)

▲ pyrazinamide (PZA)

▲ ethambutol (ETH)

▲ streptomycin (STM)

The current standard regimen is 9 months of daily INH and RMP, which is as effective in patients where resistance (see below) is not suspected as the previously standard 12- to 18-month courses. Even shorter courses (6 months) have been developed. These courses usually require close supervision because failure rates are higher if there are lapses in adherence to therapy. One example of a short course regimen is 2 months of INH, RMP, and PZA (with ETH or STM if INH resistance is possible) followed by INH and RMP daily for an additional 4 months.

Chemoprophylaxis of recent skin test converters is usually administered by giving 9 to 12 months of daily INH. There is some debate as to the utility of chemoprophylaxis in patients with a positive skin test of unknown duration. Current recommendations are to prophylax such patients if they are less than 35 years old, because of higher incidence of drug toxicity (see below) in older individuals.

Compliance with therapy is the major determinant of successful treatment of active TB. Extended periods of therapy are needed to eliminate all viable slow-growing bacteria. These long periods of therapy, especially among populations of patients with poor medical follow-up (homeless, poor) are difficult to adhere to. Early stoppage of therapy, especially as symptoms resolve, is common.

Resistance to one or more anti-TB drugs is becoming more of a problem, especially among the highest risk patients. Resistance is thought to arise by incomplete courses of treatment with insufficient numbers of drugs.

The drugs themselves have toxic **side effects** that may also limit compliance. With INH, RMP, and PZA, this toxicity is mainly hepatic, requiring monitoring of liver function during therapy.

▶ **KEY POINTS**

1. TB is a major problem among the poor, homeless, and HIV-infected populations.

2. Spread is via the respiratory route.

3. Early infection is often asymptomatic and in most patients is fully controlled.

4. Long courses of multidrug therapy is required for treatment of symptomatic disease.

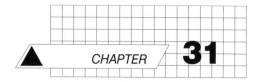

CHAPTER 31

Gastroenteritis

*G*astroenteritis refers to the inflammation of the stomach and intestinal tract, usually secondary to an infectious agent. Manifesting as **nausea, vomiting, abdominal pain**, and **diarrhea**, gastroenteritis is a common health problem in the general population and also frequently encountered in the international traveler.

► EPIDEMIOLOGY

Acute gastroenteritis can follow the ingestion of a variety of microorganisms and/or toxins produced by these agents. **Ingestion of contaminated food or drink** is generally most common, but swimming or bathing in contaminated water can also result in exposure.

Travel to areas of the world where safe food handling practices are not commonly observed is often associated with development of gastroenteritis, but **lapses in food handling** also occur in the home and in restaurants under a number of circumstances such as:

▲ undercooking of foods, in particular, ground meats

▲ failure to refrigerate foods properly (either before preparation or during storage of prepared foods)

▲ incorporation of raw ingredients (e.g., eggs) into foods that are not cooked further

▲ failure to properly clean contaminated kitchen equipment (e.g., mixing bowls, cutting boards)

▲ contamination of food by food handlers who practice poor personal hygiene

Outbreaks of gastroenteritis have occurred from environmental sources (e.g., contaminated lakes) or other point sources (e.g., a single restaurant or food packaging plant).

► ETIOLOGY AND PATHOPHYSIOLOGY

Bacteria, viruses, and **protozoans** can cause acute gastroenteritis (Table 31-1). The most commonly encountered **viral** pathogens are **rotavirus** and the **parvoviruses** (e.g., Norwalk agent). They directly infect cells of the small intestine resulting in alteration of the mucosal architecture (notably shortening or loss of the microvilli), causing diarrhea on the basis of malabsorption. The infection is readily controlled causing a short-lived (24- to 48-hour) illness.

Protozoan infections are most commonly found in travelers and people who may be exposed to untreated water (e.g., hikers). *Entamoeba histolytica* and *Giardia lamblia* are two of the most commonly encountered protozoan pathogens. The former invades the colon causing a bloody diarrhea, whereas *Giardia* colonizes the small intestine, causing a malabsorptive syndrome and an osmotic diarrhea.

Bacterial pathogens can cause gastroenteritis via several distinct **mechanisms** such as:

▲ direct invasion of the mucosa with tissue destruction and inflammation

▲ growth of the bacteria within the bowel lumen with toxin production and release

▲ adherence (but not invasion) of the bacteria to the mucosal surface with interference of the normal absorptive process without tissue destruction

▲ production of a toxin during bacterial growth in food or water which is then ingested preformed

► CLINICAL MANIFESTATIONS
History

In taking the history, it is useful to obtain **epidemiologic information** that can help determine an etiology. **Food history** should cover at least the 48 hours before the onset of symptoms. Any changes from the usual dietary habits, such as eating at restaurants or picnics, should be elicited. **Travel history** should pertain not only to other countries but to a history of camping, swimming, or other recreational activity where there can be exposure to untreated water. **History of a similar illness in others** should be taken, in particular family members or others who may have shared a particular exposure. Complete **history of antibiotic** exposure because although *Clostridium difficile*-associated diarrhea is most commonly encountered in the hospital setting, many people take courses of antibiotics as an outpatient and may not associate the onset of diarrhea with these drugs. A history of **known infection with human immunodeficiency virus (HIV)** or **HIV risk factors** should be taken because diarrhea is a common symptom in HIV-infected individuals. Some etiologic agents seen in these patients are unique and require specific methods of diagnosis and treatment (see Chapter 35).

Once a possible exposure is elicited, the incubation period before the onset of symptoms can provide a clue to the nature of the etiologic agent. Ingestion of preformed toxin (e.g., *Staphylococcus aureus* food poisoning) is followed by onset of symptoms within 12 hours. Infection with a pathogenic bacteria that needs to replicate to cause disease (e.g., *Campylobacter* or *Salmonella*) does not result in symptoms until at least 24 to 48 hours after exposure. Parasitic infections (e.g., *Giardia*) may not become symptomatic for days to weeks after exposure.

Physical Examination

The physical examination generally does little in helping determine a specific etiologic agent. **Fever** and **abdominal** pain are more suggestive of an invasive bacterial pathogen. The severity of the illness can be indicated by signs of dehydration such as **orthostatic hypotension**, **dry mucosal membranes**, and **decreased skin turgor**.

▶ DIFFERENTIAL DIAGNOSIS

The differential diagnosis of diarrhea can be found in Chapter 37.

▶ DIAGNOSTIC EVALUATION

In most cases of acute infectious diarrhea, hydration and watchful waiting are all that is necessary. However, certain variables can trigger a more extensive workup:

▲ high fever

▲ evidence of dehydration

▲ systemic toxicity

▲ bloody stool

▲ immunocompromise

▲ overseas or outdoor (e.g., hiking) travel

▲ male homosexuality

▲ recent antibiotic use

The presence of **stool leukocytes** generally suggests a bacterial pathogen. Gram stain can reveal the characteristic "gull-winged" shape characteristic of *Campylobacter*. Culture is the gold standard for identifying pathogenic bacteria. In addition to routine culture, certain organisms (*C. jejuni, Yersinia, E. coli* O157:H7) can require special media and isolation techniques to improve yield, and if these organisms are suspected, the microbiology laboratory should be notified.

If a protozoan etiology is suspected, examination of the stool for **ova and parasites** is indicated. Generally, fresh stool samples have the highest yield, but in some cases this is inconvenient and special containers with stool preservatives can be used. Generally, several samples from consecutive days are needed to increase yield.

In a patient with recent antibiotic use and diarrhea, assay for the presence of *C. difficile* toxin in stool can be diagnostic.

▶ TREATMENT

The **primary therapy in gastroenteritis** is **symptomatic**, with replacement of fluid and electrolytes lost via vomiting and diarrhea. In most cases, with symptomatic therapy, the condition will resolve on its own. Certain infections require administration of antimicrobials for clearance (see below and Table 31-1), making isolation of the etiologic agent important. For most patients, however, culture is generally reserved until symptomatic therapy fails.

In most cases of acute gastroenteritis, fluid and electrolyte management can be accomplished with **oral replacement.** For young healthy patients with mild to moderate diarrhea, oral fluids high in sugar content to facilitate passive absorption of water (fruit juices, soda, etc.) are generally sufficient along with solid food as tolerated. For more severe cases of diarrhea, especially if there are symptoms of dehydration, and for older patients, **oral rehydration solutions** that contain electrolytes and glucose should be used. Pediatric solutions such as Pedialyte and Rehydralyte can be used as well as packaged commercial rehydration packets. If there is marked dehydration, particularly in patients with underlying conditions, or if there are conditions such as intractable vomiting that make oral replacement difficult, administration of **intravenous fluids** may become necessary.

Antimotility agents such as **loperamide** and **atropine**-containing compounds (Lomotil) can be used symptomatically, particularly in cases where diarrhea can interfere with the functioning of an otherwise healthy individual. However, care must be taken when administering these agents. In cases of invasive organisms (e.g., *Salmonella*) or organisms that produce toxins (e.g., *C. difficile*), antimotility agents can be harmful.

TABLE 31-1

Causes of Gastroenteritis

Agent	Pathogenesis	Clinical/Epidemiologic Features	Therapy
Bacillus cereus	Preformed toxin	Generally causes vomiting, may also produce diarrhea, classic association with fried rice	None
Staphylococcus aureus	Preformed toxin	Vomiting with some diarrhea, found in high protein foods (meats, cream-filled cakes) also high sugar contents (custards)	None
Clostridium difficile	Toxin production in colon	Fever, abdominal pain, diarrhea, toxic megacolon, association with previous antibiotic use	Metronidazole
Escherichia coli (four main groups)			
Enterotoxigenic	Enterotoxin formation in small intestine	Voluminous watery diarrhea, fever generally absent, fecal/oral transmission	None
Enteroinvasive	Invasion of the colonic mucosa	Fever, bloody diarrhea fecal/oral transmission	Antibiotics
Enteroadherent	Adherence to small intestinal mucosa	Diarrhea, can be prolonged fecal/oral transmission	Antibiotics
Enterohemorrhagic (e.g., *E. coli* O157:H7)	Production of a cytotoxin (verotoxin) in colon	Causes hemorrhagic colitis, colitis can be followed by TTP/HUS,* from contaminated meats (especially ground meat)	Diarrhea—none, treatment of TTP/HUS is generally supportive
Campylobacter jejuni	Colonization (?invasion) of large and small bowel	Fever, watery diarrhea, abdominal pain	Antibiotics
Salmonella typhi	Invasion of small intestine, can then (via bloodstream) disseminate systemically	Protracted illness with fever, headache, malaise, splenomegaly. Constipation is more common than diarrhea, fecal/oral transmission	Antibiotics
Salmonella (non-typhi)	Invasion of small and large intestine	Fever, diarrhea, animal reservoirs, also in eggs	Antibiotics
Shigella spp.	Invasion of colon	Fever, bloody diarrhea, fecal/oral spread	Antibiotics
Vibrio cholerae	Enterotoxin	Profuse watery diarrhea, fever is rare, fecal/oral spread (often via water contamination)	Doxycycline
Entamoeba histolytica	Invasion of colon mucosa	Diarrhea, often bloody, fecal/oral spread	Metronidazole
Giardia lamblia	Colonization of small intestine	Diarrhea, secondary to malabsorption, abdominal pain, waterborne ("beaver fever")	Metronidazole

*TTP/HUS, thrombocytopenic thrombotic purpura/hemolytic uremic syndrome antibiotics; see text.

Bulk agents such as **Kaopectate** can give more form to stools but do not decrease the fluid content and thus do not prevent fluid and electrolyte loss. **Bismuth subsalicylate** (Pepto-Bismol) can decrease the volume of stool in certain cases of bacterial gastroenteritis. In addition, it possesses some antibacterial activity.

The administration of antimicrobial agents is recommended for certain documented infections in particular documented infection with the parasites *Giardia lamblia* and *Entamoeba histolytica*.

The use of antibiotics in patients with suspected or documented bacterial gastroenteritis remains controversial. In most cases, these illnesses will resolve with conservative treatment. Studies have demonstrated that for certain organisms, administration of antibiotics (generally quinolones or TMP-SMZ) can shorten the length of the diarrheal illness. Concerns about routine antibiotic use include the widespread appearance of antibiotic resistance, adverse drug reactions, and the appearance of *C. difficile*. In patients with *Salmonella* infection, the use of antibiotics can actually prolong the carrier state in some individuals whose only manifestation is gastroenteritis. For this reason, many experts recommend treatment of documented *Salmonella* infections only when there are signs of systemic illness (severe dehydration, fever).

Prevention of gastroenteritis is essential to effective management and is accomplished by adhering to proper guidelines for the safe handling of food and water. Travelers should be advised to avoid undercooked foods and any foods prepared with unpasteurized milk. Fresh fruits should be peeled by the consumer just before consumption.

Ensuring safe drinking water is important. In hotels in large cities the water may be safe, but if there is any uncertainty, the water should be boiled (at least 10 minutes) before drinking. Bottled beverages (carbonated beverages, beer, wine, and water) are generally safe, but, particularly in the case of bottled water, the traveler should ask to remove the top themselves to ensure that an empty bottle simply has not been filled with tap water.

▶ **KEY POINTS**

1. Many cases of acute diarrhea are due to infectious agents.

2. Microbes can cause diarrhea by damaging the mucosa directly, producing enterotoxin during growth in the bowel lumen or by producing a toxin that is then ingested in the form of contaminated food.

3. The primary therapy for most cases of gastroenteritis is supportive, with fluid and electrolyte replacement.

4. Antibiotics are indicated for certain parasitic infections but are generally not routinely administered for bacterial pathogens unless there are signs of systemic infection.

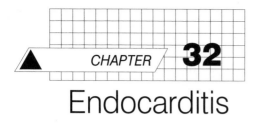

CHAPTER 32

Endocarditis

*I*nfective endocarditis (IE) is the invasion of the endothelial lining of the heart by microorganisms. Originally known as bacterial endocarditis, it can also be caused by fungi, rickettsia, and chlamydia. Before the introduction of antibiotics, it was generally a uniformly fatal disease. The introduction of antibiotics and later the development of cardiac surgery have decreased overall mortality, but IE is still associated with about a 25% mortality.

▶ EPIDEMIOLOGY AND CASE DEFINITION

In the United States there are about 10,000 to 15,000 new cases of IE each year, making it the most common form of endovascular infection. With the decrease in incidence of acute rheumatic carditis, IE has become more frequent in older patients, with a mean age of about 60 years in several recent series. IE has a higher incidence among men than women.

Infective endocarditis has been **divided into three major groups** based on host characteristics:

▲ native valve endocarditis (NVE)

▲ prosthetic valve endocarditis (PVE), further subdivided into **early,** that is, in the first month after valve surgery, and **late,** which occurs thereafter

▲ endocarditis in intravenous drug users

The etiologic organisms, management, and outcome of patients varies in each of these subdivisions.

A number of criteria for establishing the diagnosis of IE have been proposed. In 1981, the **von Reyn criteria** were proposed, which used strict case definitions based on predisposing heart disease, persistent bacteremia, vascular phenomena, and pathologic evidence of endocardial disease. More recently, investigators from Duke University proposed new diagnostic criteria (modeled after the Jones criteria for acute rheumatic fever) that incorporated two-dimensional echocardiographic findings and did not require pathology for diagnosis. The **Duke criteria** have been shown to be more useful for the **clinical diagnosis** of IE than the von Reyn criteria. The **major criteria** are:

▲ persistently positive blood cultures (at least two positive cultures separated by at least 12 hours or at least three cultures at least 1 hour apart or 70% of blood cultures positive if at least four are drawn)

▲ echocardiographic evidence of endocardial involvement (see below)

The **minor criteria** are:

▲ predisposing heart condition (see below)

▲ fever

▲ vascular phenomena (arterial emboli, septic pulmonary emboli, mycotic aneurysm, Janeway lesions)

▲ immunologic phenomena (glomerulonephritis, Osler's nodes, Roth spots, rheumatoid factor)

▲ positive blood cultures (not meeting major criteria)

▲ positive echocardiogram (not meeting major criteria)

Diagnosis of infective endocarditis requires two major criteria **or** one major plus three minor criteria **or** five minor criteria.

▶ ETIOLOGY

IE can be caused by a wide variety of microorganisms, but most (80%) cases are due to streptococci and staphylococci. Most cases of NVE are caused by *Streptococcus viridans* (50%) and *Staphylococcus aureus,* whereas most cases of IE in intravenous drug users are caused by *S. aureus.* Early PVE is thought to be due to intraoperative contamination with nosocomial pathogens, in particular *Staphylococcus epidermidis.* Late PVE is believed to be community acquired and resembles NVE in microbiology.

▶ RISK FACTORS AND PATHOGENESIS

The major risk factor for the development of IE is the presence of a **structurally abnormal heart.** Generally, this is valvular disease, but any **structural abnormality** (including iatrogenic) that leads to **turbulent blood flow within the heart** increases the risk of IE, including:

▲ mitral valve prolapse

▲ rheumatic heart disease (aortic and mitral valve)

▲ degenerative heart disease (calcifications)

3. The major risk factor for the development of endocarditis is the presence of a structurally abnormal heart.

4. Gram-positive organisms are the major cause of endocarditis and empiric therapy is directed against these organisms, adjusted for culture results including susceptibility data. Long courses of therapy are required to ensure sterilization of the infected endovascular structures.

5. Cardiac surgery, including valve replacement, may be required for severe valvular dysfunction.

6. Prophylaxis of endocarditis is recommended for patients with abnormal hearts who undergo procedures that lead to bacteremia.

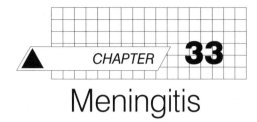

CHAPTER 33

Meningitis

Meningitis classically presents with the triad of fever, headache, and signs of meningeal irritation. There are a number of etiologies. The important distinction is between acute bacterial meningitis (ABM) and meningitis due to other causes. The term *acute aseptic meningitis syndrome* refers to meningitis for which a cause is not apparent after initial examination and routine stains and culture of the cerebrospinal fluid (CSF). Aseptic meningitis is most often viral (AVM) but can also be caused by noninfectious agents such as drugs. Although AVM and other aseptic meningitis syndromes are self-limited and uncomplicated, ABM is associated with a mortality rate of up to 30%, making its early diagnosis important.

▶ EPIDEMIOLOGY

In the United States there are an estimated 20,000 to 25,000 cases of ABM a year. Approximately 70% of these cases occur in children less than 5 years of age.

Among adults, bacterial meningitis can be divided into **community acquired** and **nosocomial.** Community-acquired meningitis generally occurs among patients greater than 50 years of age. Nosocomial meningitis is most often, but not invariably, associated with recent neurosurgery, the presence of a neurosurgical device, or altered immune state (e.g., asplenia, immunosuppressive drugs, and immune globulin deficiencies). Viral meningitis generally has a prevalence in the summer months, whereas bacterial meningitis tends to have a winter predominance.

ABM caused by *Neisseria meningitidis* is unique in that it can occur in outbreaks, often among young otherwise healthy adults who are in groups, such as college students and military recruits.

▶ ETIOLOGY

The **etiologic agents of acute bacterial meningitis** vary depending on the age of the patient and whether the condition is community acquired or nosocomial (Table 33-1). Among patients with community-acquired meningitis, about 40% are due to *Streptococcus pneumoniae* and a similar percentage of nosocomial meningitis was due to Gram-negative bacilli.

TABLE 33-1
Common Etiologies of ABM in Adults

Community Acquired	Nosocomial
Strep. pneumoniae	Gram-negative bacilli
N. meningitidis	*Staph. aureus*
L. monocytogenes	Streptococci
	Other Staphylococci

The most common **etiologic agents of aseptic meningitis** are viruses, with non-polio enteroviruses accounting for over 80% of cases for which an etiology can be identified. Other relatively common causes of aseptic meningitis include:

▲ other viruses (mumps, lymphochoriomeningitis virus, Epstein-Barr virus, cytomegalovirus, varicella-zoster virus, herpes-viruses, human immunodeficiency virus [HIV])

▲ *Mycobacterium tuberculosis*

▲ fungi (*Candida* spp., *Cryptococcus neoformans*)

▲ rickettsia (Rocky Mountain spotted fever, *Coxiella burnetii*)

▲ Spirochetes (syphilis, leptospirosis, Lyme disease)

▲ malignancy (metastatic leukemia, lymphoma, metastatic carcinomas)

▲ medications (sulfamethoxazole, nonsteroidal anti-inflammatory agents, isoniazid)

▲ vaccinations (mumps, measles)

▶ CLINICAL MANIFESTATIONS
History

The classic history of acute meningitis is that of **severe headache, fever,** and symptoms of meningeal irritation, such as **neck stiffness.** Other symptoms to inquire about include photophobia, altered mental state, seizures, and rash. An exposure history including travel, animal exposures, and ill contacts should be obtained.

Two elements of the history may help distinguish the likelihood of ABM versus AVM: patients with bacterial meningitis are more likely to be less than 5 years

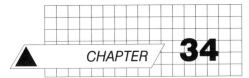
HIV Part I: Initial Care of the HIV-Infected Patient

The recognition of the human immunodeficiency virus (HIV) epidemic and the acquired immune deficiency syndrome (AIDS) in the early 1980s has resulted in a major change in the spectrum of infectious disease. As HIV has spread to virtually all patient populations, practitioners in all fields of medicine must know basic features of HIV-related conditions and how HIV infection has an impact on the care that they will give.

AIDS can be caused by HIV-1 and HIV-2. Most cases of AIDS in the United States are caused by HIV-1. HIV-2 is more closely related to a monkey virus called simian immunodeficiency virus and clinically produces a syndrome virtually identical to that caused by HIV-1. There is evidence that HIV-2-related AIDS progresses at a slower rate than AIDS due to HIV-1 infection. The remainder of the chapter focuses on HIV-1 (hereafter referred to as HIV) infection.

The clinical syndrome of AIDS has recently been redefined to include those HIV-infected individuals who either:

▲ have a CD4 count (see below) that falls below 200 cells/mm^3

▲ develop one of the so-called AIDS-defining illnesses (Fig. 34-1)

▶ EPIDEMIOLOGY

There has been a shift in the epidemiology of HIV infection in the United States. Initially recognized in young homosexual men, HIV infection has spread to other demographic groups. Rapidly rising rates of infection have been observed in African-Americans, especially if there is concomitant intravenous drug use (IVDU). In the United States, transmission via heterosexual sex has been rising (generally among prostitutes and partners of people with a history of IVDU) but not to the extent seen in other areas of the world, especially sub-Saharan Africa and regions of the Far East (e.g., Thailand).

In the United States, the peak incidence of symptomatic HIV infection occurs in those 30 to 39 years of age. Because of the association with male homosexual behavior, more men than women are infected, but as the infection continues to spread among heterosexuals, male preponderance is diminishing.

▶ ETIOLOGY AND PATHOGENESIS

HIV-1 is an RNA virus belonging to the lentivirus subfamily of retroviruses. The life cycle of retroviruses is characteristic in that their RNA genome is first transcribed into a double-stranded DNA molecule via a viral enzyme called reverse transcriptase (RT). This DNA is then integrated into the genome of the host cell where it is transcribed into RNA that codes for viral proteins as well as new RNA viral genomes. These products are then processed and packaged into new viral particles that bud from the surface of the host cell. There are several unique steps in the viral life cycle that are the target of proposed anti-HIV therapy (see below).

HIV infects cells that carry the CD4 cell marker, generally T cells of the helper subclass but other CD4-positive (CD4+) cells as well. Infection of CD4+ lymphocytes results in their eventual death. Progression of HIV infection to frank AIDS is associated with a decline in circulating CD4+ lymphocytes and may in part explain the decline in immune status.

HIV-1 is found in the highest concentrations in blood and semen but can be isolated from a number of other bodily fluids as well. Transmission commonly occurs via:

▲ unprotected sexual contact (in the United States the highest risk is with anal receptive intercourse, but transmission also occurs with vaginal intercourse and oral-genital contact)

▲ IVDU

▲ perinatal blood exchange (mother to child)

▲ transfusion of blood and blood products (accounts for about 1 to 2% of the cases in the United States to date)

Transmission has not been firmly linked to casual (social) contact. Transmission appears to require unprotected sexual contact or exchange of blood/blood products.

Primary infection with HIV is linked with the acute retroviral syndrome in approximately 50 to 60%

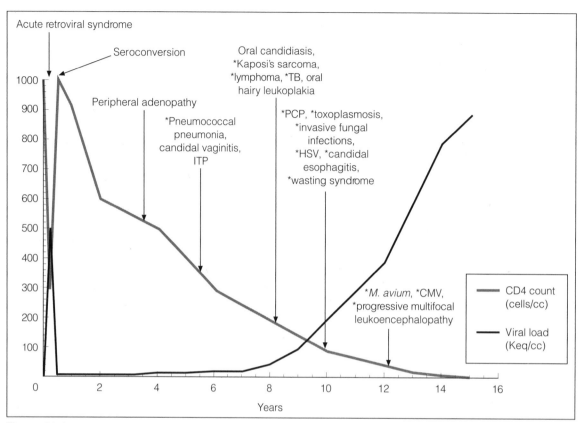

Figure 34-1 Hypothetical natural course of an HIV-infected individual.
* = AIDS-defining illness.

of cases. This manifests as a flu-like illness with fever, myalgias, rash, and headache. The CD4 count may fall acutely during the acute retroviral syndrome allowing for early appearance of opportunistic pathogens, but generally recovers to normal. High levels of viremia occur but then fall as the immune system appears to clear peripheral virus particles (see Figure 35-1).

The natural history of HIV infection then enters a phase of **clinical latency** where the patient is asymptomatic. Secondary markers of disease progression such as peripheral CD4 count and peripheral viral titers are relatively stable. What has become clear from recent studies is that despite clinical latency, there is not an accompanying viral latency. Even during the asymptomatic phase, there are very high levels of viral replication, occurring mostly in the lymphoid tissues. This viral replication is believed to cause progressive damage to the immune system, eventually leading to an inability to control the infection and the reappearance of viremia.

As the peripheral CD4 count falls, the HIV-infected individual becomes more susceptible to a va-

riety of opportunistic diseases and progression to the clinical syndrome of AIDS. The progression from HIV infection to AIDS has generally taken about 10 years in most individuals diagnosed to date.

▶ CLINICAL MANIFESTATIONS
History

The diagnosis of HIV infection is more frequently being made when patients are asymptomatic. Risk factors for HIV infection should be sought and patients with known risk factors screened (see below) for infection. Many times, screening is initiated by the patient. Physicians should inquire about HIV risk factors as part of every complete medical evaluation.

When the diagnosis of HIV infection is suspected, a **general review of systems** should be obtained, checking for:

▲ constitutional symptoms such as weight loss, fevers, night sweats, anorexia

▲ visual disturbances, persistent headache, oral lesions

▲ cough, shortness of breath, dyspnea on exertion

▲ pain or difficulty in swallowing, nausea/vomiting, diarrhea, rectal pain

▲ genital lesions, abnormal vaginal bleeding

▲ rashes, pigmented lesions, nodules

▲ new or rapidly growing nodes

Physical Examination

The baseline physical examination of a patient with newly diagnosed HIV infection should cover all organ systems, paying particular emphasis to those affected by the symptoms listed above. Women should have a complete pelvic examination including Pap smear due to the increased risk of invasive cervical cancer among HIV-infected women. Typical findings include:

▲ generalized lymphadenopathy

▲ oral candidiasis

▲ angular cheilitis

▲ pigmented lesions (Karposi's sarcoma, bacillary angiomatosis)

▲ fungal nail infections

On initial presentation, particularly in those patients diagnosed on HIV screening performed secondary to known risk factors rather than symptoms, the physical examination is entirely normal.

▶ DIAGNOSTIC EVALUATION

Testing for HIV infection is generally accomplished by a screening enzyme-linked immunoassay (ELISA) that tests for the presence of antibodies directed against the virus. If the ELISA is positive, then a follow-up Western blot is performed to test for immunoreactivity against specific viral proteins and confirm the diagnosis. The ELISA tests that are currently in use have a >99% specificity and a sensitivity of about 99.5%. When the test is used to screen the general population, even with this good test performance, there are a significant number of false positives. Thus, the Western blot is used for confirmation.

Besides the ELISA and Western blot, there are a number of other tests that can document and quantitate HIV infection. Assay for the p24 antigen of HIV is useful to detect virus before the appearance of antibody. Other direct tests for virus include detection and quantitation of viral RNA by polymerase chain reaction (PCR) and other molecular biologic assays.

When initially evaluating a patient with newly diagnosed HIV infection, the following initial tests are useful for establishing the stage of infection and the presence of possible opportunistic microorganisms:

▲ CD4 lymphocyte count

▲ complete blood count

▲ routine chemistries (electrolytes, creatinine, liver function tests)

▲ chest radiograph

▲ viral load (via PCR etc.)

▲ titers of antibodies against cytomegalovirus, *Toxoplasma gondii*, hepatitis B, hepatitis C

▲ PPD to test for tuberculosis exposure along with anergy panel

▲ RPR

▲ Pap smear for women

▶ TREATMENT

The management of the asymptomatic HIV-infected individual is twofold. The first goal is to forestall the immunologic decline due to infection. This is done via the administration of antiviral agents. The second goal is to prevent and, if unsuccessful, to initiate prompt treatment of opportunistic diseases. Prophylaxis and routine surveillance are the main tools used to accomplish this second goal.

Antiviral Agents

The first antiviral agents to be used were the nucleoside analogues. These are inhibitors of viral RT and interfere with an early stage in viral replication. Zidovudine (AZT or ZDV) was the first of the nucleoside analogues to be used. An early study showed a modest survival benefit when AZT was given to patients with advanced-stage AIDS. Other nucleoside analogues that have been developed include ddI, ddC, d4T, and 3TC. All have been used alone or in combination in a number of clinical trials. Resistance (due to mutations in RT) has arisen in viral isolates from patients on these agents and has prompted a number of different regimens of combination or rotation of these drugs (see below) when they are used for treatment of AIDS. A number of nonnucleoside inhibitors of RT have been developed and are also being studied in clinical trials.

One of the newest classes of antiviral agents to be approved for use are the protease inhibitors. These agents (saquinavir, ritonavir, and indinavir) inhibit the HIV-protease, a virally encoded protein that is necessary for proper synthesis and assembly of viral particles, thus affecting a later stage in the viral infection than the RT inhibitors.

Other drugs have been developed that target other aspects of viral replication, including soluble CD4 to block viral entry, inhibitors of viral integration (which is mediated by a virally encoded protein), and blockers of HIV surface proteins.

The current status of antiretroviral is constantly in flux as new agents become available and the results of a large number of clinical trials become available. Even a cursory review is beyond the scope of this chapter. However, there are several trends for the use of antiviral agents that are becoming accepted. First, antiretroviral therapy has generally not been started until a patient develops an AIDS-defining illness or the CD4 count falls below 500 cells/mm^3. Second, therapy generally begins with RT inhibitors. Third, combination of RT inhibitors may be more effective than single-agent therapy (perhaps by limiting resistance). Fourth, combinations of RT inhibitors and protease inhibitors may have the greatest activity against HIV. Finally, monitoring of response to antiviral therapy is via secondary markers such as CD4 count and viremia.

The time to initiate antiretroviral therapy is controversial, based on results from a number of different studies. The previous general consensus is listed above (no therapy until CD4 < 500 or AIDS-defining illness). Some experts now advocate treatment (with combination RT inhibitors ± protease inhibitors) as soon as the diagnosis of HIV infection is made, regardless of CD4 count or viral load. Others will use the CD4 count or viral load (or the rate of change of these values) to guide initiation of therapy. It remains to be seen which of these strategies will give the best long-term outcomes.

The prophylaxis and treatment of opportunistic infections is discussed in detail in the next chapter.

Most care of the asymptomatic HIV-infected patient involves careful monitoring and patient education. The patient should be encouraged to ask whatever questions they may have. Modes of transmission should be reviewed, as well as the course of progression and treatment options. For the asymptomatic patient, the psychosocial aspects of the disease are often the most difficult. Support groups and professional counseling are available and should be offered to the patient. As the disease progresses to the symptomatic stage, this support often becomes even more important.

The issue of partner notification is an ethical dilemma that needs to be faced. The patient needs to be assured that the diagnosis will remain confidential but should also be encouraged to inform others who may have been infected by them. HIV is generally not a reportable disease; therefore, the physician may be placed in a position between maintaining patient confidentiality and protecting the health of others.

Once patients have started antiretroviral therapy, they should be monitored for response and side effects. As mentioned above, response is usually measured by monitoring CD4 counts and viral load. If CD4 counts fall or viremia rises on therapy, consideration should be given to altering therapy, either by switching to different agents or adding other agents, particularly one of a different class. Development of opportunistic diseases can also be considered to be a sign of progression on therapy.

The most frequently encountered side effects of the most commonly used antivirals are listed in Table 34-1.

▶ **KEY POINTS**

1. HIV is the etiologic agent of AIDS characterized by a progressive decline in immune function that leads to an increased susceptibility to a variety of opportunistic infections and conditions.

2. HIV is transmitted by unprotected sexual contact, intravenous drug use (with shared needles), perinatally, and by blood and blood products that have failed screening.

3. After infection with HIV, there is generally a 5- to 10-year period of clinical latency where there are relatively few signs or symptoms of infection despite high rates of viral replication within lymphoid tissues.

4. The diagnosis of HIV infection is generally made by a screening ELISA test for presence of anti-HIV

TABLE 34-1

Antiviral Agents

Drug	Class	Side Effects
ZDV (AZT)	RTI	Leukopenia, anemia
ddC	RTI	Neuropathy, pancreatitis (< ddI)
ddI	RTI	Pancreatitis, neuropathy
Lamivudine (3TC)	RTI	Rash (usually with initiation of treatment)
d4T	RTI	Neuropathy
Indinavir	PI	Nephrolithiasis (esp. in setting of poor water intake)
Ritonavir	PI	GI upset
Saquinivir	PI	GI upset

RTI, reverse transcriptase inhibitor; PI, protease inhibitor.

antibodies followed by a confirmatory Western blot if the ELISA is positive.

5. The management of the asymptomatic HIV patient involves characterizing and following the progression of infection (via CD4 counts and viral load), prevention of opportunistic diseases, and attempting to forestall immunologic decline by the administration of drugs that have activity against HIV itself.

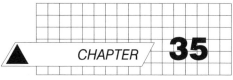

CHAPTER 35

HIV Part II: Prophylaxis and Treatment of Opportunistic Infections in HIV

7he bulk of the morbidity and mortality associated with human immunodeficiency virus (HIV) infection is due to conditions (most commonly secondary infections) that arise in the setting of the resultant immune defects. Early in the history of the HIV epidemic, most physicians waited for opportunistic diseases to arise and then attempted to treat them as best as possible. It was later demonstrated that *prophylaxis* was possible for a number of opportunistic infections—extending both the symptom-free and overall survival of HIV-infected individuals.

Given the dozens of HIV-associated opportunistic diseases, even a limited discussion of most of these is beyond the scope of this chapter. However, a few **common opportunistic diseases** are responsible for the bulk of the morbidity and mortality:

▲ *Pneumocystis carinii* pneumonia (PCP)

▲ *Mycobacterium tuberculosis*

▲ *Mycobacterium avium* complex (MAC)

▲ *Toxoplasma gondii*

▲ Recurrent *Streptococcus pneumoniae* infections

▲ Cytomegalovirus (CMV)

▲ Herpes simplex virus (HSV)

▲ Varicella-zoster virus

▲ *Cryptococcus neoformans*

▲ *Histoplasma capsulatum*

▲ *Coccidioides immitis*

▲ *Candida albicans*

▲ Lymphoma

▲ Kaposi's sarcoma

In the United States, PCP remains the most common serious opportunistic infection among HIV-infected individuals. At least half of the cases of PCP occur in persons with previously undiagnosed HIV infection.

▶ RISK FACTORS

Specific opportunistic diseases are encountered at particular degrees of immune suppression. If the CD4 count is used as a marker for immune status, certain conditions are rarely encountered until the CD4 count has fallen below a given level (see Figure in Chapter 34). For example, PCP is usually not encountered until the CD4 count is less than 200/mm³, whereas CMV disease is not seen until the CD4 count is less than 50/mm³. This has implications for both formulating a differential diagnosis for a symptomatic HIV-infected patient as well as influencing when prophylactic drugs are started.

Exposures (including remote infections) can influence the likelihood of a particular opportunistic condition. For example, CMV and central nervous system (CNS) toxoplasmosis are generally believed to be due to reactivation of latent infection and therefore would be unlikely to occur in patients without serologic evidence of past infection. The endemic fungal infections are seen in particular geographic areas (histoplasmosis in the Mississippi River Valley and coccidioidomycosis in the Southwest). Animal exposures increase risk for certain infections (e.g., cryptococcosis with pigeons and *Bartonella* with cats).

▶ CLINICAL MANIFESTATIONS
History

A given symptom complex in an HIV-infected patient can be important evidence for an opportunistic disease. The common HIV-specific differential for various symptoms include:

▲ **Constitutional symptoms (fever, weight loss, fatigue)**—mycobacterial infection (tuberculosis [TB] and MAC), HIV wasting syndrome, lymphoma, *Bartonella* infection;

▲ **Visual changes, eye, pain**—CMV retinitis, ophthalmic varicella-zoster;

▲ **Headache, mental status changes**—toxoplasma encephalitis, CNS lymphoma, cryptococcal meningitis, progressive multifocal leukoencephalopathy;

▲ **Cough, shortness of breath**—PCP, tuberculosis, recurrent bacterial pneumonia, influenza;

▲ **Oral lesions**—thrush, oral hairy leukoplakia, aphthous ulcers, HSV;

▲ **Odynophagia, dysphagia**—candidal esophagitis, CMV esophagitis, HSV esophagitis;

▲ **Chronic diarrhea**—cryptosporidiosis, isosporiasis;

▲ **Genitourinary symptoms**—recurrent HSV infection, syphilis, cervical cancer;

▲ **Skin lesions**—Kaposi's sarcoma, molluscum contagiosum, *Bartonella* infection (bacillary angiomatosis), scabies;

▲ **Enlarged lymph nodes**—lymphoma, mycobacterial infection, HIV lymphadenopathy, *Bartonella*.

Physical Examination

The physical examination of the symptomatic HIV-infected patient should be broad. In addition to examination of symptomatic regions, particular attention should be paid to:

▲ Mucosa (oral candidiasis, oral ulcers, genital lesions);

▲ Retina (retinopathy);

▲ Skin (pigmented lesions, rashes, ulcers);

▲ Lungs (consolidation, crackles);

▲ Lymph nodes (new or tender nodes, bulky adenopathy);

▲ Liver and spleen (hepato/splenomegaly).

▶ MANAGEMENT

The treatment of opportunistic diseases in HIV can be divided into:

▲ **Primary prophylaxis**—lifestyle modifications and administration of drugs designed to prevent the appearance of an opportunistic disease;

▲ **Treatment**—specific therapy to cure or control an opportunistic disease;

▲ **Secondary prophylaxis**—continued drug therapy that is designed to prevent active recurrence of an opportunistic disease once initial treatment has been completed.

The U.S. Public Health Service and the Infectious Diseases Society of America recently published guidelines on the prevention of opportunistic infections. They reviewed the literature on prophylaxis for 17 major opportunistic infections and rated their recommendations based on the quality of the published evidence.

A summary of some of the major recommendations is given in Table 35-1.

Avoidance of exposure to opportunistic pathogens is desirable but not always possible. Some opportunistic infections are believed to be due to reactivation of latent disease. Complete avoidance of certain exposures requires placing limitations on lifestyle.

In general, the following **lifestyle recommendations** can be considered:

▲ **Sexual exposure**—Use of latex condoms can reduce exposure to CMV, HSV, and other sexually transmitted diseases. Latex condoms will also prevent the transmission of HIV to others. Avoidance of sexual practices that can result in oral exposure to feces may reduce the risk of infections such as cryptosporidiosis, amebiasis, hepatitis, and giardiasis.

▲ **Environmental** exposure—Certain professions can result in increased risk of certain opportunistic infections; health care or work in shelters or correctional institutions (TB), child care (giardiasis, hepatitis, CMV), animal care (toxoplasmosis, campylobacteriosis, cryptosporidiosis), gardening (cryptosporidiosis, toxoplasmosis). Pet exposure should be monitored: cats (bartonellosis, toxoplasmosis), reptiles (salmonellosis), fish (*Mycobacterium marinum*).

▲ **Food and water-related exposures**—Avoid raw or undercooked eggs, meat, seafood, and dairy products. Avoid drinking untreated water, as well as avoid swimming in lakes and rivers. Boiling of drinking water is advisable in areas with documented cryptosporidiosis.

▲ **Travel**—Exposures to any of the above-listed risks may be increased in certain geographic areas. Particular attention needs to be paid to the risk of diarrheal illnesses (traveler's diarrhea). Killed vaccines (rabies, diphtheria-tetanus) can be given as recommended for all travelers, but live vaccines (polio, typhoid) should be avoided, with the exception of measles vaccine.

In general, the potential benefits of these lifestyle modifications needs to be weighed against the hardships that may be imposed. For example, the companionship provided by a pet can be very beneficial. Provided certain preventive measures can be taken (washing hands after handling cat litter, keeping the cat indoors, and flea control), pet ownership need not be prohibited. In addition, with the exception of condom use, the data supporting most of the above recommendations is limited.

The *treatment and primary and secondary prophylaxis* for the most commonly encountered opportunistic infections is presented in Table 35-1. For most pathogens,

TABLE 35-1

Treatment and Prophylaxis of Major Opportunistic Infections in HIV-Infected Individuals

Pathogen	Treatment (alternatives)	Indications for Prophylaxis	Primary Prophylaxis (alternatives)	Secondary Prophylaxis (alternatives)
Pneumocystis carinii	TMP/SMZ (dapsone, aerosolized pentamidine, dapsone plus pyrimethamine)	CD4 count <200/μL or unexplained fever for >2 weeks or oral candidiasis	TMP/SMZ (dapsone, aerosolized pentamidine, dapsone plus pyrimethamine)	TMP/SMZ (dapsone, aerosolized pentamidine, dapsone plus pyrimethamine)
Mycobacterium tuberculosis	Isoniazid plus pyridoxine plus rifampin plus ethambutol (until sensitivity data are available)	Tuberculin test reaction >5 mm or history of positive test without treatment or contact with active case of TB	Isoniazid plus pyridoxine (rifampin)	None
Toxoplasma gondii	Sulfadiazine plus pyrimethamine plus leukovorin (clindamycin as alternative to sulfa)	IgG antibody to *Toxoplasma* and CD4 <100/μL	TMP/SMZ (dapsone plus pyrimethamine plus leukovorin)	Sulfadiazine plus pyrimethamine plus leukovorin (clindamycin plus pyrimethamine plus leukovorin)
Mycobacterium avium complex	Clarithromycin or azithromycin plus one or more of rifabutin, ethambutol, clofazimine, ciprofloxacin	CD4 <75/μL	Clarithromycin (azithromycin, rifabutin)	Clarithromycin or azithromycin plus one or more of rifabutin, ethambutol, clofazimine, ciprofloxacin
Influenza virus	None	All patients	Influenza vaccine	None
Streptococcus pneumoniae	Penicillin, cephalosporins	All patients	Pneumococcal vaccine	Pneumococcal vaccine
Cytomegalovirus	IV ganciclovir (Foscarnet)	IgG antibody to CMV and CD4 <50/μL	Oral gancyclovir (limited data)	IV gancyclovir (IV foscarnet, oral gancyclovir)
Herpes simplex virus	Acyclovir (famciclovir)	Not recommended	Not recommended	Acyclovir (famciclovir) for frequent and/or severe relapses
Herpes (varicella) zoster virus	Acyclovir (famciclovir)	Exposure to person with acute chickenpox or zoster	Varicella-zoster immune globulin	Acyclovir (famciclovir) for frequent and/or severe relapses
Candida spp.	Fluconazole (ketoconazole)	CD4 <50/μL	Fluconazole (ketoconazole)	Generally reserved for frequent or severe recurrences—fluconazole (ketoconazole, itraconazole, clotrimazole troches, nystatin)
Cryptococcus neoformans	Fluconazole (ketoconazole)	CD4 <50/μL	Fluconazole (ketoconazole)	Fluconazole (itraconazole, weekly IV amphotericin)
Histoplasma capsulatum	Itraconazole (fluconazole)	CD4 <50/μL and endemic area	Itraconazole (fluconazole)	Itraconazole (weekly IV amphotericin, fluconazole)
Coccidioides immitis	Fluconazole (itraconazole)	CD4 <50/μL and endemic area	Fluconazole (itraconazole)	Fluconazole (itraconazole, weekly IV amphotericin)

TMP/SMZ, trimethoprim/sulfamethoxazole.

alternative regimens exist, generally used in the setting of adverse drug reactions to the primary regimen.

There is currently no prophylaxis available to prevent secondary malignancies (lymphoma, Kaposi's sarcoma, cervical cancer). The treatment of these diseases is generally undertaken in consultation with an experienced oncologist.

The standard of care for HIV-infected individuals is in a constant state of change. In general, it appears that a combination of antiviral therapy along with monitoring and prophylaxis for opportunistic diseases will provide the best long-term outcome. The specific recommendations are changing; consultation with an infectious disease specialist can help ensure that the most recent recommendations are known.

▶ KEY POINTS

1. Opportunistic diseases cause most of the morbidity and mortality attritutable to HIV infection.

2. Opportunistic infections are the most frequently encountered opportunistic diseases. Of these, *Pneumocystis carinii* pneumonia is the most common in the United States.

3. A given opportunistic infection tends to occur at specific degrees of immune suppression. The CD4 count is used to quantify immune suppression.

4. Prophylactic antibiotic regimens have been developed that decrease the risk of certain opportunistic infections.

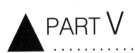

PART V

Gastrointestinal

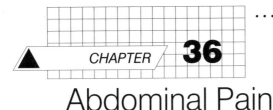

CHAPTER 36

Abdominal Pain

*T*he key feature of evaluating the patient with abdominal pain is to distinguish medical causes from surgical causes. This chapter discusses the evaluation of acute abdominal pain in the adult. Causes of chronic abdominal pain (e.g., **peptic ulcer disease**, irritable bowel syndrome) are discussed in subsequent chapters.

Abdominal pain is caused by obstruction, perforation, ischemia, infection, or metabolic disturbances. Abdominal pain referred from the hollow **viscera** travels via the splanchnic (sympathetic) nerves. It is dull, vague, and poorly localized. Diseases involving the **parietal** peritoneum produce sharp, stabbing, well-localized pain.

▶ DIFFERENTIAL DIAGNOSIS

The differential diagnosis of abdominal pain can be divided according to predominant location of the pain:

Diffuse or periumbilical

▲ Abdominal aortic aneurysm (AAA)

▲ Ischemic bowel*

▲ Bowel obstruction, especially small bowel

▲ Pancreatitis

▲ Gastroenteritis

▲ Metabolic disturbances (see below)

Right upper quadrant

▲ Cholecystitis

▲ Biliary colic

▲ Hepatitis

Right lower quadrant

▲ Appendicitis

▲ Nephrolithiasis

▲ Crohn's disease of terminal ileum

---

*Ischemic bowel may refer to chronic ischemia ("intestinal angina") or acute ischemia. For this chapter, ischemia bowel refers to the latter syndrome. In general, ischemia of the bowel is secondary to underlying atherosclerotic disease or arterial embolism (from atrial fibrillation or valvular disease). However, ischemia may also be caused by vasculitis (Henoch-Schönlein purpura, polyarteritis nodosa; see Chapter 59) or by a crisis in sickle cell anemia.

Left upper quadrant

▲ Splenic rupture

Left lower quadrant

▲ Diverticulitis

▲ Nephrolithiasis

▲ Inflammatory bowel disease

Gynecologic sources of pain (pelvic inflammatory disease, ovarian torsion, ectopic pregnancy) should be considered in all women with abdominal pain, especially lower quadrant pain.

Certain metabolic diseases may present with abdominal pain. Although these are uncommon causes, they should be considered in the differential diagnosis:

▲ Acute intermittent porphyria;

▲ Diabetic ketoacidosis (DKA);

▲ Familial Mediterranean fever.

Acute intermittent porphyria is an autosomal dominant deficiency in hydroxymethylbilane synthase (formerly known as porphobilinogen deaminase), an enzyme in the heme synthesis pathway. **Familial Mediterranean fever** is an autosomal recessive disease, more common in people of Middle Eastern descent. It is characterized by recurring bouts of fever and inflammation of the peritoneum (serositis).

▶ CLINICAL MANIFESTATIONS
History

Certain diseases often present with a typical pattern of pain. **Appendicitis** usually begins as vague, cramp-like abdominal pain that moves to the right lower quadrant, becoming sharper in quality and more intense. **Biliary colic** is characterized by severe, steady, aching pain in the right upper quadrant or epigastrium, lasting about 1 to 4 hours. Pain may be associated with a meal, and often occurs at night. More persistent pain, associated with fever, is seen in **acute cholecystitis**, which may also be referred to the right scapula.

Pancreatitis is epigastric/periumbilical in location and is a steady and boring pain, radiating to the back and relieved with sitting. Recent alcohol ingestion may be present. **Bowel ischemia** is often sudden and severe in onset. Patients often have history of atrial fibrillation, placing them at risk for arterial embolism. **Bowel obstruction** presents as crampy, midabdominal pain, occurring in paroxysms. Absence of recent bowel movement or passage of flatus is another indicator. **Nephrolithiasis** begins gradually and then escalates to a severe pain in 20 to 60 minutes, with flank pain radiating to the groin or testicle.

Nausea and **vomiting** are commonly associated symptoms in patients with acute abdominal pain. However, these two symptoms may not help to distinguish the cause because they can be seen in pancreatitis, cholecystitis, hepatitis, bowel obstruction, and appendicitis.

Patient age may suggest a particular cause. Appendicitis is more common in younger patients; elderly patients may have vascular causes (AAA, bowel ischemia) or diverticulitis.

Physical Examination

Fever occurs in infectious causes of abdominal pain but may also be present in inflammatory etiologies, such as acute pancreatitis. Jaundice is often seen in hepatitis and is usually absent in cholecystitis and biliary colic unless obstruction of the bile duct occurs. Evidence of vascular disease, such as diminished peripheral pulses, should increase the suspicion of bowel ischemia or AAA.

The abdominal examination should begin with assessing the **presence** of **bowel sounds** (often absent in pancreatitis, bowel ischemia; high pitched in bowel obstruction). **Rebound tenderness** indicates peritoneal irritation and requires immediate surgical evaluation. Although many conditions may demonstrate abdominal tenderness, **point tenderness** usually occurs in appendicitis, diverticulitis, and cholelithiasis. Pain at McBurney's point is classic for appendicitis. This point is one-third of the way between the right anterior superior iliac spine and the umbilicus. Murphy's sign (pain upon palpation of right upper quadrant with inspiration) is associated with cholecystitis. **Palpable masses** include an aortic aneurysm and a large dilated loop of bowel.

A rectal examination should be performed to examine for tenderness and the presence of occult blood. Conditions that are notable for **severe pain but relatively normal abdominal examinations** (pain out of proportion to findings) are ischemic bowel, pancreatitis, and acute intermittent porphyria.

▶ DIAGNOSTIC EVALUATION

The extent of diagnostic testing depends on the history and physical examination. The well-appearing patient will show classic symptoms of gastroenteritis (diffuse abdominal pain, diarrhea, nausea), and a benign examination may only need observation. The acutely ill patient with peritoneal signs and suspicion of perforation should go directly to the operating room for exploration. Physical examination and early testing should distinguish the surgical causes of abdominal pain from the nonsurgical causes.

The **abdominal plain film** may show free intraperitoneal air, seen under the diaphragm on an upright film, indicating perforation of a hollow viscus. Bowel obstruction reveals distended small bowel (>2.5 cm in diameter), large bowel (>9 to 10 cm), or both. Absence of air in the distal gastrointestinal tract distinguishes bowel obstruction from adynamic ileus. However, residual air may be present in early bowel obstruction. Edematous bowel loops or "thumb printing" may be seen in bowel infarction. Most renal stones (>80%) and a smaller percentage of gallstones (15%) can be seen on a plain film.

Serum electrolytes may show an **anion gap acidosis** in bowel infarction, DKA, or severe pancreatitis. **Hyperkalemia** is seen in bowel infarction and represents tissue necrosis. Leukocytosis is a nonspecific finding and is seen in many causes of abdominal pain. All women of reproductive age should have **human chorionic gonadotropin beta-subunit** sent to rule out pregnancy-related conditions. Serum **amylase** is markedly elevated in pancreatitis, although moderate elevation may be seen in biliary disease, bowel obstruction, DKA, and bowel ischemia. **Liver function tests** (LFTs) show marked elevations in transaminases in hepatitis and elevation in alkaline phosphatase in cholecystitis. LFTs may be normal in biliary colic.

Urinalysis should be sent to evaluate for hematuria (nephrolithiasis). Mild amounts of pyuria may be seen in diverticulitis and appendicitis. Ketones are detected in the urine in most patients who have not been eating due to the abdominal pain; however, large amounts of ketones raise the suspicion of DKA.

Ultrasonography may be used to evaluate the liver and biliary tree in patients with upper quadrant pain. However, the presence of stones in the gallbladder does not confirm cholecystitis because many patients have asymptomatic stones. About 5 to 10% of patients with cholecystitis will have **acalculus** cholecystitis;

no stones will be visualized in these patients. **Sonographic findings of cholecystitis** include:

▲ gallbladder wall thickening

▲ sonographic Murphy's sign (tenderness with pressure applied by probe over gallbladder)

▲ pericholecystic fluid

Abdominal ultrasound can also show an aortic aneurysm or reveal a dilated ureter in nephrolithiasis.

Computed tomography (CT) is not needed in most evaluations of abdominal pain. However, it is very sensitive in detecting inflammation in the pancreas (pancreatitis) and large bowel (diverticulitis). Splenic rupture or laceration may be seen with abdominal CT. Bowel wall edema, as seen in bowel ischemia, can also be detected.

The **Watson-Schwartz test** is used to detect elevated levels of hydroxymethylbilane synthase seen in attacks of acute intermittent porphyria. This test can be performed in patients with a suspicious history or findings of a neuropathy in addition to the abdominal pain.

▶ TREATMENT

Surgery should be performed immediately in patients with suspected appendicitis, bowel infarction, ruptured AAA, or splenic rupture. Surgery is usually delayed 24 to 72 hours in the stable patient with cholecystitis while antibiotics are given. Treatment of medical causes of abdominal pain is discussed in Chapters 24, 39, and 43.

▶ KEY POINTS

1. Pregnancy or ectopic pregnancy should be considered in all women of reproductive age with abdominal pain.

2. Vascular causes of abdominal pain (bowel ischemia, AAA) should be considered in elderly patients.

3. Point tenderness is suggestive of appendicitis, diverticulitis, and cholecystitis.

4. Abdominal plain film should be obtained in patients with suspected obstruction or perforation.

5. Diabetic ketoacidosis can produce abdominal pain, vomiting, ketonuria, and an anion gap acidosis.

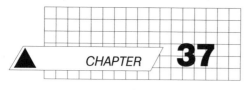

CHAPTER 37

Diarrhea

Adults normally produce about 150 g stool/day. Diarrhea is the increase in volume of stool and is often accompanied by increased stool fluid content and frequency. There are four basic **pathophysiologic causes of diarrhea:**

1. Increased secretion of electrolytes and water into the bowel lumen;
2. Increased osmotic load within the intestine, leading to water retention in the bowel lumen;
3. Inflammation leading to exudation of protein and fluid from the intestinal mucosa;
4. Altered intestinal motility, leading to rapid transit times.

In addition to classification based on pathophysiology, diarrhea can also be divided into **acute,** which usually has a sudden onset and often has a benign self-limited course, and **chronic,** which may persist for weeks to years, sometimes with a waxing and waning course.

▶ DIFFERENTIAL DIAGNOSIS

Causes of diarrhea can be grouped according to the pathogenic mechanisms presented above:

Increased secretion

▲ cholera toxin

▲ clostridial endotoxin (e.g., *Clostridium difficile* after antibiotic use)

▲ noninvasive microbial gastroenteritis (e.g., viral gastroenteritis)

▲ carcinoid syndrome

▲ vasoactive intestinal peptide-secreting tumor

▲ villous adenoma

Increased osmotic load

▲ sorbitol ingestion ("sugar-free candy diarrhea")

▲ bile salt malabsorption

▲ pancreatic insufficiency

▲ lactase deficiency ("lactose intolerance")

▲ malabsorption (e.g., celiac sprue)

▲ postantrectomy rapid gastric emptying ("dumping syndrome")

▲ magnesium-containing laxatives

Inflammation

▲ ulcerative colitis

▲ Crohn's disease

▲ radiation-induced enteritis

▲ invasive microbial gastroenteritis (e.g., *Shigella, Entamoeba*)

Altered intestinal motility

▲ thyrotoxicosis

▲ irritable bowel syndrome

▲ neurologic disease (e.g., diabetes-associated enteropathy)

▶ CLINICAL MANIFESTATIONS
History

History helps to determine whether the illness is acute or chronic and provides hints as to the underlying etiology. For example, infectious diarrhea often occurs in outbreaks associated with particular foods or environmental exposures, such as swimming or drinking of stream water. The nature of the stool can give important clues to etiology:

▲ watery (secretory)

▲ bulky, greasy (osmotic)

▲ bloody ± leukocytes (inflammatory)

A medication history is important because many drugs, including antibiotics, antihypertensives, anti-inflammatory agents, and diuretics, can cause diarrhea. Laxative abuse is a very common cause of chronic secretory diarrhea.

Other important historical features to obtain include the presence of fever, abdominal pain, flatulence, and extraintestinal symptoms such as arthritis, rashes, weight loss, or edema. Association with meals or fasting should be investigated.

Physical Examination

Important elements of the physical examination are the degree of hydration, the presence of abdominal tenderness, rectal mass or blood, and characterization of bowel sounds. Along with providing etiologic clues, these elements indicate the severity of the illness.

▶ DIAGNOSTIC EVALUATION

The approach to diagnostic testing is based on whether the diarrhea is acute or chronic. Because acute diarrhea (if not associated with drugs) is often infectious (see Chapter 31), examination of the stool coupled with culture are the principal tests used. Not every patient who presents with diarrhea needs to be evaluated with these expensive and time-consuming tests. If the patient is clinically well, watchful waiting and symptomatic therapy with oral fluids are all that may be necessary. However, certain **clinical features** should trigger a stool examination:

▲ high fever

▲ evidence of dehydration

▲ systemic toxicity

▲ bloody stool

▲ immunocompromise

▲ overseas or outdoor (e.g., hiking) travel

▲ male homosexuality

▲ recent antibiotic use

The presence of blood and/or leukocytes in the stool suggests an invasive microbial (e.g., *Shigella*, *Campylobacter*, or *Entamoeba*) rather than a viral or toxin mediated cause. It is important to also consider the possibility of ulcerative colitis, Crohn's disease, and other inflammatory diarrheas when blood and/or leukocytes are found in the stool.

Culture for bacterial pathogens and **examination for parasites** can identify etiologic organisms. If *Campylobacter* or *Yersinia* is suspected, the microbiology laboratory should be notified because these organisms often will not grow on routine culture media.

Chronic diarrhea is usually not inflammatory in nature. Exceptions include inflammatory bowel disease and radiation enteritis, but history usually suggests these causes of chronic diarrhea. Often, evaluation of chronic diarrhea centers on the differentiation between an osmotic diarrhea and a secretory diarrhea. A simple and useful diagnostic test is to assess the clinical change resulting from fasting. Osmotic diarrhea (which is generally due to some sort of malabsorption syndrome) improves with fasting, whereas secretory diarrhea persists during fasting.

Another rapid way to distinguish between secretory and osmotic diarrhea is to calculate the stool osmotic gap using the formula:

osmotic gap

$$= \text{stool osmolality} - 2(\text{stool Na} + \text{stool K})$$

Stool osmolality is usually estimated using the measured plasma osmolality. An osmotic gap greater than 50 mOsmol/kg H_2O suggests an osmotic diarrhea.

Further diagnostic testing is generally only necessary in the workup of chronic diarrheas. **Endoscopy**, either sigmoidoscopy or full colonoscopy with biopsy, can reveal a number of findings that are suggestive or diagnostic of a particular etiology:

▲ inflammation with pathology indicative of inflammatory bowel disease

▲ melanosis coli in laxative abuse

▲ villous adenoma

▲ pseudomembranous colitis (*C. difficile*)

▲ flask-shaped ulcers in amebiasis

If initial workup reveals an osmotic diarrhea, there are **studies** that can be used to check for the presence of a number of **malabsorption syndrome**s.

▲ ᴅ-Xylose test (measures absorptive capacity of the proximal small bowel)

▲ Schilling test (evaluates the terminal ileum)

▲ bile salt breath test (evaluates the terminal ileum)

▲ measurement of pancreatic secretions (to test for maldigestion from pancreatic insufficiency)

▲ lactose challenge (to test for lactase deficiency)

When further diagnostic tests fail to reveal an organic cause for chronic diarrhea, the diagnosis of **irritable bowel syndrome** can be tested for and treated by the combination of diet (avoidance of "trigger foods," caffeine), addition of fiber and bulk agents (psyllium), drugs (antispasmodics), and psychological management (stress reduction).

▶ KEY POINTS

1. Diarrhea is the increase in stool volume (usually with increased fluid content and frequency).

2. The four major pathogenic mechanisms for diarrhea are increased secretion, osmotic load, inflammation, and altered intestinal motility.

3. Inflammatory diarrhea is characterized by the presence of blood and/or leukocytes in the stool.

4. Osmotic and secretory diarrhea can be distinguished by calculation of stool osmolar gap or response to fasting.

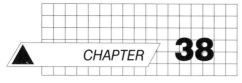

CHAPTER 38

Peptic Ulcer Disease and Gastritis

*D*yspepsia, or epigastric discomfort, is a common complaint. Ulcer disease and gastritis are two important causes of dyspepsia and are the focus of this discussion.

▶ EPIDEMIOLOGY

Most people experience transient episodic epigastric pain, but only 10 to 15% of the U.S. population is estimated to have chronic dyspepsia. Of these, about half will be found to have peptic ulcers. The lifetime incidence of peptic ulcer disease (gastric and duodenal ulcers) in the United States is 5 to 10%, making it a common clinical problem.

The incidence of duodenal ulcers is twice as high in men, whereas the incidence of gastric ulcer is only slightly higher among men. The peak age of incidence of duodenal ulcers is the fifth decade. Gastric ulcers also increase in incidence among older patients with a slight male predominance.

It is important to note that the above epidemiology holds for the United States and other industrialized countries. The epidemiology varies worldwide with hygiene and socioeconomic status, which are important factors for infection with *Helicobacter pylori* (see below).

Gastritis, the **inflammation of the gastric mucosa**, occurs in a variety of settings and as such is not a single disease (see below).

▶ ETIOLOGY AND PATHOPHYSIOLOGY

In gastritis, inflammation is limited to the gastric mucosa. It can be an acute or chronic disease, each with a particular pathogenesis. In **acute gastritis**, there is erosion and damage to the gastric mucosa and a brisk inflammatory infiltrate. This damage can be diffuse or patchy in distribution. Acute gastritis generally occurs in the setting of a serious systemic illness, such as trauma, burns, sepsis, liver and renal failure, and shock, or with certain drugs, such as nonsteroidal anti-inflammatory drugs (NSAIDs), ethanol, steroids (high doses), and strong alkali and acid agents.

Chronic gastritis is characterized by mononuclear cell infiltrates and lack of mucosal erosions. Chronic infection with *H. pylori* is associated with at least three types of chronic gastritis: **chronic active gastritis, atrophic gastritis**, and so-called **type B gastritis**. Atrophic gastritis is believed to be a precursor to some gastric cancers.

In contrast to gastritis, **ulcers** are focal areas of **deep erosion** through the mucosa and, in some cases, through the submucosa. They commonly occur in the stomach and the duodenum. There are some differences between the pathogenesis of gastric and duodenal ulcers. In **duodenal ulcers, excess gastric acid** is necessary for ulcer formation (hence the dictum, "no acid, no ulcer"). In contrast, patients with **gastric ulcer** tend to have **normal or even reduced gastric acid** secretion.

H. pylori infection appears to be associated with greater than 90% of duodenal ulcers and 70 to 80% of gastric ulcers. The precise pathogenesis of *H. pylori* infection resulting in peptic ulcer is not clear but appears to involve both bacterial and host factors. Only about one of six individuals who are infected with *H. pylori* develops ulcers.

H. pylori infection is also associated with the development of gastric cancer and low-grade non-Hodgkin gastric lymphoma. Only a small (< 1 to 2%) number of *H. pylori*-infected individuals develop gastric cancer, and it appears that those who have gastric ulcers are more prone to develop cancer than those who have duodenal ulcers.

Complications of peptic ulcer include:

▲ bleeding (may be occult or frank melena or hematemesis)

▲ perforation

▲ obstruction

▲ weight loss

▶ RISK FACTORS

Besides *H. pylori* infection, other risk factors for the development of peptic ulcer are:

▲ male sex

▲ first-degree relatives with duodenal ulcer (risk for duodenal ulcer)

▲ stress

▲ cigarette smoking

▲ aspirin and NSAID use

▶ CLINICAL MANIFESTATIONS
History

The most common symptom in peptic ulcer disease is **epigastric pain**. The patient commonly reports a **gnawing, burning**, or **aching** discomfort. In patients with duodenal ulcer, the pain typically occurs within 2 to 3 hours of a meal (presumably reflecting increased acid and pancreatic enzyme load in the duodenum). The pain awakens the patient in the middle of the night, but pain occurring before breakfast is rare. Food and antacids generally provide prompt relief. The relationship between food and pain in the setting of gastric ulcer is more variable; food may actually aggravate gastric ulcer pain.

Other symptoms that can be seen in peptic ulcer disease are nausea, vomiting, early satiety and emesis of undigested food (in the setting of obstruction), melena, hematemesis, and back or shoulder pain (often in the setting of posterior penetration of a duodenal ulcer).

In patients with gastritis, pain is often less prominent. Occult or frank gastrointestinal bleeding (with melena or hematemesis) is often the only finding.

Physical Examination

On physical examination, the most common finding is epigastric tenderness. Other findings that are usually seen in the setting of complications include:

▲ "succussion splash," a sound produced by air and fluid in a distended stomach several hours postprandially due to gastric outlet obstruction

▲ peritoneal signs (rigid abdomen, diminished bowel sounds, rebound tenderness) in the setting of perforation

▲ occult blood on rectal examination

▶ DIFFERENTIAL DIAGNOSIS

The differential of epigastric pain, variably associated with food ingestion, includes:

▲ pancreatitis

▲ gastroesophageal reflux disease

▲ myocardial ischemia

▲ cholecystitis

▲ nonulcer dyspepsia

▶ DIAGNOSTIC EVALUATION

The main techniques by which peptic ulcers can be diagnosed are **radiographic studies** (barium swallow) and **endoscopy**. The diagnosis of gastritis can generally only be made by endoscopy.

Barium studies have a sensitivity for peptic ulcer disease of about 80 to 90% compared with greater than 90% for an experienced endoscopist. There are no firm guidelines as to which study should be performed for initial diagnosis. Barium studies have traditionally been the initial method. In some patients with a typical history and no evidence of complication or malignancy, a therapeutic trial of medical therapy (see below) can be diagnostic. In the setting of acute severe bleeding, endoscopy is preferred, because it can be therapeutic (via cautery) and diagnostic.

The diagnosis of possible *H. pylori* infection can be accomplished by a number of means, all of which have a sensitivity of greater than 90%:

▲ culture of biopsy specimen (the gold standard)

▲ serology (high sensitivity, lower specificity)

▲ direct urease test (requires endoscopic biopsy)

▲ urease breath test

▶ TREATMENT

The medical treatment of peptic ulcers is designed to relieve symptoms and to accelerate the healing of the ulcer. Treatment of gastritis involves the same, along with removal of the inciting insult. One **nonpharmacologic therapy** used in this disease is an avoidance of NSAIDs and aspirin. Cessation of smoking is another important intervention.

Traditional pharmacologic treatment, designed to inhibit or neutralize gastric acid or protect the mucosa, has been shown to relieve symptoms and to promote ulcer healing, particularly for duodenal ulcers. The major classes of drugs used are:

▲ H_2-**receptor antagonists** (cimetidine, ranitidine, famotidine, nizatidine)—limits both basal and stimulated acid secretion;

▲ **antacids** (aluminum hydroxide, magnesium hydroxide, calcium carbonate, and others)—neutralize gastric acid and provide relatively prompt relief of symptoms once started;

▲ **proton pump inhibitors** (omeprazole)—most potent antisecretory agent which limits the terminal step in acid secretion;

▲ **sucralfate**—mucosal protectant without significant antacid effect.

A typical treatment regimen for peptic ulcer disease involves 4 to 6 weeks of an H_2-receptor antagonist or omeprazole along with antacid use as needed for symptoms. Treatment can be extended if there is incomplete response. Treatment for gastritis generally involves shorter periods of antacid treatment along with sucralfate and elimination of the underlying etiology.

The realization that *H. pylori* infection is the underlying etiology in most ulcers has changed the nature of treatment. Treatment of concomitant *H. pylori* infection is believed by many to be a necessary component of therapy for patients with ulcer disease. A number of effective antibiotic regimens have been developed. One of the first shown to be efficacious is the combination of tetracycline, metronidazole, and bismuth, given for 2 weeks. Other regimens using proton-pump inhibitors (omeprazole) and antibiotics such as clarithromycin and amoxicillin have subsequently been developed. Cost, patient compliance, and side effects are considerations when choosing between the various regimens with proven efficacy.

The high prevalence of *H. pylori* infection in the setting of ulcer disease has prompted some physicians to recommend empiric antibiotic treatment for patients with the complaint of dyspepsia. Others recommend antibiotic treatment only for patients with proven *H. pylori* infection. These various recommendations are currently being studied without clear consensus.

If patients are unable to obtain relief from medical therapy and endoscopy fails to yield another complication such as a malignancy, surgery may be an option. Surgery is also performed in an emergency setting of perforation, obstruction, and uncontrolled bleeding.

Generally, a vagotomy (partial or selective) is combined with a pyloroplasty or antrectomy for untraceable duodenal ulcer disease. Vagotomy with or without a partial gastrectomy is the common procedure for unresponsive gastric ulcer disease. With treatment for *H. pylori*, surgery is required much less often than in the past, before the role of *H. pylori* infection was known.

Patients who have partial gastrectomies are prone to a number of **postgastrectomy syndromes**, including "dumping syndrome," pernicious anemia, and diarrhea. Patients with duodenal ulcer disease traditionally have a high rate of recurrence. These patients previously required maintenance antisecretory therapy. It has since been shown that adequate treatment for *H. pylori* infection greatly decreases recurrence of duodenal ulcers.

▶ KEY POINTS

1. Peptic ulcer disease (gastric and duodenal ulcers) generally manifests as chronic epigastric pain.

2. Gastritis is superficial mucosal inflammation as opposed to the deeper damage seen in ulcer disease.

3. Infection with *Helicobacter pylori* increases the risk of developing peptic ulcer disease.

4. Therapy of peptic ulcers involves antacid therapy ± mucosal protective agents to increase the rate of healing.

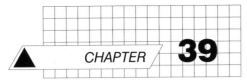

CHAPTER 39

Inflammatory Bowel Disease

*7*he inflammatory bowel diseases (IBDs), ulcerative colitis and Crohn's disease, are both idiopathic, chronic, inflammatory conditions of the bowel, but their clinical and pathologic features are quite different.

Ulcerative colitis

▲   Involves only the colon (large intestine), with 95% involving the rectum;

▲   Disease is limited to the mucosa;

▲   Uniform and continuous involvement of affected areas.

Crohn's disease

▲   May involve any part of the gastrointestinal (GI) tract from mouth to anus;

▲   About 30% affects small intestine only, 30% affects large intestine only, and 40% affects both;

▲   Only about 50% of Crohn's disease involves the rectum;

▲   Disease may involve entire bowel wall (transmural);

▲   Diseased bowel may be separated by healthy bowel ("skip lesions").

▶ EPIDEMIOLOGY

Both types of IBD occur more often in whites than blacks and in men more often than women. These diseases most often present between the ages of 15 and 35, but there is a second peak in patients 60 to 70 years old.

▶ ETIOLOGY

The underlying pathophysiology of IBD remains unknown. The increased incidence of disease in relatives of IBD patients suggests a genetic predisposition. No infectious agents have been isolated, but the effectiveness of antibiotics in treatment is suggestive of an infectious etiology. Finally, the pathology of the disease with inflammation and granuloma formation supports the concept of an immune mechanism.

▶ CLINICAL MANIFESTATIONS
History

The patient with ulcerative colitis often presents with **bloody diarrhea** and **abdominal pain**. There may also be a complaint of tenesmus, or painful urgency to move bowels. A travel history (dysentery) and recent antibiotic use (*Clostridium difficile*) should be obtained to evaluate other possible etiologies.

Crohn's disease presents with similar symptoms, but the pain may be more cramp-like, with accompanying **fever** and **weight loss**. Acute ileitis (inflammation of ileum) may mimic appendicitis with right lower quadrant pain.

Patients with **irritable bowel syndrome** may have many similar symptoms, including abdominal pain, bloating, and diarrhea. However, with irritable bowel syndrome, symptoms have often been prolonged, and there is an absence of bleeding and weight loss.

Physical Examination

Vital sign abnormalities are present in the severely ill patient with IBD, such as tachycardia, orthostatic hypotension, and fever. On abdominal examination, abdominal tenderness is often present, but rebound tenderness necessitates consideration of appendicitis, perforation, or other causes of a surgical abdomen (see Chapter 36). Patients with Crohn's disease may have fullness or palpable masses, representing adherent loops of bowel. Rectal fistulas in Crohn's disease may present as a perirectal abscess.

Skin examination may show the characteristic **pyoderma gangrenosum**, an ulcerating lesion usually located on the trunk, or **erythema nodosum**, violaceous subcutaneous nodules located most often on the lower legs. Aphthous ulcers of the oral cavity occur in 5 to 10% of patients. Finally, uveitis and arthritis may be associated with IBD (see Chapter 57).

▶ DIFFERENTIAL DIAGNOSIS

In the patient with **lower GI bleeding**, consider diverticulosis, colon cancer or polyps, arteriovenous malformations, or hemorrhoids. In the patient with **bloody diarrhea**, consider infectious etiologies such as *Yersinia*, *Campylobacter*, *Shigella*, *Salmonella*, amebiasis, or *C.*

difficile. In the **elderly patient** with a presentation suggesting IBD, consider the above diagnoses and diverticulitis or ischemic bowel.

▶ DIAGNOSTIC EVALUATION

Helpful initial studies include a complete blood count, serum albumin, and alkaline phosphatase. They may reveal signs of inflammation (leukocytosis, increased erythrocyte sedimentation rate) or malabsorption (decreased albumin). Anemia is often multifactorial and causes include iron, folate, and B_{12} deficiencies or chronic disease.

Increased alkaline phosphatase may represent underlying liver disease, which occurs at a higher frequency in patients with IBD. **Hepatobiliary diseases** include:

▲ sclerosing cholangitis (mostly ulcerative colitis)

▲ cholelithiasis (mostly Crohn's disease)

▲ fatty liver

▲ granulomatous hepatitis

▲ cholangiocarcinoma

Definite diagnosis in IBD is made by direct visualization of the colon and biopsy. **Sigmoidoscopy** or **colonoscopy** reveals erythematous, friable mucosa with longitudinal ulcerations (**cobblestone** appearance) in Crohn's disease, or regeneration of the mucosa around a diseased colon that gives the appearance of **pseudopolyps** in ulcerative colitis.

Biopsy in Crohn's disease shows involvement of entire bowel wall with **granuloma formation** or lymphoid aggregates. Ulcerative colitis is limited to the mucosa but may have **crypt abscesses**.

▶ TREATMENT

The natural history of IBD varies with the type of disease and severity of the initial presentation. In ulcerative colitis, disease limited to the rectum has a relatively benign course. In fact, 20% of patients with ulcerative colitis are relapse free a decade after the initial presentation. Crohn's disease, however, tends to be more severe, with frequent relapses. Only 10% of patients are relapse free 2 years after initial presentation.

Initial treatment for IBD consists of medical therapy to keep disease in remission. Surgery is reserved for:

▲ intractable disease

▲ obstruction

▲ perforation

▲ prophylactic resection to prevent colon cancer (in ulcerative colitis)

Removal of the entire colon will cure ulcerative colitis but will leave the patient with a colostomy. However, new surgical techniques strip the mucosa off the rectum while leaving the sphincter intact. An ileoanal anastomosis is then performed to avoid colostomy. Surgery in Crohn's disease is never curative. The disease will recur around the surgical resection.

Sulfasalazine remains as a first-line treatment for ulcerative colitis. This compound consists of a sulfapyridine moiety and 5-aminosalicylate (5-ASA), also known as mesalamine. The active drug is the 5-ASA, which is liberated in the colon by enzymatic cleavage. Sulfasalazine (4–6 g/day in divided doses) is effective in treatment of mild to moderate ulcerative colitis and in maintaining remissions in these patients. It is less effective in treatment of Crohn's disease because the drug is not active in the small intestine. **Side effects** of sulfasalazine include:

▲ nausea

▲ headache

▲ allergic reactions

▲ hepatitis

▲ bone marrow suppression

Recognition that the last three side effects are due to the inactive sulfa moiety has led to the development of **5-ASA dimers** (olsalazine) that are not degraded in the proximal bowel and **mesalamine enemas** for distal disease.

Prednisone is commonly used for controlling moderate to severe IBD, often in doses of 40–60 mg/day. However, because side effects (bone loss, hyperglycemia, cataracts) are common with chronic use and steroids are not effective at maintaining remission, they should be tapered off when possible.

Patients who become steroid dependent may benefit from **immunomodulators**. Examples (with side effects) include:

▲ azathioprine, 6-mercaptopurine (bone marrow suppression, pancreatitis)

▲ methotrexate (diarrhea, stomatitis, bone marrow suppression, hepatic fibrosis)

▲ cyclosporin A (hypertension, renal dysfunction, seizures)

A treatment unique to Crohn's disease is the use of antibiotics, such as **metronidazole**. This drug can control mild to moderate Crohn's disease and increase

TABLE 39-1

Diagnosis and Treatment of Inflammatory Bowel Disease

	Crohn's Disease	Ulcerative Colitis
Location	Entire GI tract Mostly small intestine and colon	Limited to colon
Rectal involvement	Often spared	Almost always involved
History	Abdominal pain, weight loss	Bloody diarrhea
Colonoscopy	Skip lesions Cobblestone mucosa	Continuous involvement, pseudopolyps
Treatment	Metronidazole Immunomodulators	Sulfasalazine or 5-ASA drugs Immunomodulators
Complications	Bowel obstruction Fistulas	Toxic megacolon Colon carcinoma

healing of perianal disease. Recently, ciprofloxacin has been used in these situations. There is no evidence that antibiotics are effective in ulcerative colitis.

Patients with IBD may develop several different complications, which should be suspected in patients with acute deterioration. **Enteric fistulas** or **bowel obstruction** may occur in 20 to 30% of patients with Crohn's disease. Fistulas may be interintestinal, enterovaginal, or enterovesicular. **Toxic megacolon** in ulcerative colitis may present with fever, pain, and a distended colon (>6 cm on abdominal x-ray). There may be air in the bowel wall. Treatment is conservative at first, with bowel rest, parenteral nutrition, steroids, empiric antibiotics, and surgery only if needed.

Finally, patients with diffuse ulcerative colitis are at extremely high risk for **colon carcinoma** after 10 years of active disease. Patients should be screened with colonoscopy every 1 to 2 years depending on the clinical course. Colectomy is recommended if colonoscopy reveals high-grade dysplasia or any dysplasia associated with a mass. Although patients with Crohn's disease are at increased cancer risk as well (although not as high as ulcerative colitis), optimum treatment and best approach to surveillance remain to be defined.

The key features of diagnosis and treatment of inflammatory bowel disease are summarized in Table 39-1.

▶ KEY POINTS

1. Crohn's disease involves the entire GI tract, mostly the small intestine and colon, whereas ulcerative colitis is limited to the colon.

2. The rectum is often spared in Crohn's disease but is almost always involved in ulcerative colitis.

3. Abdominal pain and weight loss mark Crohn's disease, whereas bloody diarrhea marks ulcerative colitis.

4. Colonoscopy reveals skip lesions and cobblestone mucosa in Crohn's disease and continuous involvement and pseudopolyps in ulcerative colitis.

5. Crohn's disease is treated with metronidazole and immunomodulators and ulcerative colitis with sulfasalazine or 5-ASA drugs and immunomodulators.

6. Complications of Crohn's disease include bowel obstruction and fistulas; complications of ulcerative colitis include toxic megacolon and colon carcinoma.

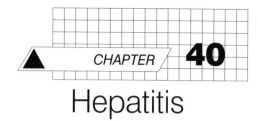

CHAPTER 40

Hepatitis

$\mathcal{H}$epatitis refers to inflammation of the liver parenchyma that can be caused by a variety of infectious and noninfectious etiologies. This inflammation can be acute or chronic. By convention, chronic hepatitis is defined as hepatitis that persists for greater than 6 months.

▶ ETIOLOGY AND PATHOPHYSIOLOGY

A number of **viruses** can cause hepatitis. Overall, viral hepatitis (both acute and chronic) is the most common type of hepatitis encountered in the United States and worldwide. The hepatitis viruses differ regarding the nature of their genome, transmission, ability to cause chronic infection, and severity of disease (Table 40-1). Hepatitis D virus (HDV) is unique in that it is a defective virus and requires coexisting hepatitis B virus (HBV) infection to establish a productive infection.

Hepatic injury due to hepatitis virus infection is believed to be a result of the **host immune response against infected hepatocytes**. The viruses (with the possible exception of hepatitis C virus [HCV]) are not believed to be directly cytotoxic themselves. In chronic viral hepatitis due to HBV, HCV, and HDV, the host immune response is insufficient to clear the infection, and there is **ongoing viral replication**. Despite the inability of the immune system to clear the infection, there is continued immune-mediated hepatic injury. A number of host and viral factors influence the development of chronic hepatitis, including age of infection (the younger the age at which infection in acquired, the higher chance of developing chronic disease); hepatitis virus type (HCV most commonly becomes chronic); and immunosuppression (increased risk of chronic disease).

In addition to the hepatitis viruses, other viral infections can cause hepatic damage, including **cytomegalovirus**, **herpes** simplex virus, and **coxsackie viruses**. Various **drugs** can cause acute and chronic hepatitis:

▲ Oxyphenisatin (a laxative, no longer used in the United States; one of the first drugs proven to cause chronic hepatitis);

▲ Halothane (causes a rare, idiosyncratic, severe acute hepatitis);

▲ Isoniazid (about 10% of adults on isoniazid will have transient liver function test (LFT) elevations, due to a toxic metabolite; in <1%, an acute hepatitis can result, which can be fatal);

▲ Methyldopa (associated with chronic hepatitis);

▲ Azole antifungals (ketoconazole and fluconazole have been associated with acute hepatitis).

Alcohol can cause a severe, even fatal, acute hepatitis. Chronic alcohol use can lead to a condition known as **alcoholic fatty liver** and eventually **cirrhosis** (see Chapter 41).

There is a rare idiopathic form of chronic hepatitis known as **autoimmune chronic active hepatitis** (ACAH). As suggested by the name, this disease is characterized by chronic hepatic inflammation and the production of a number of autoantibodies. Three-fourths of patients with this disease are women of childbearing age. Patients with ACAH have a higher than normal incidence of other autoimmune disorders.

A chronic form of hepatitis is associated with the **hereditary disorders** Wilson's disease, hemochromatosis, and alpha-1-antitrypsin deficiency. When unrecognized, these diseases can progress to cirrhosis (see Chapter 41).

▶ CLINICAL MANIFESTATIONS
History

Patients who present with **acute hepatitis** generally report the following:

▲ jaundice

▲ dark-colored urine (from bilirubin in urine)

▲ abdominal pain or discomfort (often in the right upper quadrant)

▲ fever

▲ nausea/vomiting

Other associated symptoms can include fatigue, malaise, headache, myalgias, and arthralgias. Patients who present with severe **fulminant acute hepatitis**

TABLE 40-1

Features of Viral Hepatitis

	Viral Genome	Epidemiology	Acute Mortality (%)	Chronic Disease (%)	Laboratory Markers
HAV	ssRNA	Fecal-oral	0.2	None	HAV antigen, anti-HAV, HAV RNA
HBV	dsDNA	Parenteral, sexual, perinatal	0.2–1.0	2–7	HBsAg, HBcAg, HBeAg, anti-HBsAg, anti-HBcAg, anti-HBeAg, HBV DNA
HCV	ssRNA	Parenteral, ?sexual	0.2	50–70	HCV antigen, anti-HCV
HDV	ssRNA	Parenteral, ?sexual	2–20	?50	HDV antigen, anti-HDV
HEV	ssRNA	Fecal-oral	0.2	None	HEV Ag, anti-HEV

can present with signs of **liver failure**, such as encephalopathy, coagulopathy, ascites, and renal failure. Patients with mild cases of acute hepatitis can be **minimally symptomatic** or entirely **asymptomatic**.

The clinical presentation of **chronic hepatitis** is commonly insidious. A few patients with chronic viral hepatitis may recall an acute episode of jaundice (especially with hepatitis B). In many other cases, nonspecific symptoms such as **fatigue, malaise, anorexia,** and **arthralgias** are the only presenting complaints. Many times the diagnosis is only entertained when screening liver function tests (see below) reveal chronic elevated transaminases. Other patients with chronic hepatitis are only diagnosed when they present with cirrhosis and end-stage liver disease.

Physical Examination

Findings in **acute hepatitis** generally include:

▲ jaundice

▲ hepatomegaly (often tender)

▲ splenomegaly

▲ adenopathy

More severe cases can present with complications from **hepatic failure** such as ascites, edema, encephalopathy (e.g., asterixis), or gastrointestinal bleeding.

In **chronic hepatitis,** the physical examination is often unrevealing unless significant hepatic impairment is present, at which time findings of chronic liver failure are present (see Chapter 41).

▶ DIFFERENTIAL DIAGNOSIS

For **acute hepatitis,** the major differential diagnosis is between the etiologies listed above and other conditions that can cause direct (toxic) hepatic injury and/or result in cholestasis:

▲ biliary tract disease (acute cholecystitis, cholangitis, obstructing common duct stone)

▲ drug-induced cholestasis (see Chapter 42)

▲ direct hepatotoxins (acetaminophen overdose, mushroom [*Amanita*] poisoning, carbon tetrachloride)

▲ right-sided heart failure (due to hepatic congestion)

The differential diagnosis for **chronic hepatitis** includes:

▲ chronic biliary tract disease (primary biliary cirrhosis, primary sclerosing cholangitis)

▲ nonalcoholic steatohepatitis (a condition characterized by fatty deposits and inflammation throughout the hepatic lobule seen in obese females with hyperlipidemia)

▶ DIAGNOSTIC EVALUATION

Hepatitis leads to **hepatocyte necrosis** and release of hepatic enzymes. Clinically, increases in the serum levels of the **aminotransferases** aspartate aminotransferase (AST) and alanine aminotransferase (ALT) have proven to be useful in detecting hepatocellular necrosis. Excretion, and to a lesser extent, conjugation of bilirubin is also impaired by hepatocyte injury, leading to elevation of the **serum bilirubin** level.

The **pattern of aminotransferase elevation** may give clues to the underlying etiology. In general, acute viral hepatitis causes a greater absolute elevation than alcoholic hepatitis. Furthermore, in **alcoholic hepatitis,** the serum AST is usually elevated out of proportion to the ALT, leading to an AST/ALT ratio > 2. A single measurement of aminotransferase level, however, is a poor indicator of the absolute degree of hepatic damage.

The diagnosis of **viral hepatitis** is aided by the availability of specific **serologic tests** that detect specific viral proteins and/or host antibodies directed against these viral proteins (Table 40-1). There are multiple serologic tests available, but for the most commonly encountered situations, the following recommendations for their use can be made:

For the diagnosis of presumed **acute viral hepatitis**:

▲ IgM anti-hepatitis A virus (HAV)

▲ IgM anti-HBcAg

▲ HBsAg

▲ anti-HCV (variably present in acute disease, may need serial serology)

If HBsAg is present, test for coexisting HDV by anti-HDV is appropriate, particularly if there are risk factors (intravenous drug use or exposure to blood or blood products).

For the diagnosis of presumed **chronic viral hepatitis**:

▲ HBsAg

▲ anti-HCV

Again, testing for HDV is appropriate if HBsAg is present.

The presence of anti-HBsAg (IgG) indicates **distant resolved infection** with HBV. Patients with chronic HBV infection do not develop anti-HBsAg, which is protective and also develops in response to successful immunization against HBV (see below). In contrast, the development of anti-HCV simply indicates infection with HCV; the development of anti-HCV is seen in patients with chronic HCV infection, and these antibodies are not protective.

In chronic viral hepatitis, the degree of viral replication can be determined by the measurement of HBV DNA or HCV RNA (using a polymerase chain reaction-based assay).

In patients in whom a diagnosis of **autoimmune chronic active hepatitis** is suspected (e.g., a woman with chronically elevated aminotransferases and without serologic evidence of chronic viral hepatitis), measurement of **autoantibody** titers can be useful:

▲ antinuclear antibody, primarily in a homogeneous pattern

▲ anti-smooth muscle antibody

▲ anti-liver-kidney microsomal antibodies

▲ anti-cytokeratin antibodies

When present in high titers, these autoantibodies can be useful in making the diagnosis of ACAH, but they are not invariably present. Another common laboratory abnormality seen in ACAH is **hyperglobulinemia**.

Percutaneous liver biopsy can be performed in cases where the diagnosis remains uncertain. Done in consultation with a gastroenterologist, the procedure is relatively safe and yields important diagnostic information, because specific causes of hepatitis have characteristic histologic appearance.

An assessment of the **degree of hepatocellular impairment** can be determined by measurement of:

▲ prothrombin time

▲ serum albumin

▲ serum ammonia level

▶ TREATMENT

For **acute viral hepatitis**, there is **no specific therapy**. In many cases, close outpatient follow-up with laboratory monitoring to document resolution of hepatic injury is sufficient. Hospitalization for closer monitoring may be required in more severe cases. For drug- or alcohol-related hepatitis, therapy involves removal of the offending agent followed by supportive care.

The treatment of **chronic viral hepatitis** (generally HBV and HCV) has been revolutionized by the recognition that an insufficient immune response appears to be a factor in continued productive viral infection. The administration of interferon-alpha to bolster the immune response and allow clearance of the virus has proven to be successful in about 50% of patients with chronic stable HBV or HCV. Unfortunately, about 50% of patients with HCV who respond to interferon therapy relapse after discontinuation of the interferon, compared with about 1 to 2% of patients with HBV who respond to therapy.

Interferon therapy should not be administered to patients with chronic HBV or HCV who have evidence of decompensated liver disease because interferon therapy actually results in increased hepatic inflammation, which can be extremely harmful in this case.

In cases of severe alcoholic hepatitis (as judged by marked hyperbilirubinemia and prothrombin time prolongation), there is the suggestion that administration of glucocorticoids may increase survival, but this finding is still somewhat controversial.

For patients with autoimmune chronic active hepatitis, administration of glucocorticoids is the treatment of choice. Up to 80% of patients will respond with symptomatic, biochemical, and histologic improvement and with an increase in survival. It is not clear if the development of cirrhosis is prevented by steroid therapy.

Patients who are diagnosed with acute HBV or HCV infection should be followed for the development of chronic hepatitis. For HBV, resolution of infection is marked by the appearance of anti-HBsAg and normalization of transaminase levels. For HCV, recovery is marked by normalization of transaminases alone, because there is no serologic marker of recovery.

For patients with fulminant acute hepatitis or chronic hepatitis that progresses to end-stage liver failure, orthotopic liver transplantation is a limited, but potentially lifesaving, option.

Prophylaxis against some forms of viral hepatitis is available: HAV immune globulin (all preparations of immune globulin have some anti-HAV activity), HAV vaccine, HBV recombinant HBV vaccine, and hepatitis B immune globulin (recommended for postexposure prophylaxis, e.g., needle-stick, in a nonimmunized individual).

▶ KEY POINTS

1. Hepatitis, acute or chronic inflammation of the liver, can be caused by infectious and noninfectious causes.

2. Hepatitis viruses are responsible for most cases of acute and chronic hepatitis seen worldwide.

3. Noninfectious causes of hepatitis include drugs, hereditary disorders such as Wilson's disease, and an idiopathic disorder called autoimmune chronic active hepatitis.

4. Chronic hepatitis (both infectious and noninfectious) can lead to cirrhosis and end-stage liver failure.

5. Treatment of acute hepatitis is mainly supportive. Some cases of chronic viral hepatitis will respond to interferon therapy. Corticosteroids are the treatment of choice for autoimmune chronic active hepatitis.

6. Immunoprophylaxis is available for hepatitis A and hepatitis B virus infection.

Infectious
    Hepatitis A, B, C, D

Non-Infectious

① Heriditary
    . Wilson's
    . Hemachromatosis
    . α_1-antitrypsin

② Alcohol

③ Auto-immune chronic active Hepatitis.

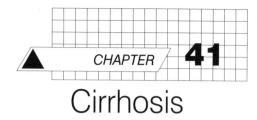

CHAPTER 41

Cirrhosis

*C*irrhosis is defined as irreversible hepatic injury, characterized by fibrosis and regenerative nodules in the liver. The normal **function of the liver** includes:

▲ production of protein

▲ filtering of mesenteric blood flow

▲ metabolism of endogenous (e.g., bilirubin) and exogenous (e.g., drugs) substances

Loss of these functions in cirrhosis leads to the common complications of ascites, portal hypertension, jaundice, and encephalopathy.

▶ ETIOLOGY

The underlying **causes of cirrhosis** include:

▲ alcohol

▲ chronic hepatitis B or C

▲ biliary disease (sclerosing cholangitis, primary biliary cirrhosis)

▲ cardiac disease

▲ autoimmune hepatitis

▲ inherited diseases (hemochromatosis, Wilson's disease, α-1 antitrypsin [α-1AT] deficiency)

In the United States, alcoholism is the most common cause of cirrhosis; viral hepatitis (mostly hepatitis B) is the number one cause worldwide. Biliary disease is discussed in Chapter 42.

Inherited Disorders

Hemochromatosis is an autosomal recessive disorder of increased iron absorption and results in excess deposition of iron in certain organs. It is characterized by liver, heart, and gonadal failure. Pancreatic failure, leading to glucose intolerance, combined with increased skin pigmentation has resulted in hemochromatosis being described as "bronze diabetes." Secondary hemochromatosis (in contrast to hereditary) may occur in patients who are transfusion dependent, such as in thalassemia major.

Wilson's disease is an autosomal recessive disorder of copper excretion, resulting in increased accumulation of copper in the liver and brain. Patients may present with fulminant or chronic hepatitis, cirrhosis, psychiatric involvement, or neurologic disease (tremor, rigidity).

α-1AT deficiency is an autosomal recessive disorder characterized by abnormal alleles of serum α-1AT. This disease often presents as early emphysema and asymptomatic cirrhosis.

▶ PATHOPHYSIOLOGY

Mortality and morbidity in cirrhosis is usually due to its complications. **Ascites** is the accumulation of fluid within the peritoneal cavity. It is the result of multiple factors, including increased capillary hydrostatic pressure (portal hypertension), decreased plasma oncotic pressure (hypoalbuminemia), and increased sodium reabsorption by the kidney.

Esophageal varices develop from portal vein hypertension that is transmitted to systemic collateral veins in the gastroesophageal junction. Rupture of these veins and the resultant bleeding are dependent on the size of the varices and the extent of portal hypertension. Bleeding from esophageal varices usually presents as painless massive hematemesis and/or melena. Because other etiologies of upper gastrointestinal (GI) bleeding are also common in cirrhotics (gastritis, peptic ulcer disease), variceal bleeding should be confirmed with endoscopy (even in the patient with known varices).

Hepatic encephalopathy is characterized by confusion, personality changes, and asterixis and may progress to obtundation and coma. The etiology is unknown; increased ammonia levels have been implicated in the pathogenesis but remain unproved. Recent evidence suggests that increased levels of γ-aminobutyric acid may have an etiologic role.

▶ CLINICAL MANIFESTATIONS

History

The patient with end-stage liver disease often has no specific complaint except fatigue and malaise. However, failure of liver function may result in leg edema, easy bruisability, and increased abdominal girth (from ascites).

Evaluation for possible causes of cirrhosis should include a detailed alcohol history (which the patient may deny), past episodes of hepatitis, or risk factors for hepatitis (intravenous drug use, high-risk sexual behavior, blood transfusions). Family history may suggest an inherited liver disease; however, because most are autosomal recessive, the patient's parents are usually unaffected.

Physical Examination

The abdominal examination in cirrhosis usually reveals a firm or nonpalpable liver. Flanks may be bulging due to ascites and shifting dullness may be present. Portal hypertension will lead to splenomegaly, internal hemorrhoids, and caput medusae (prominent periumbilical veins).

Skin findings in cirrhosis include jaundice and spider telangiectases. Examination of the hand may reveal:

▲ clubbing

▲ palmar erythema

▲ Dupuytren's contracture (permanent flexion of third or fourth metacarpal phalangeal joint)

A sign of hepatic encephalopathy is asterixis, an unintentional contraction of the wrist when the wrists are held in complete extension (as if stopping traffic).

▶ DIFFERENTIAL DIAGNOSIS

In the patient presenting with ascites, consider:

▲ abdominal malignancy (pancreatic, ovarian)

▲ nephrotic syndrome

▲ cardiac failure (especially constrictive pericarditis)

▲ peritoneal tuberculosis

▲ peritoneal mesothelioma

See Chapter 42 for the differential of the patient presenting with jaundice.

▶ DIAGNOSTIC EVALUATION

The following laboratory findings are seen in cirrhosis:

▲ hyponatremia, due to decreased delivery of sodium to distal nephron and resulting in increased in antidiuretic hormone secretion

▲ decreased blood urea nitrogen, due to malnutrition and decreased protein production

▲ decreased albumin

▲ increased bilirubin (mostly direct)

Hematologic abnormalities include:

▲ increased prothrombin time due to decreased production of vitamin K-dependent clotting factors

▲ macrocytic anemia (mean cell volume > 100) due to increased red blood cell membrane in liver disease, which may also be due to concomitant alcohol use or folate deficiency

▲ thrombocytopenia secondary to splenomegaly

Inherited diseases may be diagnosed by the following tests:

▲ hemochromatosis: increased ferritin and increased iron-total iron binding capacity ratio (>55%)

▲ Wilson's disease: decreased ceruloplasmin (<20 mg/dL)

▲ α-1AT deficiency: absence of alpha-globulin spike on immunoelectrophoresis and decreased serum α-1AT

These hereditary diseases are then confirmed by liver biopsy.

Patients with new onset ascites should undergo paracentesis to determine the etiology of ascites and rule out infection. Two useful tests on ascitic fluid are a cell count and an albumin level. The difference between the serum albumin and ascites albumin level, the so-called *serum-ascites albumin gradient* (SAAG), is the most specific test to differentiate between causes of ascites.

SAAG < 1.1	SAAG > 1.1
Malignancy	Cirrhosis
Tuberculosis	Hepatic metastases
Pancreatitis	Budd-Chiari syndrome
Nephrotic syndrome	Cardiac disease
	Myxedema

An absolute polymorphonuclear count of greater than 250 cells/mL is consistent with spontaneous bacterial peritonitis and should be treated (see below). Ascitic fluid should be inoculated into blood culture bottles at the bedside to improve sensitivity.

▶ TREATMENT

The most important intervention in the patient with cirrhosis is complete abstinence from alcohol. Patients who continue to drink after diagnosis have an extremely poor prognosis. The patient should be monitored for the complications of cirrhosis, which include:

▲ bleeding esophageal varices

▲ ascites

▲ hepatic encephalopathy

Prognosis in cirrhosis is influenced by the development of these complications and has been summarized by the Child's criteria (Table 41-1).

Liver transplantation is usually indicated when the patient has refractory ascites, recurrent encephalopathy, recurrent variceal bleeding, or progressive malnutrition. Absolute contraindications to transplantation include:

▲ infection outside of hepatobiliary system (including AIDS)

▲ metastatic liver disease

▲ uncorrectable coagulopathy

The 5-year survival rate for liver transplantation is about 70%.

Therapeutics
Treatment of Ascites

1. Sodium restriction(< 2g NaCl).

2. Diuretic therapy: **potassium-sparing diuretics** (spironolactone, amiloride, triamterene) are the drugs of choice to counteract high aldosterone state in cirrhosis. Urinary sodium should exceed urinary potassium during therapy. Some patients may require the addition of furosemide.

3. Large volume **paracentesis**: removal of 6 to 8 liters of peritoneal fluid is an effective and prompt method to decrease ascites. Concerns about precipitating hypotension and renal failure have led to the practice of transfusing albumin during the procedure, although randomized trials have not demonstrated much benefit.

4. Peritoneovenous (Leveen) shunt: this plastic shunt connects the peritoneum to the vena cava. Although effective in decreasing ascites, complications include thrombosis or infection of shunt and disseminated intravascular coagulation.

Patients with ascites may develop **spontaneous bacterial peritonitis** due to low amount of albumin and bacteriostatic proteins in the ascitic fluid. Symptoms may include fever, abdominal pain, and worsening mental status, but often symptoms are minimal (such as malaise, anorexia). If paracentesis confirms the diagnosis, treatment directed at gram-negative enteric organisms (*Escherichia coli, Klebsiella*) and *Streptococcus pneumoniae* should be started. The empiric drug of choice is cefotaxime. Patients who fail to improve or appear seriously ill warrant treatment for Enterococcus and anaerobic organisms (<10% of all cases) with a drug such as ampicillin/sulbactam. Aminoglycosides should be avoided in patients with cirrhosis because of the increased risk of nephrotoxicity.

Treatment of Esophageal Varices

1. Replacement of blood products and coagulation factors if needed.

2. Intravenous **vasopressin**: constricts portal blood flow and controls bleeding in about 80% of cases. Side effects include hypertension and hyponatremia. Hypertension may be countered by intravenous nitroglycerin.

3. Intravenous **somatostatin**: as effective as vasopressin with a similar mechanism of action.

4. Endoscopic **sclerotherapy** (injection) or **band ligation** of varices: immediate treatment reduces rebleeding rates, and follow-up treatments are required to obliterate varices. Both are very effective, although band ligation has gained recent preference because of a lower rebleeding and complication rates.

As a treatment of last resort, balloon tamponade may be used as a temporizing measure with a Sengstaken-Blakemore tube.

Treatment of Hepatic Encephalopathy

1. Correction of precipitating factors, including infection, gastrointestinal bleeding, excess dietary protein, hypokalemia, hypovolemia, alkalosis, drugs (especially narcotics and benzodiazepines).

2. Lactulose (30 mL two to four times daily): a nonabsorbable disaccharide that decreases ammonia absorption; dose is adjusted until diarrhea occurs.

3. Neomycin (500 mg every 6 hours): a broad-spectrum antibiotic that decreases ammonia production from bacteria in GI tract. Although systemic absorption is minimal, its use may still be limited by nephrotoxicity.

TABLE 41-1

Child's Criteria

	A	B	C
Bilirubin (mg/dL)	<2.3	2.3–2.9	>2.9
Albumin (g/dL)	>3.5	3.0–3.5	<3.0
Ascites	None	Easily controlled	Poorly controlled
Encephalopathy	None	Mildly	Advanced
Nutrition	Excellent	Good	Fair

Continued Care

Portosystemic Shunts

Shunt procedures are reserved for patients refractory to standard treatments or recurrent variceal bleeding. The **transjugular intrahepatic portosystemic shunt (TIPS)** is a relatively noninvasive method to treat the complications of portal hypertension. A radiologist places a stent from the inferior vena cava through the liver parenchyma into the portal system, decompressing the portal system. Complications include hepatic encephalopathy (20 to 30% of patients) and shunt thrombosis or stenosis. A more permanent solution is **distal splenorenal shunt**, which connects the splenic vein to the distal left renal vein. However, in addition to perioperative mortality and morbidity, this surgery may increase the risk of hepatic encephalopathy (although lower than earlier portocaval shunts).

Hepatocellular Cancer

Cirrhosis is the most important predisposing risk factor for hepatocellular cancer (HCC), and HCC should be suspected in the stable cirrhotic with new clinical deterioration. Alpha-fetoprotein may be elevated in HCC, but its use as a screening test is limited because of its relatively low sensitivity and specificity. Treatment is surgical resection for localized disease in patients who are eligible for surgery. Hepatic artery embolization or chemoembolization are options for other patients.

▶ KEY POINTS

1. Alcohol consumption is the primary cause of cirrhosis in the United States.

2. The patient with ascites due to cirrhosis should have a serum-ascites albumin gradient > 1.1 g/dL. Causes of a low gradient (< 1.1 g/dL) include malignancy, pancreatitis, and tuberculosis.

3. The patient with spontaneous bacterial peritonitis should be empirically treated with an antibiotic, such as cefotaxime, that covers enteric gram-negative rods and streptococcus.

4. In the patient with new onset hepatic encephalopathy, an underlying precipitant should be suspected, including infection, GI bleeding, hypokalemia, and drugs.

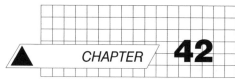

CHAPTER 42

Cholestatic Liver Disease

*B*ile is formed in the hepatic lobules, secreted into bile canaliculi, and then flows into bile ducts. These ducts drain into the common hepatic duct, which is joined by the cystic duct of the gallbladder to form the common bile duct. Obstruction of normal bile flow from the liver at any of these sites results in cholestasis.

Diseases that cause cholestasis are classified as intrahepatic or extrahepatic obstructions. This distinction must be made early in the evaluation because treatment strategies differ greatly. Cholecystitis (inflammation of the gallbladder) and cholelithiasis (gallstones) do not cause obstruction of biliary flow and are not discussed in this chapter.

▶ EPIDEMIOLOGY

Some etiologies of cholestasis involve particular populations. Primary biliary cirrhosis (PBC) affects predominantly middle-aged women, whereas primary sclerosing cholangitis (PSC) affects mostly men.

▶ ETIOLOGY AND RISK FACTORS

Both PBC and PSC seem to have an autoimmune etiology. PSC is associated with inflammatory bowel disease (especially ulcerative colitis) in up to 90% of cases (see Chapter 52).

Many drugs are known to cause cholestatic liver disease, and space does not allow for a complete listing. Some of the more well-known agents include:

▲ erythromycin

▲ oral contraceptives and estrogen

▲ anabolic steroids

▲ sulfonamides

▲ chlorpromazine

▶ CLINICAL EVALUATION
History

Symptoms of cholestatic liver disease include:

▲ pruritus

▲ fatigue

▲ steatorrhea

▲ jaundice

Malabsorption of fat-soluble vitamins (A, D, E, K) may lead to symptoms as well (see Chapter 51). Patients with pancreatic carcinoma may present with the classic triad of jaundice, weight loss, and back or abdominal pain. Patients with extrahepatic bile duct obstruction may also present with signs of ascending cholangitis:

▲ fever and chills

▲ right upper quadrant pain

▲ jaundice

▲ nausea and vomiting

Physical Examination

In early cholestatic disease, the physical examination may be completely normal. Later, jaundice and scleral icterus appear. Splenomegaly, ascites, telangiectasia, and lower extremity edema are signs of cirrhosis that may be seen in advanced cases of PBC or PSC.

▶ DIFFERENTIAL DIAGNOSIS

Cholestasis must be differentiated from other causes of jaundice, such as:

▲ hepatocellular injury

▲ hemolysis

The differential of cholestasis may be divided into extrahepatic bile duct obstruction:

▲ pancreatic carcinoma

▲ cholangiocarcinoma

▲ bile duct strictures

▲ choledocholithiasis

and intrahepatic duct obstruction:

▲ primary biliary cirrhosis

▲ sclerosing cholangitis

▲ drug reactions

▶ DIAGNOSTIC EVALUATION

Elevation of alkaline phosphatase is almost always seen in cholestatic liver disease. Because bone disease also increases alkaline phosphatase, the hepatic source of the elevation is confirmed by an elevated **5′-nucleotidase** or **gamma glutamyl transpeptidase (GGT)**. **Bilirubin**, predominantly direct (conjugated), may also be increased and indicates more advanced obstruction. Serum transaminases (aspartate aminotransferase and alanine aminotransferase) are usually mildly elevated. This pattern of liver function tests is in contrast to hemolysis (indirect hyperbilirubinemia) and hepatocellular dysfunction (transaminases elevated more than alkaline phosphatase).

After determining that the patient has evidence of cholestasis, the next step is to classify the problem as intrahepatic or extrahepatic. **Ultrasound** is the initial test. Bile duct dilation indicates obstruction at or below the common bile duct (extrahepatic obstruction). Gallstones may be visualized in the common bile duct. However, obstruction may not produce duct dilation during the first 24 hours.

In the patient with extrahepatic obstruction, a cholangiogram must then be performed to localize the obstruction. **Endoscopic retrograde cholangio-pancreatography** (ERCP) is one technique used to visualize the bile ducts. If a common bile duct stone proves to be the cause of obstruction, removal may be achieved through a papillotomy (opening of the pancreatic ampulla). Biopsy or brushings may be performed during ERCP to diagnose pancreatic or biliary malignancy. Percutaneous hepatic cholangiogram is another diagnostic alternative but has a higher incidence of complications.

Abdominal computed tomography may be useful to:

▲ visualize bile ducts if ultrasound is inadequate

▲ look for pancreatic masses as a cause of obstruction

▲ identify common bile duct stones

▲ stage pancreatic carcinoma or cholangiocarcinoma (hepatic metastasis)

In the patient without bile duct dilation, diagnosis depends on blood tests and possibly liver biopsy. **Antimitochondrial antibody** (AMA) is positive in 95% of patients with PBC. AMA is not present in PSC, although 60% of PSC cases have the peripheral pattern of **antineutrophil cytoplasmic antibody** (p-ANCA). PSC may also be diagnosed by the narrow beaded appearance of both intra- and extrahepatic ducts on ERCP. If the diagnosis remains in doubt, **liver biopsy** is used to confirm the diagnosis and assess prognosis.

▶ TREATMENT

Treatment is determined by the nature of the obstruction. Extrahepatic obstruction will require an intervention to relieve the obstruction, whereas intrahepatic obstructions are treated medically.

Intrahepatic Obstruction

For drug hepatitis, removal of all possible offending agents is indicated. Liver enzymes usually return to normal, although continued worsening may occur. In PBC, medical treatment may slow the progression of disease. **Ursodiol** (ursodeoxycholic acid), 13–15 mg/kg/day, has been shown to decrease liver function test abnormalities and decrease pruritus in PBC. It presumably decreases the accumulation of toxic bile salts. Long-term results also suggest that treatment with ursodiol delays need for liver transplantation. Medical treatment is less successful for PSC. Balloon dilation of a predominant stricture is sometimes used for PSC, but this does not change the natural history of the disease.

Extrahepatic Obstruction

Discovery of a common duct stone necessitates early removal to prevent continued obstruction and possible cholangitis. ERCP has become the preferred method of stone extraction, although surgery is occasionally necessary. In patients with pancreatic carcinoma or cholangiocarcinoma, surgical resection may be considered, but the malignancy has almost always spread by time of diagnosis. In cases of advanced malignancy, endoscopically placed stents will relieve symptomatic obstruction but do little to change the course of disease.

Cholestyramine, a bile acid resin, is often used to control symptoms of pruritus in patients with long-standing cholestasis. Patients should also be followed for development of **deficiencies of fat-soluble vitamins:**

▲ vitamin D (osteoporosis, hypocalcemia)

▲ vitamin A (night blindness)

▲ vitamin K (increased prothrombin time)

▲ vitamin E (ataxia, neuropathy)

Given the young age at which PBC and PSC often occur, patients with end-stage liver disease should be considered for **liver transplantation**. Transplantation is usually indicated when the patient has refractory ascites, recurrent encephalopathy, recurrent variceal bleeding, or progressive malnutrition.

Absolute **contraindications to transplantation** include:

▲ **infection** outside of hepatobiliary system (including **AIDS**)

▲ **metastatic liver disease**

▲ **uncorrectable coagulo**pathy

The 5-year survival rate for liver transplantation is about 70%.

▶ KEY POINTS

1. Laboratory findings in cholestatic liver disease include **increased alkaline phosphatase** with **normal** to slightly elevated **transaminases** (alanine and aspartate).

2. A **hepatic source** of an **elevated alkaline phosphatase** is confirmed by an elevated 5′-nucleosidase or **GGT**.

3. The **initial test** in evaluating cholestatic liver disease is the **right upper quadrant ultrasound** to determine whether the **obstruction is intra-** or **extrahepatic**.

4. **Primary biliary cirrhosis** occurs mostly in **middle-aged women** and often presents with **pruritus** or asymptomatic **elevations in alkaline phosphatase**; **antimitochondrial antibody** is present in most cases.

5. **Primary sclerosing cholangitis** is usually seen in association with **inflammatory bowel disease**; patients may present with **ascending cholangitis** (fever, right upper quadrant pain, jaundice).

▲ Chronic pancreatitis—seen most often as a consequence of alcohol-induced or idiopathic pancreatitis. Symptoms included recurrent pain and malabsorption. Diagnosis confirmed by ERCP, showing beaded dilated pancreatic duct ("chain of lakes"). Treatment mainly symptomatic with pancreatic enzyme replacement if needed. In severe cases, diabetes may develop as well. Ductal stenting has relieved pain in some patients.

▶ KEY POINTS

1. Alcohol and biliary tract disease are the underlying etiologies in most cases of pancreatitis; metabolic causes and drugs should be ruled out.

2. Diagnosis is based on the typical picture of abdominal pain associated with an increased amylase and lipase. Imaging studies, such as x-ray and ultrasound, may be used to rule out other abdominal pathology.

3. Treatment is mainly supportive with intravenous fluids and analgesia.

4. Complications, such as pseudocyst or abscess, are detected by CT.

5. Pancreatic abscess requires surgical treatment.

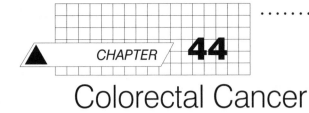

CHAPTER 44

Colorectal Cancer

*C*olorectal cancer ranks fourth in cancer incidence and second in cancer-associated mortality in the United States, making primary prevention, screening, diagnosis, and therapy of concern to most physicians who care for adults.

▶ EPIDEMIOLOGY

In the United States, there are an estimated 140,000 new cases of colorectal cancer diagnosed each year with about 55,000 deaths related to the disease. The overall lifetime risk is about 6% for the general population. Men have a slightly higher age-adjusted death rate than women. The incidence of colorectal cancer increases with age, beginning to rise after age 40 and then significantly after age 55.

Worldwide, colorectal cancer rates vary depending on geographic location. The United States (with a rate of 14/100,000 population) is near the upper end of a broad range. Rates in Australia and several European countries are higher (up to 30/100,000 in the Czech republic), whereas rates in most Asian and South American countries are much lower (3/100,000 in Ecuador). Environmental factors are suggested to play a role because persons from an area of low incidence assume a significantly higher risk when they migrate to areas of high incidence.

▶ ETIOLOGY

The current hypothesis is that most colorectal cancers arise from preexisting benign adenomatous polyps that undergo sequential malignant transformation. Adenomas are neoplastic lesions that display abnormal cellular differentiation and are of varying architecture, size, and shape. Histologically, **adenomas** can be classified as:

▲ tubular (80 to 85% of all adenomas)

▲ tubulovillous (8 to 16%)

▲ villous (3 to 15%)

Although adenomatous polyps are considered to be premalignant lesions, only about 5% are estimated to develop into cancer.

Factors associated with malignant transformation are:

▲ increasing size (< 1% of polyps smaller than 1 cm diameter develop into frank malignancies, whereas about 10% of those larger than 2 cm will)

▲ villous histology

At the molecular level, neoplastic and malignant transformation are believed to be due to **accumulation of damage to the DNA** of the mucosal cells of the colon. Two key events are believed to be the activation of the *ras* oncogene and the inactivation of one or more of the so-called tumor-suppressor genes (e.g., *dcc* and p53). The DNA damage can be due to **exogenous agents** (e.g., oxidizing and alkylating products of cellular metabolism) or **endogenous agents** (e.g., carcinogens, viruses, and radiation).

Cancers can initially be confined to the mucosa (carcinoma in situ) and then progress to the submucosa, muscularis propria, and adjacent tissues. Once the cancer invades past the mucosa, it can metastasize to regional lymph nodes and distant sites. Invasive cancer involving the rectum differs from other colon cancers in that local recurrences after resection are more common.

▶ RISK FACTORS

A number of **risk factors** have been associated with the development of colorectal cancer:

▲ history of adenomatous polyps

▲ inflammatory bowel disease (ulcerative colitis > Crohn's disease)

▲ familial disorders (familial polyposis, hereditary nonpolyposis syndrome)

▲ personal history of another malignancy (ovarian, endometrial, breast)

▲ family history of colon cancer in first-degree relatives

A number of studies have looked at dietary and lifestyle risk factors, with conflicting and inconclusive results. The strongest positive associations are as follows:

▲ high animal fat consumption (red meat)

▲ low fiber consumption (lack of fruits and vegetables)

▲ obesity

▲ ethanol

▲ refined sugar

▲ cigarette smoking

Additionally, there is the suggestion that regular use of aspirin may **lower** the incidence of colorectal cancer.

▶ CLINICAL MANIFESTATIONS
History

Most neoplastic colorectal lesions present without symptoms. Symptoms generally occur in more advanced disease. For this reason, screening (see below) is advocated for the detection of neoplasms in asymptomatic patients. When present, the most common **symptoms** of colorectal cancer are:

▲ gastrointestinal bleeding (may be occult and variably associated with iron-deficiency anemia)

▲ change in bowel habits (narrowed caliber of stool, chronic diarrhea, constipation)

▲ abdominal pain

▲ anorexia/weight loss (generally late, with advanced, metastatic cancers)

Physical Examination

In a manner similar to history, patients with colorectal cancer generally have few specific physical examination findings. A mass may be found on external palpation of the abdomen or on digital rectal examination, but this is uncommon.

▶ DIAGNOSTIC EVALUATION

The main studies used for screening and diagnosis of colorectal cancer are:

▲ the fecal occult blood test (FOBT)

▲ barium enema (BE)

▲ sigmoidoscopy

▲ colonoscopy

Screening is generally done with FOBT and sigmoidoscopy, whereas BE and colonoscopy are generally reserved for diagnosis in patients with a positive screening test (Table 44-1).

▶ TREATMENT

The overall management of colorectal cancer involves both primary prevention, by reducing the potential risk factors listed above, and secondary prevention, by screening to detect and treat asymptomatic cancers and premalignant precursors. Several organizations have published guidelines for the surveillance of colorectal cancer using the above methods (Table 44-2).

TABLE 44-1

Tests for Colorectal Neoplasms

Test	Characteristics	Advantages	Disadvantages
Fecal occult blood testing	Screening test with sensitivity and specificity about 50%; certain foods (rare red meat, radishes, broccoli) can give false-positive results; false negatives due to intermittent nature of blood loss	Inexpensive; easy to do	Poor sensitivity and specificity; does not localize source of blood loss (upper GI vs lower GI)
Sigmoidoscopy	Screening examination; 60-cm flexible scope (formerly a 20–25 cm rigid scope was used)	Allows direct visualization and biopsy/removal of lesions; safer than colonoscopy; can be performed in office without need for sedation/anesthesia	Inability to demonstrate lesions in the proximal colon; therefore, lower sensitivity compared with barium enema and colonoscopy
Barium enema	Sensitivity of 80–90% for lesions larger than 1 cm; sensitivity of 50–75% for lesions smaller than 1 cm	Allows visualization of proximal and distal colon; minimal discomfort to patient	Lower sensitivity for potentially clinically important but smaller lesions; no ability to biopsy/remove lesions
Colonoscopy	Gold standard for diagnosis; sensitivity of about 95%, near 100% sensitivity	Allows visualization of proximal and distal colon; allows direct visualization and biopsy/removal of lesions	High cost; increased risk to patient (sedation, possibility of perforation); uncomfortable for patient and requires extensive bowel preparation

TABLE 44-2

Guidelines for Colorectal Cancer Screening

Risk Factor	Recommendation
None	Starting at age 50, annual FOBT, DRE; flexible sigmoidoscopy every 3–5 yr
Ulcerative colitis	Colonoscopy after 8–10 yr of disease, then surveillance colonoscopy every 1–2 yr
Adenomatous polyps	Surveillance colonoscopy every 3–5 yr after excision—every 1–3 yr if multiple, large (>1 cm), villous, malignant (noninvasive)
Familial polyposis disorder (suspected)	Screening flexible sigmoidoscopy by age 20
Familial nonpolyposis disorder (suspected)	Screening colonoscopy or barium enema by age 35–40, then surveillance every 3–5 yr
Positive family history	Screening as for average risk; consider barium enema or colonoscopy

DRE = digital rectal exam.

Polyps and carcinoma in situ are detected and then subsequently cured by excisional biopsy with sigmoidoscopy or colonoscopy. If invasive cancer is detected, the next step is to determine the local extent of the tumor and the presence of metastatic disease. Abdominal computed tomography is generally of use for this staging.

Colectomy is the treatment modality of choice for invasive colon cancer. Adjuvant therapy with chemotherapy and/or radiation therapy is added if the clinical situation warrants, generally, if there are nodal metastases. Colon cancer with nodal metastases is gener-ally treated with postoperative 5-fluorouracil (5-FU) and levamisole. Because of the higher risk of local recurrences, rectal cancers characterized by invasion through the muscularis with or without nodal disease, and all tumors with nodal involvement are treated with surgery plus postoperative 5-FU and high dose pelvic irradiation.

Once colorectal neoplasms are discovered and treated, monitoring for recurrence must be maintained because the patient is now at higher than average risk for future neoplasms. This includes both patients who are discovered to have benign polyps as well as malignant disease.

▶ **KEY POINTS**

1. Colorectal cancers are believed to arise from malignant transformation of benign adenomatous polyps.

2. Environmental and dietary factors are believed to play a role in the development of colorectal neoplasms, and primary prevention may be possible.

3. Fecal occult blood testing, sigmoidoscopy, barium enema, and colonoscopy are the commonly available screening and diagnostic tests.

4. Early detection via screening, the intensity of which is tailored to relative risk, may result in significant decreases in mortality.

5. Surgery, followed by chemotherapy and/or radiation for more extensive disease, is the therapy of choice for invasive disease.

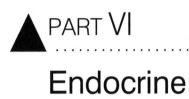

PART VI

Endocrine

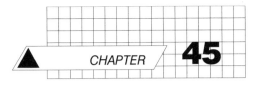

CHAPTER 45

Weight Loss

*A*t steady state, a normal individual balances food intake and energy expenditure to maintain a stable weight. **Energy expenditure** can be divided into:

▲ Basal metabolism—the amount of energy required to maintain the structural and functional integrity of the body while at rest; about 50% of the ingested energy.

▲ Physical activity—energy expended in excess of that required to breath while supine. Includes energy required to sit or stand upright without any other movement. A normal nonsedentary individual will expend about 40% of the ingested energy in physical activity.

▲ Dietary thermogenesis—energy that is associated with the absorption of food and is released as heat.

A **change in body mass** reflects a **change in the balance** between food intake and energy expenditure. It is not clear whether there is an endogenous "set point" that controls body mass. The control of hunger and satiety, however, appears to reside in the hypothalamus and other sections of the central nervous system. These **hunger and satiety control centers can be influenced by a number of factors:**

▲ nutritional

▲ endocrine

▲ emotional

▲ gastrointestinal

Weight gain is generally caused by **excess caloric intake.** Occasionally, endocrine disorders such as Cushing's syndrome, hypothyroidism, hypogonadism, and insulinomas are the cause of unanticipated weight gain, but this is exceedingly rare. **Unexpected weight loss,** however, is often associated with a specific **pathologic process.** An individual has conscious control over food intake and exercise, but in the absence of deliberate dieting or increase in physical activity, unexpected weight loss should trigger a search for an underlying cause.

▶ DIFFERENTIAL DIAGNOSIS

The **mechanisms of pathologic weight loss** include:

▲ Decreased intake: most serious illnesses are accompanied by anorexia and may also trigger malaise and depression that can further limit food intake;

▲ Decreased absorption: digestion and/or absorption of food are impaired;

▲ Accelerated metabolism: many illnesses increase basal metabolic energy expenditure; it appears that endocrine factors, especially inflammatory cytokines, play a major role in mediating this increased energy demand.

Given these mechanisms for altering the energy balance, there are a number of conditions that can cause significant weight loss.

Malignancy

Occult malignancy is often the cause of weight loss in the absence of other signs and symptoms. A combination of accelerated metabolism mediated by cytokines and anorexia (which also can been docrine mediated) are the usual mechanisms. The cytokine tumor necrosis factor, produced in response to certain malignancies, was originally called cachexin because of its effect on body mass. Cancers directly involving a segment of the gastrointestinal (GI) system can interfere with thedigestion and/or absorption of food.

Gastrointestinal Disease

Several GI diseases cause wasting in the face of normal or increased food intake due to defects in absorption:

▲ celiac disease (gluten intolerance)

▲ pancreatic insufficiency

▲ liver and biliary tract disease

▲ short bowel syndrome/postgastrectomy syndrome (due to surgical removal of significant sections of the GI tract)

▲ intestinal hypomotility with bacterial overgrowth (e.g., amyloidosis, scleroderma)

▲ heart failure (with visceral congestion)

Intra-abdominal masses (e.g., splenomegaly, tumors, ascites) can also cause weight loss by compression of the GI tract. Strictures and other **obstructing lesions** can limit the intake of food.

A number of chronic infectious diseases are classically associated with weight loss:

▲ endocarditis

▲ tuberculosis

▲ endemic fungal infections

▲ HIV

Inflammatory cytokines and resultant increased metabolic activity are believed to be responsible. This also appears to be the mechanism behind weight loss associated with conditions such as the collagen vascular diseases.

A number of metabolic derangements result in weight loss in patients with insulin-dependent diabetes:

▲ Insulin deficiency and glucagon excess result in a net catabolic state due to increased lipolysis and proteolysis in the setting of impaired protein and lipid synthesis;

▲ Glycosuria results in calorie wasting, which can be quite significant in patients with poor glucose control and/or renal impairment;

▲ GI disturbance: autonomic dysfunction as a result of the neuropathy associated with chronic hyperglycemia can lead to abnormal GI motility and malabsorption.

With endocrine disease, **hyperthyroidism** is the most commonly encountered endocrine cause of weight loss. Both basal metabolic rate and physical activity are increased by the hyperthyroid state. Other causes of endocrine-mediated weight loss are **pheochromocytomas** (due to increased metabolism from catecholamines) and **adrenal insufficiency** (due to anorexia from cortisol deficiency).

Although **anorexia nervosa** is commonly considered to be one of the major psychiatric illnesses leading to weight loss, among the elderly, **depression** is by far the most common cause. Other psychiatric illnesses can lead to decreased food intake as well.

▶ CLINICAL MANIFESTATIONS
History and Physical Examination

Evidence for etiologies can usually be found with a careful history and physical. **Constitutional symptoms** such as fever, malaise, and anorexia often ac-

company chronic infections and malignancies. GI disorders can be accompanied by signs and **symptoms of malabsorption** such as increased flatulence, steatorrhea, and abdominal pain after meals. **Signs of depression** should be sought, particularly in the elderly patient. Among this population, depression is approximately as frequent a cause of unexplained weight loss as an occult malignancy.

▶ DIAGNOSTIC EVALUATION

Provided a specific cause is not readily apparent after a thorough history and physical, it is reasonable to send the following **initial screening tests**:

▲ Complete blood count (with differential);

▲ Erythrocyte sedimentation rate (usually significantly elevated with malignancies, chronic infections, and chronic inflammatory conditions);

▲ Albumin (can provide an assessment of the degree of malnutrition);

▲ Liver function tests;

▲ Screening thyroid function tests (see Chapters 46 and 47);

▲ Fasting glucose.

These tests are relatively inexpensive and can detect a variety of conditions that may cause weight loss. Additional diagnostic tests should be performed only to confirm a diagnosis suggested by the preliminary workup.

▶ TREATMENT

If a specific cause is found, correction of this etiology, if possible, is of obvious importance. **Calorie supplementation** to promote the restoration of body mass may also be appropriate while correcting the underlying abnormality. This can be accomplished by enteral or parenteral means. In the absence of complicating conditions (e.g., aspiration risk, obstructing lesions), the enteral route is generally preferred. Parenteral therapy requires the placement of an indwelling catheter with its attendant risks. In patients with anorexia, a number of pharmacologic agents can be used to improve appetite, including cannabinoid derivatives and certain stimulants.

▶ KEY POINTS

1. Body mass is normally maintained by a balance between food intake and energy expenditure; weight loss is therefore a reflection of decreased

food intake (and/or absorption) and/or increased metabolic demand.

2. Malignancy and chronic infections are the most common causes of increased metabolic demand, leading to unexplained weight loss.

3. Increased metabolic activity appears to be mediated by cytokines.

4. A number of gastrointestinal diseases can affect the digestion and absorption of food and cause weight loss despite apparently adequate food intake.

5. Given the wide variety of underlying etiologies, the diagnosis of unexplained weight loss requires an orderly assessment beginning with a history, physical, and basic laboratory testing.

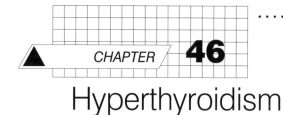
Hyperthyroidism

Hyperthyroidism is characterized by oversecretion of thyroid hormone. Elevated levels of free thyroxine (FT4) or T3 feedback to the pituitary gland, resulting in suppression of thyroid stimulating hormone (TSH). Hyperthyroidism can result from autonomous nodules, diffuse overproduction (Grave's disease), or damage to the thyroid (subacute thyroiditis).

▶ EPIDEMIOLOGY

Hyperthyroidism tends to occur more often in women. Grave's disease is the primary cause of hyperthyroidism in younger individuals, and multinodular goiter is more common in the elderly.

▶ ETIOLOGY

Subacute thyroiditis is subdivided into granulomatous and lymphocytic thyroiditis. Granulomatous thyroiditis, also known as DeQuervain's or painful thyroiditis, is most likely viral in origin, often following a flu-like syndrome. Lymphocytic thyroiditis (painless or silent thyroiditis) appears to be an autoimmune process. It is often seen in postpartum women. **Grave's disease** is another autoimmune thyroid disease. The production of antibodies to the thyroid TSH receptor results in stimulation of the receptor, leading to hyperthyroidism.

▶ CLINICAL FINDINGS
History

Symptoms of hyperthyroidism are:

▲ heat intolerance

▲ palpations

▲ weight loss

▲ nervousness

▲ loose bowel movements

The elderly are more likely to present with **apathetic hyperthyroidism**, characterized by weight loss, anorexia, and fatigue.

Neck pain is a prominent feature in DeQuervain's thyroiditis. An abrupt onset of symptoms may follow an upper respiratory illness.

The history should also investigate the possibility of **ingestion of excess exogenous thyroid hormone**. This can occur several ways, the most obvious being iatrogenic overreplacement with levothyroxine for other thyroid diseases. However, patients may also ingest excess bovine thyroid hormone by eating ground beef prepared from neck muscles. Finally, some patients surreptitiously abuse levothyroxine, usually as a method of weight loss. Health care professionals with medical knowledge and access to drugs may be more likely to do this than other patients.

A **recent iodine exposure** (such as a diagnostic study with intravenous contrast material) may precipitate hyperthyroidism in the patient with a multinodular gland. This is known as the Jod-Basedow effect.

Physical Examination

Tachycardia is present in most patients and an irregular pulse may be a sign of atrial fibrillation. Fever can be present in subacute thyroiditis.

Signs of the high metabolism seen in hyperthyroidism include:

▲ warm, moist skin

▲ lid lag (upper eyelid does not cover sclera above iris with downward gaze)

▲ tremor

Thyroid exam reveals an enlarged, painless thyroid in Grave's disease. In granulocytic thyroiditis, the gland is exquisitely tender. Nodules may be palpated in thyroid adenoma (single) or multinodular goiter (multiple). Patients taking excessive exogenous hormone will have nonpalpable glands.

Two other findings are seen exclusively in Grave's disease. **Proptosis** is visible protusion of the eye and believed to be secondary to an autoimmune reaction in the retroorbital space. **Pretibial myxedema** is a brawny thickening of skin in lower extremities. Although the name "myxedema" suggests it is seen in hypothyroidism, it is a feature of hyperthyroidism.

Differential Diagnosis

The differential diagnosis of **hyperthyroidism** can be divided physiologically by iodine uptake on thyroid scan (see below).

High uptake:

▲ Grave's disease

▲ toxic multinodular goiter

▲ solitary adenoma

▲ TSH-secreting pituitary tumor (rare)

Low uptake:

▲ subacute thyroiditis

▲ exogenous thyroiduse

▲ struma ovarii (rare)*

Laboratory Studies

The initial step in diagnosing hyperthyroidism is the presence of an increased **FT4** in association with a **decreased TSH** (<0.05). Free T4 is preferred to total T4, which is influenced by increases in thyroid-binding globulin (TBG). If FT4 is normal (but TSH low), the patient may have T3 thyrotoxicosis (elevated T3 levels) or subclinical hyperthyroidism.

A **thyroid scan** is used to evaluate uptake of radioactive iodine (RAI) in the thyroid gland. The RAI used is I^{123}, different from the I^{131} used to ablate the thyroid gland (see treatment). Normal uptake is 30%. Low uptake (<5%) in the setting of hyperthyroidism indicates either damage to the gland or an ectopic source of T4 (see Differential Diagnosis above).

Antimicrosomal antibody is present in autoimmune thyroid diseases (Grave's, lymphocytic thyroiditis). Antithyroglobulin antibody is also seen in Grave's disease. An **electrocardiogram** may show atrial fibrillation or sinus tachycardia.

▶ MANAGEMENT
Management Strategy

Patients with **thyroiditis** improve on their own in a few weeks. Management consists of treating the hyperthyroid symptoms (tachycardia, nervousness) with beta-blockers (see below) until hyperthyroidism resolves. In DeQuervain's (painful) thyroiditis, a short course of glucocorticoids (prednisone 20 to 40 mg daily) results in prompt resolution of the pain and inflammation.

In diseases characterized by **overproduction of thyroid hormone** (e.g., Grave's, adenomas), treatment is aimed at **reducing T4 production** by:

▲ radioactive iodine

▲ antithyroid drugs (methimazole, propiothiouracil)

▲ surgery

*Struma ovarii is an ovarian teratoma that produces thyroid hormone.

Radioactive iodine has the advantage of being highly effective, but will usually require life-long replacement therapy due to destruction of the thyroid gland. Overactive thyroid adenomas may preferentially take up iodine, destroying the adenoma and leaving the normal gland intact.

In subclinical (asymptomatic) hyperthyroidism, the optimum treatment is unknown. Some advocate treating elderly patients because they are at increased risk for atrial fibrillation and osteoporosis with long-standing subclinical hyperthyroidism.

Therapeutics

RAI is used to ablate an overactive thyroid. The dose given to the patient will depend on the size and iodine uptake of the gland. It should *not* be used in pregnant women because of the risk of fetal hypothyroidism. Despite earlier concerns, there appears to be no long-term risk of increased cancer in patients treated with RAI. RAI has become a popular treatment for Grave's disease given the simplicity of the regimen (one dose) and success rate. The risk of hypothyroidism, however, following RAI approaches 90%.

Antithyroid drugs interfere with the production of T4. In Grave's disease, these drugs are associated with a remission rate of 30 to 50%. Features of the two antithyroid drugs used (methimazole and propiothiouracil) are listed in Table 46-1. Methimazole has the advantage of once daily dosing, although it is a second-line agent in pregnancy due to early reports of an increased incidence of scalp defects (aplasiacutis) in newborns.

Major side effects of antithyroid drugs include:

▲ agranulocytosis

▲ hepatitis

Fever or sore throat may be the first sign of agranulocytosis in patients taking these medications. They should be instructed to seek medical attention if these symptoms occur.

Propranolol (20 to 40 mg two to four times daily) may be used to control symptoms of hyperthyroidism.

TABLE 46-1

Antithyroid Drugs

	Usual Initial Dose	Half-life	Use in Pregnancy
Propiothiouracil	100 mg qd	1–3 hrs	Yes
Methimazole	30 mg tid	6–8 hrs	Maybe

Although any beta-blocker may be used, propranolol has the added benefit of preventing conversion of T4 to the more active T3.

Continued Care

Patients recovering from hyperthyroidism should be monitored for a recurrence of, or change to, hypothyroidism. This is very frequent after RAI treatment and is permanent. It may also occur after subacute thyroiditis, although patients usually recover normal thyroid function after weeks to months.

▶ KEY POINTS

1. Hyperthyroidism is diagnosed by the presence of increased T4 with a suppressed TSH. The exceptions are the rare case of a TSH-producing pituitary adenoma (TSH high) and T3 thyrotoxicosis (T3 high and T4 normal).

2. A thyroid scan is useful to differentiate the etiologies into high uptake and low uptake causes.

3. Important causes of low uptake and hyperthyroidism include thyroiditis and surreptitious use of thyroid hormone.

4. Hyperthyroidism may be treated by RAI or antithyroid drugs. Most patients treated with RAI will eventually become hypothyroid.

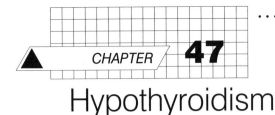

CHAPTER 47

Hypothyroidism

Hypothyroidism is characterized by underproduction of thyroid hormone. Low levels of thyroid hormone result in an increased production of thyroid stimulating hormone (TSH) by the pituitary. In the United States, hypothyroidism is often due to an autoimmune disease (i.e., Hashimoto's thyroiditis) or iatrogenesis (following radiation treatment). The most common cause worldwide is iodine deficiency.

Although hypothyroidism is often suspected in patients with common complaints such as fatigue and weight gain, many patients with hypothyroidism are completely asymptomatic. On the other hand, profound hypothyroidism may present with **myxedema coma**. These patients have severe depression of all organ systems, including the cardiac, respiratory, and central nervous systems.

► EPIDEMIOLOGY

Hashimoto's thyroiditis occurs more often in **women**, typically presenting between the ages of 30 and 50. However, Hashimoto's thyroiditis is also a common cause of hypothyroidism in the **elderly**. The incidence of hypothyroidism (both overt and subclinical) has been reported to be between 2% and 10%. Iodine deficiency is rare in the United States and Europe, but it is still prevalent in parts of Africa and Asia.

► RISK FACTORS

Patients with a history of other "autoimmune" diseases are at increased risk for hypothyroidism. These diseases include diabetes mellitus, Addison's disease, pernicious anemia, and vitiligo. A family history of thyroid disease also increases a patient's risk.

► CLINICAL FINDINGS

History

Symptoms of hypothyroidism include:

▲ cold intolerance

▲ weight gain

▲ fatigue

▲ constipation

▲ hoarseness

▲ dry skin

In the elderly, symptoms of hypothyroidism are often incorrectly ascribed to "aging." Patients may also present for evaluation of a condition associated with hypothyroidism, such as **carpal tunnel syndrome**, **sleep apnea**, or **anemia**. Patients with a history of head and neck **irradiation** are at risk for hypothyroidism, due to either primary thyroid failure (neck radiation) or panhypopituitarism (cranial irradiation). **Lithium ingestion** impairs secretion of thyroid hormone and may cause hypothyroidism in certain individuals.

Physical Examination

Diastolic blood pressure is often mildly elevated in hypothyroidism. In severe cases, bradycardia and hypothermia are present. Some patients will have dry skin, coarse hair, and thinning of the lateral third of the eyebrows.

A **goiter**, or enlarged thyroid, is often present in patients with Hashimoto's thyroiditis. The gland is firm and sometimes lobulated. The gland may not be palpable after radiation or ablative therapy.

Neurologic examination may be notable for a **delayed relaxation of deep tendon reflexes**. Patients with myxedema coma have a characteristic edematous face with periorbital edema and **macroglossia**.

Differential Diagnosis

The causes of **hypothyroidism** include:

▲ Hashimoto's (chronic lymphocytic) thyroiditis

▲ iodine deficiency

▲ lithium ingestion

▲ postradiation or postablative therapy

▲ recovery from subacute thyroiditis (transient)

▲ panhypopituitarism

Laboratory Studies

The characteristic laboratory values for hypothyroidism are a **low or low-normal free T4**, in association with an **elevated TSH** (greater than 5). The exception to this pattern is central hypothyroidism, as seen in panhypopituitarism. TSH in these patients is low to normal (see Chapter 51). Patients with an elevated TSH but normal free T4 are said to have subclinical (or compensated) hypothyroidism.

Nonthyroid studies that can be abnormal in hypothyroidism include:

▲ hypercholesterolemia

▲ elevated creatinine phosphokinase

▲ abnormal electrocardiogram (decreased voltage, T-wave flattening)

Thyroid autoantibodies (**thyroid microsomal antibody** and **thyroglobulin antibody**) are found in Hashimoto's thyroiditis and are useful in confirming the autoimmune diagnosis. They are negative, however, in a small percentage of patients with autoimmune thyroid disease.

► MANAGEMENT

Management Strategy

Treatment in hypothyroidism is based on the severity of symptoms and the degree of hypothyroidism. Patients with subclinical hypothyroidism may be followed without treatment. About 5% of these patients each year progress to symptomatic hypothyroidism. When treatment is instituted, therapy consists of exogenous thyroid hormone, since the underlying cause of hypothyroidism is usually not correctable (with the exception of iodine deficiency). The **speed of the replacement** is dependent on the patient's age and medical condition. In the elderly and in patients with known coronary artery disease, replacement should be advanced slowly over months. Patients with myxedema coma are rapidly treated with intravenous thyroid hormone (300 to 500 μg bolus, followed by 50 μg daily).

An important caveat is needed for patients with suspected **panhypopituitarism**. Since these patients are usually adrenally insufficient, thyroid replacement may increase the metabolism of the small amount of the body's remaining cortisol, thereby precipitating an **adrenal crisis**. Therefore, patients with known or highly suspected panhypopituitarism should always begin hydrocortisone treatment prior to thyroid replacement therapy.

Therapeutics

Levothyroxine is the treatment of choice because of its long half-life (one week) and once daily dosing. The typical dose is 1.7 μg/kg body weight, with most patients controlled between 100 and 150 μg daily. As stated above, patients at risk for decompensation with rapid replacement may be started on a low dose (25 μg) and increased in 25 μg increments every few weeks.

Continued Care

Levothyroxine therapy should be monitored by following **serum TSH**. Initially, TSH should be measured every 4 to 6 weeks (reflecting the time required to achieve a steady state of the replacement). Patients often feel least symptomatic when TSH is on the low end of normal. However, overreplacement increases the risk of atrial fibrillation and excessive bone loss. Once a stable replacement dose is achieved, TSH can be monitored every 6 months.

Patients with a history of radiation exposure are at increased risk for **thyroid cancer**, and physical examination should concentrate on the presence of new nodules that may represent cancer. Patients with Hashimoto's thyroiditis have an increased incidence of **thyroid lymphoma**, which usually presents as an enlarging thyroid mass. Radioactive iodine does *not* apparently increase the risk of thyroid malignancy.

► KEY POINTS

1. Hashimoto's thyroiditis is an autoimmune disease that is the most common cause of hypothyroidism in the United States. Most patients have antithyroid antibodies.

2. Patients with a low T4 and low-to-normal TSH may have central (pituitary) hypothyroidism. Replacement of thyroid hormone may cause adrenal crisis by increasing the metabolism of cortisol.

3. Levothyroxine therapy is monitored by following TSH levels. TSH takes weeks to months to respond to a new dose of levothyroxine. Replacement should be instituted slowly in the elderly and patients with coronary artery disease.

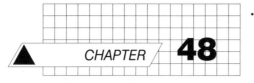
Diabetes Mellitus

*D*iabetes mellitus is the abnormal regulation of glucose, resulting in hyperglycemia. Although the serum glucose concentration varies throughout the day depending on activity and dietary intake of nutrients, patients with diabetes are unable to properly respond to these normal fluctuations.

Diabetes is generally divided into type I (insulin-dependent diabetes mellitus [IDDM]), in which there is an **absence of insulin produced** by the pancreas, and type II (non-insulin-dependent diabetes mellitus [NIDDM]), in which the defect is in **peripheral response to intrinsically produced insulin**.

► EPIDEMIOLOGY

In the United States there are about 10 million type II diabetics, accounting for 80 to 90% of all patients with diabetes. Generally, patients with NIDDM are over the age of 40 years. IDDM usually presents in the first two decades of life. It has become clear that IDDM and NIDDM can present in both the pediatric and adult populations.

► PATHOPHYSIOLOGY

In IDDM, there is an absolute lack of insulin production. Unless exogenous insulin is supplied, patients with IDDM eventually develop **ketoacidosis**. There is some evidence that IDDM results from autoimmune destruction of the pancreatic islet cells that produce insulin, perhaps triggered by a viral infection.

In NIDDM, there is an abnormal response to endogenously produced insulin. Because patients with NIDDM still produce insulin, they are not prone to ketosis. The response of various tissues to insulin is blunted, so-called "insulin resistance." Early in NIDDM, **hyperinsulinemia** may be present as the pancreas tries to overcome peripheral insulin resistance. In patients with long-standing NIDDM, there is eventually decreased insulin secretion that worsens the hyperglycemia. Patients with NIDDM also have notable disturbances in lipid metabolism, including low levels of high-density lipoprotein and elevated levels of intermediate density lipoprotein (IDL), β-very-low-density lipoprotein, and triglycerides.

A number of poorly defined metabolic abnormalities are believed to result in insulin resistance. **Obesity** clearly aggravates these metabolic abnormalities, and weight loss can ameliorate them.

Although acute ketoacidosis in the setting of IDDM can be fatal, most morbidity of IDDM and NIDDM results from the secondary effects of long-term hyperglycemia on the **vascular system**:

▲ retinitis

▲ nephropathy

▲ neuropathy

▲ coronary artery disease

▲ peripheral vascular disease

▲ hypertension

The first three represent **microvascular** damage, whereas the last three are manifestations of **macrovascular** injury.

NIDDM patients may develop **nonketotic hyperosmolar coma**, a syndrome of profound dehydration that results from sustained hyperglycemic diuresis in a patient who is unable to take in enough fluids to offset urinary losses. Generally, this is seen in debilitated older diabetics who, often in the setting of another insult such as infection or stroke, are unable to maintain water intake. Mortality in this condition can approach 50%.

► CLINICAL MANIFESTATIONS
History

Patients who present with IDDM often do so in a dramatic fashion with acute diabetic ketoacidosis. In contrast, patients with NIDDM often present with asymptomatic hyperglycemia. **Symptomatic patients** may present with polyuria, polydipsia, polyphagia, fatigue, blurred vision, and candidal vaginitis. Patients who have not routinely sought medical attention present with **symptoms relating to end-stage vasculopathy**, such as gastrointestinal dysfunction, postural dizziness (secondary to autonomic dysfunction), impotence, numbness in a "stocking/glove" distribution, and chest pain.

Physical Examination

When the diagnosis of NIDDM is made, a complete physical examination should be performed, in particular looking for signs of end-organ damage, such as retinopathy, S4 gallop (hypertension), peripheral neuropathy, and poor distal perfusion.

▶ DIFFERENTIAL DIAGNOSIS

Other conditions that can result in hyperglycemia that is not a result of IDDM or NIDDM include:

▲ high-dose steroid therapy

▲ pancreatitis

▲ administration of dextrose-containing intravenous fluids

▲ pancreatectomy

▲ drugs (e.g., thiazide diuretics)

▲ stress (via catecholamine release)

▶ DIAGNOSTIC EVALUATION

To make the diagnosis of NIDDM, the following criteria have been proposed: fasting glucose greater than 140 mg/dL (normally <115 mg/dL) or an abnormal glucose tolerance test. The **glucose tolerance test** is done as follows: patient must fast for 10 to 16 hours (and refrain from caffeine and cigarettes), 75 g of a glucose solution is administered orally (40 g/m^2), and blood is sampled at 0, 0.5, 1.0, 1.5, and 2.0 hours for serum glucose measurement.

The diagnosis of diabetes is made when 2-hour value and at least one other is greater than 200 mg/dL (normally <160 mg/dL at 1 hour and <140 at 2 hours). Patients who have values that fall in between the normal range and those defined for frank diabetes are said to have **impaired glucose tolerance**. About 1 to 5% of such patients will progress to frank diabetes each year. An important measure of persistent hyperglycemia is the **glycosylated hemoglobin** (HgA1c). Normally, 3.8 to 6.3% of the total hemoglobin is glycosylated, and this proportion rises directly with the average blood glucose level. Given the average lifespan of a red blood cell at 120 days, measurement of HgA1c gives an indication of the level of blood glucose control over a 3-month period.

An assessment of renal function with urinalysis and measurement of serum creatinine is necessary.

▶ TREATMENT

Diabetic management is twofold: restore glycemic control and monitor for and treat complications of long-term diabetes. An important development in the management of diabetes is the demonstration that the closer a patient comes to achieving **euglycemia** (so-called "tight" control), the less likely the rate of microvascular complications. This was demonstrated in patients with IDDM, but most experts believe this also pertains to patients with NIDDM.

Despite the finding that tight control leads to fewer long-term microvascular complications, a physician must determine whether maintenance of euglycemia is a realistic goal for the individual patient. In young patients with IDDM or NIDDM, euglycemia is generally the goal because they stand to gain the most from tight control. With the elderly patient, especially those with complications or other comorbid conditions, the problems associated with tight control, such as inconvenience and the greater risk of hypoglycemia (see below), may outweigh any potential benefit.

In **IDDM**, administration of exogenous insulin is mandatory to prevent ketoacidosis. In **NIDDM**, lifestyle modifications (diet, exercise), oral hypoglycemia drugs (sulfonylureas and biguanides), and insulin are the therapeutic options. **Diet** coupled with an **exercise program** with the goal of **weight reduction** is the initial priority. Many patients, particularly early in the course of their disease, can often be adequately controlled by weight loss alone. Even if weight loss is not sufficient, it will make subsequent pharmacologic treatment easier by decreasing the amount of drug that is required to achieve good control. In addition, diet and exercise can improve the lipid profile, decreasing the risk of subsequent coronary and peripheral vascular disease.

If lifestyle modifications alone are not sufficient, the next step is generally to add an oral hypoglycemic agent, usually a **sulfonylurea**. The sulfonylureas act primarily by stimulating insulin release from the pancreatic beta cells.

Hypoglycemia is the most common side effect of sulfonylureas. Although less common than with insulin, **sulfonylurea**-induced hypoglycemia tends to be more severe and prolonged (due to the longer half-life of these drugs).

The **biguanides** are oral agents that are believed to lower blood glucose by inhibiting hepatic gluconeogenesis. Phenformin was removed from the market in the United States because of a rare association with severe lactic acidosis. Metformin has been commonly used outside of the United States and has been recently introduced here.

Subcutaneous insulin is the treatment of choice for patients with IDDM and is necessary for the adequate control of many patients with NIDDM, particularly later in the disease when levels of endogenous insulin production fall.

A variety of insulin is available. They differ in their formulation such that the pharmacokinetics (rate of onset, peak effect, and length of duration) are tailored for specific uses:

▲ Short-acting (e.g., regular, crystalline zinc insulin)—used in diabetic emergencies and routine treatment. Onset of action within 1 hour and peak effect at about 3 to 5 hours.

▲ Intermediate-acting (e.g., neutral protamine Hagedorn, lente)—used for routine treatment. Onset of action in 2 to 3 hours with peak effect at 8 to 10 hours.

▲ Long acting (e.g., ultralente)—used in some routine treatment regimens to provide a low basal level of insulin.

Insulin administration schedules have been developed to differ in the number of injections and the formulations of insulin used. The different schedules are tailored to the degree of control that is desired. Commonly, regimens use a combination of 1 or 2 daily injections of intermediate insulin with two or more injections of short-acting insulin to cover meals. For some patients (highly motivated patients with IDDM), continuous subcutaneous insulin infusion via a pump is an option. These devices administer continuous low levels of regular insulin with boluses (either preprogrammed or manually entered) before meals.

Patients on insulin need to **self-monitor their capillary blood glucose.** This is done with fingerstick blood draws and then placing a drop of blood on a colorimetric reagent strip that can be read manually or with a small portable instrument. More frequent monitoring is required for attempted tighter management, given the greater risk of hypoglycemia.

All diabetics who are on drug treatment, either with insulin or oral hypoglycemics, need to be educated about the **signs** and **symptoms of hypoglycemia.** These are due to the **release of epinephrine,** which is released in response to hypoglycemia, and **central nervous system dysfunction due to hypoglycemia,** because the central nervous system uses only glucose as an energy source. Symptoms of **epinephrine release** are:

▲ tachycardia

▲ diaphoresis

▲ tremor/anxiety

▲ dizziness

Symptoms of **central nervous system dysfunction** are:

▲ headache

▲ blurred vision

▲ confusion

▲ blunted mental acuity

▲ seizures

▲ loss of consciousness

Rapid drops in blood glucose levels (e.g., after administration of regular insulin without a subsequent meal) tends to produce more adrenergic symptoms, whereas more gradual falls can produce more central nervous system symptoms without adrenergic ones. Diabetics should be instructed to always carry sugar with them to be taken if they have any of the symptoms of hypoglycemia. This sugar can be in the form of candy or prepackaged high-glucose gels or tablets. After taking sugar, they should check a fingerstick glucose if possible. Diabetic management also needs to be altered in the setting of other illnesses, especially infection, or if the patient's diet is to be drastically changed, as in fasting before surgery.

▶ KEY POINTS

1. There are two main types of diabetes, distinguished by the absolute requirement for exogenous insulin (IDDM) or the relative resistance to the action of endogenous insulin (NIDDM).

2. The main complications (retinopathy, nephropathy, coronary artery disease, peripheral vascular disease) of both IDDM and NIDDM are related to vascular pathology that arises with long-term elevation of blood glucose.

3. The development of microvascular disease can be prevented by normalization of blood glucose levels via pharmacologic and/or lifestyle intervention.

4. The diagnosis of NIDDM is made by abnormally elevated fasting blood glucose or abnormal response to an orally administered glucose challenge (glucose tolerance test).

5. Treatment of IDDM requires the administration of exogenous insulin, whereas NIDDM is treated by a combination of lifestyle modification (diet/exercise) and, when needed, oral hypoglycemic drugs and/or insulin.

6. All diabetics who are on pharmacologic treatment need to be educated on the signs and treatment of hypoglycemia.

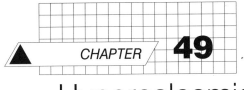

CHAPTER 49

Hypercalcemia

*U*nder normal circumstances, serum calcium is tightly regulated by **parathyroid hormone** (PTH), which stimulates bone resorption and decreases renal excretion of calcium. PTH also increases activation of **vitamin D,** which assists in increasing calcium reabsorption from the gut. Therefore, disorders involving increased bone destruction, decreased renal excretion, increased gastrointestinal absorption, or unregulated secretion of PTH may manifest as hypercalcemia.

► ETIOLOGY AND DIFFERENTIAL DIAGNOSIS

The two most common causes of hypercalcemia are **primary hyperparathyroidism** and **malignancy,** accounting for 90% of all cases. Primary hyperparathyroidism occurs when increased PTH is secreted. The etiologies of **primary hyperparathyroidism** are:

▲ solitary parathyroid adenoma (85% of primary hyperparathyroidism)

▲ parathyroid hyperplasia (15% of cases, may be associated with hereditary causes, such as the MEN syndromes)

▲ rare cases of mixed type or multiple adenomas

Malignancy may cause hypercalcemia by two mechanisms. In **humoral hypercalcemia** of **malignancy** (HHM), a PTH-like protein is secreted by the tumor. Cancers most likely to cause HHM include:

▲ lung cancer (especially squamous cell)

▲ head and neck cancer

▲ renal cancer

▲ T-cell leukemia (associated with the virus HTLV-1)

The other mechanism is **direct bone destruction,** believed to be mediated by an osteoclast activating factor. Cancers involved in bone destruction include multiple myeloma and breast cancer.

Although most cases of hypercalcemia are caused by primary hyperparathyroidism or malignancy, other causes include:

Vitamin D mediated

▲ increased vitamin D ingestion

▲ granulomatous disease (e.g., sarcoid, tuberculosis)

Increased bone turnover

▲ hyperthyroidism

▲ immobilization (usually in association with underlying high bone turnover, as in Paget's disease)

▲ vitamin A intoxication

Decreased renal excretion of calcium

▲ thiazide diuretics

▲ milk-alkali syndrome

Milk-alkali syndrome may be caused by excessive ingestion of antacids. The resulting alkalosis leads to greater renal absorption of calcium, which in turn induces volume depletion. The cycle then continues, with more alkalosis and calcium reabsorption, perpetuating decreasing renal function.

Lithium intake and familial hypocalciuric hypercalcemia (FHH) are additional causes of mild to moderate hypercalcemia that involve increased PTH secretion (but are not primary hyperparathyroidism). FHH is a rare autosomal dominant disorder in which urine calcium excretion remains low (< 100 mg/day) despite hypercalcemia. This is in contrast to primary hyperparathyroidism, where hypercalciuria occurs.

► CLINICAL MANIFESTATIONS

History

Symptoms due to hypercalcemia are nonspecific and include **fatigue, anorexia,** and **drowsiness;** with higher elevations of calcium, confusion and stupor occur. Gastrointestinal complaints include nausea, vomiting, and constipation. Inhibition of renal concentrating ability leads to polyuria. Patients with primary hyperparathyroidism and chronic hypercalcemia may give a history or recurrent nephrolithiasis or peptic ulcer disease.

The etiology of hypercalcemia may be assisted by a history of weight loss and heavy tobacco use (malignancy), drug ingestion (lithium, thiazides, antacids), or excess vitamin ingestion (A or D). A positive family history may be discovered in multiple endocrine neoplasia (MEN) or familial hypocalciuric hypercalcemia (FHH).

Physical Examination

Physical examination is usually unrevealing but should include a search for findings suggestive of malignancy, such as adenopathy or abnormal masses.

▶ DIAGNOSTIC EVALUATION

The most helpful test in differentiating the cause of hypercalcemia is the **PTH assay**. If elevated, this points toward primary hyperparathyroidism. This is the cause in most (90%) asymptomatic patients, especially if the hypercalcemia is chronic. Other causes to consider with a normal to high PTH include FHH (see above) and lithium ingestion. If the PTH is low or undetectable, malignancy is most likely.

Malignancy is usually apparent on initial testing, which should include:

▲ **chest x-ray** (lung cancer)

▲ **urine for red cells** (renal cancer)

▲ **mammogram** (breast cancer)

▲ **serum** and **urine immunoelectrophoresis** (multiple myeloma)

If these initial tests are unrevealing and cancer is still suspect, computed tomography of chest or abdomen may be performed.

X-rays in hypercalcemia may show either the consequence of the disease or the etiology. Metastatic cancer or myeloma may appear as lytic lesions on bone films. Long-standing primary hyperparathyroidism may result in the following **bone manifestations**:

▲ osteitis fibrosa cystica

▲ subperiosteal reabsorption in phalanges

▲ chondrocalcinosis with associated pseudogout (see Chapter 54)

Cardiac manifestations of hypercalcemia present as a **shortened QT interval** on electrocardiogram.

▶ TREATMENT

The initial goal of treatment is to return the calcium to normal range to prevent neurologic and cardiac dysfunction. The intensity of treatment depends on the level of calcium. After initially controlling calcium level, therapy is aimed at treating the underlying etiology.

The first treatment for moderate to severe hypercalcemia (>12 to 13 mg/dL) is **intravenous saline**, which restores the depleted intravascular volume and increases renal calcium excretion. Rates of infusion are often 200 to 400 mL/hour. Once volume status has been returned to normal, loop diuretics (e.g., furosemide) may be added to further increase calcium excretion.

After restoring volume and maximizing calcium excretion, sustained control of serum calcium via inhibition of bone resorption is the next priority. **Calcitonin** can be administered subcutaneously every 6 hours and reduces calcium levels within hours. However, continued use results in tachyphylaxis and limits the use of this drug. The **biphosphonates** (etidronate, pamidronate, and alendronate) are synthetic analogues of pyrophosphate and inhibit osteoclast resorption of bone. They may be given intravenously and will lower calcium over the next 2 to 3 days. Of the three agents, pamidronate (45–60 mg intravenously) seems to be the preferred choice. Although not useful in the first few hours of hypercalcemia, the biphosphonates may maintain normocalcemia for several weeks after a single dose. Other agents, such as gallium nitrate or plicamycin, have been limited by side effects.

Once calcium homeostasis is achieved, the focus turns to the underlying disease. In the case of drugs or vitamin D excess, the calcium will normalize with removal of the offending agent. For malignancy-related hypercalcemia, cases of improvement have been reported after successful treatment of the cancer. Unfortunately, this is not usually possible due to the advanced nature of many of these cancers. Patients with malignancy-related hypercalcemia survive an average of 6 months after diagnosis of hypercalcemia.

For symptomatic primary hyperparathyroidism, surgery should be performed. A single adenoma may be removed, or if hyperplasia is present, three and one-half glands are removed. The remaining tissue is sometimes implanted in the forearm to ensure easy access in case of recurrent hypercalcemia.

For **asymptomatic hyperparathyroidism**, surgery is recommended for patients under age 50. For older patients, surgery should be recommended if there is:

▲ a calcium level greater than 1.5 mg/dL above normal

▲ history of life-threatening hypercalcemia

▲ nephrolithiasis or reduction in creatinine clearance

▲ bone density 2 or more standard deviations below controls

If surgery is deferred, patients should be instructed to maintain adequate hydration. Calcium intake should be moderate. High intake could worsen hypercalcemia; a deficient diet could further stimulate PTH production and worsen bone loss.

If surgery is performed, one must monitor for **postoperative hypocalcemia**. This may be secondary to:

▲ hypoparathyroidism (too much gland removed or ischemic injury)

▲ "hungry bone syndrome," which is rapid bone formation after gland removal results in excessive calcium loss from bloodstream. Usually only seen with severe osteitis fibrosa cystica

Signs of hypocalcemia include muscle twitching and spasm.

▶ **KEY POINTS**

1. The two most common etiologies of hypercalcemia are primary hyperparathyroidism and malignancy.

2. Parathyroid hormone can successfully discriminate these two etiologies.

3. Immediate treatment consists of hydration and perhaps loop diuretics. Long-term control is achieved by treating the underlying disease or by using biphosphonates.

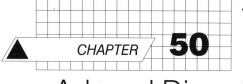

CHAPTER 50

Adrenal Disorders

*7*he **adrenal cortex** is responsible for the synthesis of three major steroid hormones:

▲ mineralocorticoids (e.g., aldosterone)

▲ glucocorticoids (e.g., cortisol)

▲ androgens (e.g., dehydroepiandrosterone [DHEA])

The **adrenal medulla** produces catecholamines, primarily epinephrine and norepinephrine. The main stimulus for catecholamine secretion is the sympathetic nervous system.

Corticotropin releasing hormone (CRH) produced by the hypothalamus stimulates **adrenocorticotropin** (ACTH), which in turn stimulates cortisol secretion. Aldosterone secretion is controlled by the renin–angiotensin axis (Fig. 50-1). **Renin** (produced in the kidney's juxtaglomerular cells) converts angiotensinogen to angiotensin I, which is then metabolized to **angiotensin II** by angiotensin converting enzyme (ACE). Angiotensin II, in addition to being a potent vasoconstrictor, stimulates aldosterone. Aldosterone is also stimulated to a lesser extent by hyperkalemia and ACTH. Aldosterone increases sodium reabsorption and potassium excretion in the distal renal tubule.

Adrenal gland disorders may be classified into disorders of hyperfunction:

▲ Cushing's syndrome (cortisol)

▲ primary aldosteronism*

▲ pheochromocytoma (catecholamines)

and the disorder of adrenal insufficiency (Addison's disease).

▶ ETIOLOGY

Cushing's syndrome (cortisol excess) may arise from the adrenal gland itself or from stimulation by ACTH. The main causes are:

▲ pituitary adenoma (mostly microadenomas)

▲ adrenal tumor

▲ ectopic ACTH production (usually from small-cell lung cancer)

Primary aldosteronism is the result of a unilateral adrenal adenoma or bilateral adrenal hyperplasia. Pheochromocytoma follows "the rule of 10":

▲ 10% are located outside the adrenal gland (mainly sympathetic nerve ganglia)

▲ 10% are bilateral

▲ 10% are malignant

Pheochromocytomas may be associated with the **multiple endocrine neoplasia (MEN) syndrome type II**. Other features of this syndrome are medullary carcinoma of the thyroid and either parathyroid hyperplasia (type IIa) or ganglioneuromas (type IIb).

Addison's disease is usually related to an **autoimmune** etiology. It can be associated with other autoimmune diseases such as Hashimoto's thyroiditis, type I diabetes mellitus, and premature ovarian failure; this combination is known as the **polyglandular autoimmune syndrome** (type II). Other causes of Addison's disease are tuberculosis and adrenal hemorrhage.

▶ CLINICAL FINDINGS

History

About two-thirds of patients with pheochromocytoma will have the classic **spells**, consisting of headache, sweating, palpitations, pallor, or flushing. These spells often last 10 to 60 minutes. Patients with hyperaldosteronism are usually asymptomatic, although hypertension may be the initial presenting problem.

The presentation of adrenal insufficiency is variable; patients often have nonspecific symptoms such as weight loss, nausea, and abdominal pain. Cortisol excess, as in Cushing's disease, presents as weight gain, amenorrhea, muscle weakness, and sometimes depression.

Physical Examination

Hypertension is a common feature in pheochromocytoma and hyperaldosteronism. Hypertension may occur only during spells in 40% of patients with pheochromocytoma. Orthostatic hypotension is associated with adrenal insufficiency, but may also be seen in pheochromocytoma due to the volume depletion.

---

*Many conditions (such as renal artery stenosis) may secondarily increase plasma aldosterone. For this chapter, the term *hyperaldosteronism* refers to aldosterone excess generated from the adrenal glands (primary aldosteronism).

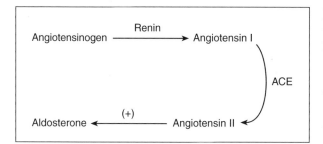

Figure 50-1 The renin–angiotensin axis.

Physical findings in Cushing's syndrome include:

▲ truncal obesity

▲ excess fat deposition on cervical spine ("buffalo hump") and face ("moon facies")

▲ abdominal stria and thinning of skin

▲ hirsutism

Differential Diagnosis

Consider the diagnosis of pheochromocytoma in the patient with hypertension and spells as well as:

▲ thyrotoxicosis

▲ cardiac arrhythmias

▲ anxiety disorder

▲ labile essential hypertension

Hyperaldosteronism often presents as hypertension and hypokalemia. Other etiologies with a similar presentation include:

▲ Cushing's syndrome

▲ renovascular hypertension

▲ malignant hypertension

▲ secondary hyperaldosteronism (e.g., heart failure)

Laboratory Studies

Electrolytes

The hallmark of hyperaldosteronism is hypertension in association with **hypokalemia**. Hyperglycemia may be present in all the adrenal excess syndromes, but is most common in Cushing's syndrome. Primary adrenal insufficiency has the characteristic pattern of **hyperkalemia** and **hyponatremia**.

Adrenal Insufficiency

The ACTH stimulation test is described in Chapter 2.

Hyperaldosteronism

The initial step in the patient with hypokalemia and hypertension is to look for a suppressed renin level (from excess aldosterone production). A standing plasma renin activity (PRA) of < 3.0 ng/ml/hr or a ratio of aldosterone/PRA of greater than 20 is suggestive of primary aldosteronism. Attempts are then made to suppress the excess aldosterone level with a high sodium diet. Continued high aldosterone levels (on urine collection) confirm the diagnosis.

Pheochromocytoma

Urine levels for catecholamines and their metabolites (metanephrines, vanillylmandelic acid [VMA]) will be elevated in patients with pheochromocytoma. No single test is usually adequate; sensitivity and specificity depend on the specific laboratory and range of normal values. In general, urinary catecholamines are the most sensitive, metanephrines the most specific, and VMA the least useful. Plasma levels of these substances are greatly affected by stress or position and are not useful.

Cushing's Disease

This initial screening test in Cushing's disease is the **overnight dexamethasone suppression test**. In normal individuals, administration of 1 mg of dexamethasone at midnight suppresses the next morning's (8 A.M.) cortisol to less than 5 μg/dl. Failure to suppress cortisol occurs in Cushing's disease, but false-positive tests also occur in obesity, depression, and alcoholism. The diagnosis of cortisol excess is confirmed by a **low-dose dexamethasone suppression test** (0.5 mg of dexamethasone every 6 hours for 2 days). A 24-hour urine for free cortisol will continue to demonstrate increased levels in patients with Cushing's syndrome. A **high-dose dexamethasone suppression test** (2 mg every 6 hours) will usually result in cortisol suppression of a pituitary adenoma, but not in adrenal hyperplasia or ectopic ACTH production. Serum **ACTH levels** are elevated in both ectopic ACTH production and pituitary adenomas.

Imaging Studies

Computed tomography (CT) of the abdomen will usually locate the adrenal masses in pheochromocytoma, adrenal adenomas, and adrenal carcinomas. Since asymptomatic adrenal masses ("incidentalomas") are quite common (1% of individuals), an abdominal CT should not be routinely ordered unless the above disorders are confirmed biochemically. **Magnetic resonance imaging** of the brain is the test of choice for detecting pituitary adenomas in Cushing's disease (see Chapter 51), and a chest X-ray or CT may be needed in ectopic ACTH production to look for a small cell carcinoma or bronchial adenoma.

▶ MANAGEMENT

Management Strategy

Surgical resection is the treatment for pheochromocytomas and adrenal adenomas. Prior to surgery for pheochromocytomas, combined alpha- and beta-blockade is required. Alpha-adrenergic blockade is instituted with an agent such as phenoxybenzamine. Then, low-dose beta-blockade (propranolol 10 mg two to four times daily) is begun and slowly increased to control tachycardia.

Patients with idiopathic hyperaldosteronism do not benefit from unilateral adrenalectomy. Instead, medical treatment with an aldosterone antagonist (e.g., spironolactone) is indicated.

Therapeutics

Spironolactone is indicated for bilateral adrenal hyperplasia, with a dosage of 100 to 400 mg daily. Side effects include gynecomastia, menstrual irregularities, and impotence.

Amiloride is another potassium sparing agent and the preferred choice for men with bilateral adrenal hyperplasia, with a dosage of 10 to 30 mg daily.

Maintenance therapy in patients with adrenal insufficiency consists of approximately 7.5 mg of **prednisone** daily (often divided as 5 mg in the morning and 2.5 mg in the evening to mimic normal circadian rhythms). Side effects from excess replacement include osteoporosis, weight gain, and hyperglycemia.

Fludrocortisone is the mineralocorticoid replacement for patients with primary adrenal insufficiency. The average dose is 0.05 to 0.10 mg daily. Side effects include hypokalemia, hypertension, and fluid retention.

Continued Care

Although blood pressure often improves following resection, hypertension may persist after treatment for pheochromocytoma or hyperaldosteronism. For a malignant pheochromocytoma, urine metanephrines should be periodically checked to test for recurrence.

Patients with adrenal insufficiency require stress dose steroids at times of surgery or severe illness. The usual recommended dose is 100 mg of hydrocortisone three times daily.

▶ KEY POINTS

1. Pheochromocytoma is characterized by oversecretion of catecholamines, resulting in spells of diaphoresis and palpitations and sustained or paroxysmal hypertension.

2. Primary hyperaldosteronism presents as the combination of hypertension and hypokalemia. Plasma renin activity is suppressed and aldosterone is elevated. Abdominal CT reveals a unilateral adrenal adenoma in about 60% of cases.

3. Cushing's syndrome (cortisol excess) may be due to a pituitary adenoma, adrenal tumor, or ectopic ACTH production. The initial screening test is the overnight dexamethasone suppression test.

4. Primary adrenal insufficiency is usually autoimmune in etiology. Symptoms include weakness, weight loss, and abdominal pain. Hyponatremia and hyperkalemia are often present.

CHAPTER 51

Pituitary Disorders

*T*he anterior pituitary gland produces six hormones; the posterior pituitary gland stores and releases two hormones. These hormones and their major functions are listed in Table 51-1. The anterior pituitary hormones are stimulated by hormones produced in the hypothalamus. The one exception is prolactin, which is chronically inhibited by **dopamine**. Drugs that block dopamine elevate prolactin levels.

Diseases of the pituitary may be classified as disorders of oversecretion or undersecretion of these hormones. Oversecretion of pituitary hormones occurs in **pituitary adenomas**. Undersecretion of all anterior hormones occurs in **panhypopituitarism**, and undersecretion of vasopressin produces **diabetes insipidus**.

▶ EPIDEMIOLOGY

Pituitary adenomas are uncommon diseases, with an annual incidence of 1 in 100,000 individuals. A pituitary adenoma is classified by the predominant hormone which is secreted. Most pituitary adenomas are nonfunctioning (although they produce the alpha subunit of luteinizing hormone [LH], follicle stimulating hormone [FSH], and thyroid stimulating hormone [TSH]); the most common functioning adenomas are **prolactinomas**, followed by adenomas that produce growth hormone (leading to **acromegaly**) and those that produce adrenocorticotropin (ACTH) (causing **Cushing's disease**).

▶ RISK FACTORS

Pituitary adenomas may occur in association with the **multiple endocrine neoplasia (MEN) syndrome type** I. Associated diseases include parathyroid hyperplasia and pancreatic islet cell tumors.

▶ CLINICAL FINDINGS

History

Hypogonadism (amenorrhea in women; impotence in men) along with **galactorrhea** may be seen in prolactin-secreting adenomas. Galactorrhea is defined as milk production outside of the postpartum period; it is not usually seen in men. Amenorrhea may also be seen in other hormone excesses (such as ACTH and growth hormone [GH]), and in hypopituitarism.

The physical changes related to excess growth hormone are slow to develop and often go unnoticed by the patient. Instead, complaints in acromegaly are nonspecific, such as fatigue, arthralgias, or headaches. Hypersomnulence (due to sleep apnea) and increased sweating can also be seen.

Symptoms of Cushing's disease are discussed in Chapter 50. Nonfunctioning adenomas and gonadotropin-producing adenomas usually produce local, not systemic, symptoms such as **visual defects** and **headaches**. TSH-producing adenomas are rare and mimic symptoms of hyperthyroidism (see Chapter 46).

Symptoms of **hypopituitarism** are related to the lack of pituitary hormones. Loss of axillary and pubic hair, impotence, fatigue, and weight loss or gain are all seen. Polyuria and polydipsia suggest diabetes insipidus. Lack of lactation following pregnancy may be the first suspicion of **Sheehan's syndrome** (postpartum infarction of the pituitary, often due to hypotension during delivery).

Physical Examination

Hypertension is often seen in acromegaly and Cushing's disease. Orthostatic hypotension may be seen in panhypopituitarism.

Skin exam is notable for:

▲ hirsutism (Cushing's disease, acromegaly)

▲ moist, doughy skin (acromegaly)

▲ purple stria (Cushing's disease)

Widening of the spaces between teeth, macroglossia, and coarse facial features are also seen in acromegaly.

The proximity of the pituitary to the optic chiasm may result in visual field deficits due to compression from a large adenoma. By compressing the chiasm itself, the adenoma primarily affects the optic fibers that cross over the midline (temporal visual fields), resulting in the classic **bitemporal hemianopsia**.

Differential Diagnosis

Causes of **hypopituitarism** include:

▲ large pituitary adenomas

TABLE 51-1
Hormones and Their Major Functions

Hormone	Function
Growth hormone (GH)	Regulation of growth and metabolism
Adrenocorticotropin (ACTH)	Controls secretion of glucocorticoids
Luteinizing hormone (LH)	Controls gonadal function
Follicle stimulating hormone (FSH)	Controls gonadal function
Prolactin	Necessary for lactation
Thyroid stimulating hormone (TSH)	Regulates thyroid function
Oxytocin	Necessary for milk secretion in lactation
Vasopressin	Regulates water excretion

▲ hypothalamic tumors (e.g., craniopharyngioma)

▲ granulomatous disease (sarcoidosis, tuberculosis)

▲ postpartum necrosis (Sheehan's syndrome)

▲ radiation

▲ infiltrative diseases (hemochromatosis, amyloidosis)

In the patient with **amenorrhea** and **hirsutism**, consider:

▲ pituitary disorders (Cushing's disease, acromegaly)

▲ polycystic ovary syndrome

▲ congenital adrenal hyperplasia

Always remember to rule out pregnancy in women with amenorrhea.

Laboratory Studies
Pituitary Adenomas
Prolactin levels will be elevated in patients with prolactinomas, usually levels above 150 μg/L. Mild elevations in prolactin may be seen with nonfunctioning pituitary adenomas (due to stalk compression), dopamine antagonists (such as phenothiazines), pregnancy, and hypothyroidism. GH is difficult to measure due to its pulsatile secretion, and therefore **somatomedin-C**, produced by the liver in response to GH, is measured instead. Elevated levels of somatomedin-C are found in acromegaly. Cushing's disease may be screened for by an **overnight dexamethasone suppression test** and confirmed by elevated levels of free cortisol in the urine. These tests are discussed further in Chapter 50.

Magnetic resonance imaging is the radiologic test of choice for pituitary abnormalities. The pituitary as well as the optic chiasm is well visualized. Pituitary tumors are classified as microadenomas (<10 mm) and macroadenomas (>10 mm).

Panhypopituitarism
Laboratories reveal deficiencies in multiple peripheral hormones (thyroxine, testosterone or estrogen, cortisol) without an increase in the respective pituitary hormones. These patterns include:

▲ low free T4 (thyroxine) and T3 in the setting of low or low-normal TSH

▲ low testosterone or estrogen with low FSH and LH

▲ suboptimal Cortrosyn stimulation test (may still be normal in hypopituitarism of recent onset such as Sheehan's syndrome)

Note that since prolactin secretion is under chronic inhibition, prolactin level may be normal or slightly elevated.

Diabetes Insipidus
This disorder is suggested by **low urine osmolality** in the setting of **high serum osmolality**. Under direct supervision, the patient is restricted from fluid intake until serum osmolality is greater than 295 mOsm/kg. Patients fail to increase the urine osmolality; improvement with administration of vasopressin confirms a central etiology (pituitary or hypothalamic) to the disorder.

▶ MANAGEMENT
Management Strategy
Pituitary Adenomas
Management of adenomas is directed at correcting the oversecretion of hormone and mass effects. In most cases, this goal is accomplished by resection of the pituitary adenoma. **Transsphenoidal surgery** is the standard of care and if performed well, can lead to remission in 70 to 80% of patients. Surgery is less successful for larger tumors.

The exception to this approach is prolactin microadenomas, which may remain stable for years. These patients may be conservatively followed or treated medically (especially women wishing for pregnancy or resuming menses to prevent osteoporosis). Medical treatment is listed below (therapeutics).

Conventional radiation therapy has been used in the past, but side effects of hypopituitarism and overall lack of efficacy have relegated this technique to an adjunctive role in refractory patients. Newer techniques, such as "gamma knife" and heavy particle therapy, show higher success rates.

Panhypopituitarism

Patients with large adenomas should have a resection as above. Most patients have irreversible causes, and treatment consists of hormone replacement therapy. Daily medications include prednisone (5 to 7.5 mg) and levothyroxine (0.05 to 0.15 mg). Replacement of estrogen in women and testosterone in men relieve symptoms of hypogonadism. Cortisol should be the first hormone replaced, and stress doses (hydrocortisone 100 mg tid) are indicated during surgery.

Therapeutics

Bromocriptine, a dopamine agonist, is the treatment of choice for most prolactin microadenomas. Menses returns and fields improve in 80% of patients. Side effects are orthostasis, nausea, and vomiting.

Somatostatin, an inhibitor of GH, is effective in only 50% of patients with acromegaly. It is given subcutaneously; side effects are cramps, diarrhea, and gallstones. It is used primarily as an adjunct.

Desmopressin (dDAVP), a synthetic vasopressin, is used for central diabetes insipidus. It is given intranasally twice daily.

Continued Care

Patients with pituitary tumors should have a formal examination of visual fields and those with deficits followed closely for worsening. Blood levels of hormones may be followed during treatment or after surgery to assess response. Patients undergoing surgery or radiation should be monitored for the development of hypopituitarism or diabetes insipidus. Patients with acromegaly have an increased rate of colonic polyps and should be screened with colonoscopy.

▶ KEY POINTS

1. Most pituitary adenomas are "nonfunctioning"; the most common functioning adenomas are prolactinomas.

2. Prolactinomas often present as amenorrhea and galactorrhea in women. Diagnosis is confirmed by an elevated prolactin (>150 µg/L) and treatment in most cases is bromocryptine.

3. Acromegaly (excess GH) often presents as fatigue and arthralgias, sometimes in association with common disorders such as diabetes, hypertension, or carpal tunnel syndrome. Somatomedin-C levels are elevated.

4. Hypopituitarism is suspected in patients with hypogonadism who have low levels of FSH and LH. TSH is also low or normal. Causes include large nonfunctioning adenomas and radiation exposure.

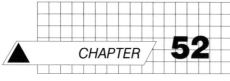

CHAPTER 52

Nutritional Disorders

*N*utritional disorders can be grouped on the basis of the nutrient involved: protein, carbohydrates, and fats (structural/energy nutrients), vitamins, and trace elements. Regarding structural/energy nutrients, both deficiency (protein-calorie malnutrition) and excess (obesity) are commonly encountered. Vitamin deficiencies are only rarely seen in clinical practice, even in developing countries. In fact, syndromes caused by vitamin excess (hypervitaminosis) are more frequent than deficiencies. Both deficiency and toxic states are encountered with trace elements.

▶ ENERGY-STRUCTURAL NUTRIENTS
Protein-Calorie Malnutrition

Protein-calorie malnutrition (PCM) is a common and severe nutritional problem in developing countries. PCM has traditionally divided into two distinct clinical syndromes:

▲ Kwashiorkor, caused by **protein deficiency in the setting of adequate energy intake**. The classic clinical picture is of a child with limb wasting, edema, and abdominal distension from hepatomegaly and ascites.

▲ Marasmus, caused by **deficiency in both calories and protein**. Patients with marasmus exhibit generalized wasting without edema and organomegaly.

In industrialized countries, these distinct syndromes are rarely encountered. However, PCM is still a common condition, encountered in severe systemic illness (e.g., heart failure, renal failure, malignancy, HIV infection), psychiatric patients, substance abusers (drug and alcohol), and children and the elderly (particularly of low socioeconomic class).

PCM leads to abnormalities in virtually every organ system; however, defects in **immune function** (leading to increased risk of infection) and **wound healing** are of primary clinical concern. Both contribute to mortality in systemically ill patients. Prevention of PCM by **formal assessment of energy requirements** should be undertaken in all ill patients who are admitted to the hospital or diagnosed with a systemic illness.

Patients who are found to have PCM or who are at increased risk for its development can be treated by **calorie supplementation** (see Chapter 45).

Obesity

One measure of obesity is the body mass index (BMI), which is defined as weight (in kg) ÷ height (in m²). The patient's BMI can be compared with tables of normal values. There is no set level at which an individual is considered obese, but a BMI above the 85th percentile has been shown to be **associated with a health risk**.

The significance of obesity lies in the association with a number of disorders:

▲ Type II (non-insulin-dependent) diabetes mellitus is three times more common in obese patients. In the United States, 85% of type II diabetics are obese. Obesity appears to predispose to the development of diabetes via a number of mechanisms; **insulin resistance** (see Chapter 47) associated with obesity apparently plays a significant role.

▲ Hypertriglyceridemia and, to a lesser extent, hypercholesterolemia ensue. Hypertriglyceridemia may be a manifestation of the hyperinsulinemia that results from insulin resistance.

▲ Hypertension: although the mechanism is not known, obesity increases the chance of developing hypertension. Weight loss in obese individuals leads to reductions in the degree of systemic hypertension.

▲ Respiratory disturbances: severe obesity can lead to significant hypoventilation with cyanosis and hypercapnia (pickwickian syndrome). Sleep apnea also appears to occur in obese individuals. Chronic hypoventilation can lead to pulmonary hypertension and cor pulmonale.

▲ Cardiovascular disturbances: due to a number of factors, including hypertension, increased work load, and hyperlipidemia, obese patients are at greater risk for the development of heart failure and coronary artery disease. Cerebrovascular disease is also more common in obese individuals.

▲ Musculoskeletal disturbances: the stress of increased weight increases the incidence of degenerative joint disease. The lower back and large joints of the lower extremities are particularly affected.

▲ Gastrointestinal disease: obesity is a risk factor for the development of **cholesterol gallstones**.

The **management of obesity** is often frustrating for patients and physicians alike. A contributing factor is that the primary interventions require significant modifications of lifestyle. **Diet modification** is the key intervention in the treatment of obesity. Reduction of intake (calories) to a level below the daily expenditures (see Chapter 45) will result in the consumption of stored calories from fat. Many different diets are advertised, but there is no convincing evidence that any one has an advantage over the other. Provided that the diets are not deficient in any major nutrients, a reduction in caloric intake with one diet should produce results similar to any other.

Exercise is a useful adjunct to diet therapy in obese patients. Exercise increases the daily energy expenditure. In addition, regular exercise can increase the chances that weight loss will be maintained.

Drugs can also be used to aid in weight loss. The main drugs that are used are **anorexants** that act to decrease appetite. **Amphetamine derivatives** and the central serotonin inducing drug **fenfluramine** are among the more commonly used agents. The development of tolerance and side effects limit their use. The association between fenfluramine use and pulmonary hypertension has virtually eliminated its use in weight loss. One strategy is to use these drugs for short periods to help patients overcome a "weight plateau" but then continue with diet and exercise alone.

Surgery is used in patients who are morbidly obese and have life-threatening complications like cor pulmonale and severe apnea. **Small bowel bypass** has been traditionally used, but due to the multiple complications associated with the procedure (diarrhea, electrolyte losses, vitamin deficiencies, pseudo-obstruction, hepatic failure, arthritis), **gastric plication** has become more popular. This procedure has the advantage of being reversible. Still, surgery is reserved for patients who have severe complications from obesity.

▶ VITAMINS

Vitamins are organic compounds that serve as cofactors for enzymes or (in the case of vitamin A and the visual pigments) prosthetic groups necessary for a functional molecule. The body may be able to synthesize some vitamins at a low level; in other cases, there is an absolute dietary requirement for the vitamin. Because of the widespread availability of vitamin supplements, the classic syndromes of severe vitamin deficiency (Table 52-1) are rarely encountered in modern clinical practice. The notable exception is the high incidence of certain vitamin deficiencies that occur in the setting of alcohol abuse.

▶ TRACE ELEMENTS

The trace elements are those that are present in body fluids at concentrations less than 1 µg/g wet weight. This includes cobalt, copper, manganese, selenium, and zinc. Deficiency is commonly due to inadequate dietary intake or loss in body fluids (e.g., pancreatic fistula). Toxicity can occur due to excess of these elements and other metals (e.g., aluminum, nickel, lead). The clinical syndromes of deficiency and toxicity are varied and can affect almost any organ system. Some of the more common disorders are:

▲ iron deficiency-anemia

▲ zinc deficiency, which causes dermatitis, diarrhea, and impaired spermatogenesis

▲ aluminum toxicity, seen in patients on chronic hemodialysis, which manifests as neurologic compromise, osteomalacia, andanemia

▶ KEY POINTS

1. Protein-calorie malnutrition is commonly encountered among seriously ill patients and contributes to mortality.

2. Obesity is associated with a number of health risks, many of which are reduced with the loss of excess weight.

3. The management of obesity focuses on reduction of intake (calories) coupled with exercise.

4. In industrialized countries, vitamin toxicity (excess) is more commonly encountered than deficiency states.

TABLE 52-1

Classic Syndromes of Vitamin Deficiency or Excess

Vitamin	Function	Deficiency	Excess/Toxicity
B_1 (thiamin)	Coenzyme to carbon–carbon bond cleavage (decarboxylases, transketolases)	Most commonly due to alcoholism; clinical syndrome of beri-beri—high output heart failure and nervous system disturbances (Wernicke-Korsakoff syndrome) with ataxia, confabulation	Intravenous administration is rarely associated with an anaphylactoid reaction
B_2 (riboflavin)	Cofactor in a number of oxidation-reduction reactions	Dietary insufficiency most common; clinically manifests as angular stomatitis, glossitis, cheilosis, corneal irritation, dermatitis, delayed intellectual development	None known
B_6 (pyridoxine)	Coenzyme in the intermediate metabolism of amino acids; also involved in heme and sphingosine synthesis	Generally via dietary insufficiency; certain drugs can cause deficiency, notably isoniazid and cycloserine; clinical manifestations of weakness, dermatitis, stomatitis, glossitis, peripheral neuropathy	With extremely high doses (1000× the recommended daily allowance), sensory neuropathy has been reported
B_{12} (cobalamin)	Cofactor in carbon transfer; required for DNA synthesis	Prolonged dietary deficiency; clinically manifests as megaloblastic anemia with neurologic abnormalities (see Chapter 62)	None known
Folate	Cofactor in carbon transfer; required for DNA synthesis	Dietary deficiency; megaloblastic anemia	None known
Niacin	Coenzyme in oxidation-reduction reactions	Can be synthesized in small amounts from dietary tryptophan, deficiency secondary to diet (classic association with diet that has corn as a staple); clinical syndrome of pellagra-diarrhea, dementia, dermatitis, mucosal abnormalities	Large doses (e.g., used in therapy of hypercholesterolemia) can cause histamine release and manifest as flushing, pruritus, and gastrointestinal disturbances
C (ascorbic acid)	Involved in many oxidation-reduction reactions and collagen synthesis	Dietary deficiency; manifests as clinical syndrome of scurvy, with easy bruising (capillary fragility), purpura, bleeding gums, poor wound healing	High doses can cause gastrointestinal discomfort, false-negative guaiac test for fecal blood, predispose to formation of oxalate stones; may also exacerbate systemic acidosis in the setting of renal disease
A (retinoic acid)	Prosthetic group in visual pigments, also appears to influence development of epithelial cells	Dietary deficiency, alcoholism appears to exacerbate; night blindness is often initial symptom; can progress to conjunctival dryness and corneal ulceration and necrosis; skin dryness and hyperkeratosis can be seen	Acute toxicity can cause central nervous system effects (headaches, drowsiness, increased intracerebral pressure, papilledema); chronic excess can cause alopecia, hepatosplenomegaly, hyperostosis, joint pain
E (tocopherol)	Antioxidant	Deficiency usually results from severe malabsorption; clinically may manifest as areflexis, ophthalmoplegia, and loss of proprioception	High doses can cause gastrointestinal symptoms such as flatulence and diarrhea
D (cholecalciferol)	Involved in calcium homeostasis	Usually due to nutritional deficiency, also reduced sunlight exposure, manifests as rickets in children (bowed limbs, pathologic fractures, delayed growth) and osteomalacia in adults (bone pain, fractures, limb weakness); osteomalacia often requires bone densitometry for diagnosis	Toxicity generally results in hypercalcemia (see Chapter 49)
K	Required for the proper synthesis of coagulation factors	Synthesized by intestinal bacteria and also in diet, so clinical deficiency is rare in adults, more common in newborns; if present, manifests as bleeding tendency	None known

CHAPTER 53

Hyperlipidemia

*H*yperlipidemia consists of elevated cholesterol levels or elevated triglyceride levels. Hypercholesterolemia has been unequivocally associated with premature coronary artery disease (CAD). Hypertriglyceridemia has less of an association with heart disease but at high levels leads to pancreatitis. Recommendations on screening and treatment in this chapter are based on the recent National Cholesterol Education Program.

Serum lipids are measured in the blood as follows:

▲ Low-density lipoproteins (LDL): "bad" cholesterol, most closely associated with cardiac disease;

▲ High-density lipoproteins (HDL): "good" cholesterol, involved in removing cholesterol from tissues and protecting against CAD;

▲ Triglycerides: used as a proxy measure for very-low-density lipoproteins (VLDL) in the fasting state.

▶ EPIDEMIOLOGY

Cholesterol levels rise with age by about 2 mg/dL each year. Women have lower cholesterol levels than men until menopause, when values become more equivalent. Hypercholesterolemia is extremely common, with over 20% of adults having cholesterol levels greater than 240 mg/dL.

▶ ETIOLOGY

Genetic factors play a role in the development of hyperlipidemia, mostly through polygenic mechanisms. A few autosomal disorders account for a small number of individuals with extreme elevations in lipids. **Familial hypercholesterolemia** is characterized by a defective hepatic LDL receptor, resulting in LDL elevations. **Familial combined hyperlipidemia** is a more common disorder that may present with elevation in cholesterol, triglycerides, or both.

Dietary factors that may increase cholesterol include a high intake of saturated fats and exogenous cholesterol. Alcohol increases triglycerides by inhibiting their metabolism.

▶ RISK FACTORS

Evaluation of hyperlipidemia involves assessing for additional risk factors for CAD:

▲ men older than 45 years or women older than 55 years

▲ family history of premature CAD (men <55 or women <65)

▲ current smoking

▲ hypertension

▲ diabetes mellitus

▲ low HDL cholesterol (<35 mg/dL)

High HDL cholesterol (>60 mg/dL) is considered a protective factor; patients with high HDL are considered to have one less risk factor.

▶ CLINICAL MANIFESTATIONS

History

The history should concentrate on obtaining additional risk factors for CAD (see above) and comorbid factors that may influence treatment decisions, such as a history of diabetes, peptic ulcer, or gout.

Physical Examination

Physical examination is almost always normal in hyperlipidemia, except in cases of extreme elevation of cholesterol, as seen in hereditary disorders. Physical findings include:

▲ **tendinous xanthomas** (subcutaneous painless nodules located on extensor tendons or Achilles tendon)

▲ **eruptive xanthomas** (smaller yellowish papules occurring on buttocks and pressure-sensitive surfaces)

▲ **xanthlasmas** (yellowish plaques located on eyelids)

▶ DIFFERENTIAL DIAGNOSIS

Once the diagnosis of hyperlipidemia is made, always consider other disorders that may increase lipid levels, such as:

▲ hypothyroidism

▲ nephrotic syndrome

▲ diabetes mellitus

▲ cholestatic liver disease

▲ drugs (thiazides, beta-blockers, oral contraceptives)

▶ DIAGNOSTIC EVALUATION

The initial screening test in healthy patients should be a nonfasting total cholesterol and an HDL level. A cholesterol of less than 200 mg/dL and an HDL over 35 mg/dL are desirable values. All patients with cholesterol levels more than 240 mg/dL, all patients with HDL cholesterol less than 35 mg/dL, and patients with borderline cholesterol values (200 to 239) and two or more additional risk factors for CAD (see Risk Factors above) should return for a fasting lipid analysis. In a fasting analysis, triglycerides are measured as well, and LDL is calculated by the following equation: LDL = Total Cholesterol − (HDL) − (Triglycerides ÷ 5). This calculation is only accurate in the fasting state and if the triglyceride level is less than 400 mg/dL.

Laboratory tests to obtain to rule out secondary causes include thyroid-stimulating hormone (hypothyroidism), fasting glucose or HbA1C (diabetes mellitus), and urinalysis for protein (nephrotic syndrome).

Treatment

Treatment for hyperlipidemia is directed at lowering risk of CAD. Intensity of treatment depends on the patient's individual risk for CAD and the level of LDL (Table 53-1). Treatment may be divided into nonpharmacologic measures (diet, exercise, smoking cessation) or pharmacologic measures. Weight loss, smoking cessation, and aerobic exercise are some of the few techniques to raise HDL.

Overall, treatment is most aggressive in patients with known CAD (LDL goal below 100 mg/dL), often requiring lipid-lowering agents. On the other hand, drug therapy should be delayed in men under age 35 and premenopausal women because of the low incidence of CAD in these populations. However, patients with a strong family history and high cholesterol may have a hereditary disorder requiring more intense treatment.

Dietary therapy limits the intake of cholesterol and saturated fats. A step 1 diet is the initial recommendation and involves daily intake of less than 300 mg of cholesterol, less than 30% of calories from fat, and 8 to 10% of calories from saturated fat. All animal products contain cholesterol, and patients should substitute meat and dairy products with fruits, grains, and vegetables. If unsuccessful, a more restrictive step 2 diet may be recommended; cholesterol is limited to less than 200 mg daily with less than 7% of calories obtained from saturated fat.

Patients have varied responses to dietary intake. Those who already have well-balanced diets may show no change in their cholesterol values. On average, cholesterol will decrease by 5 to 10% of total value with a step 1 diet. The largest decrease in total cholesterol through diet is probably about 20 to 25%; therefore, if a greater decrease is desired, drug therapy may be considered early.

Drug therapy in hyperlipidemia consists of five main classes of drugs. The drugs differ in their side effects, potency, and lipid-lowering properties (Table 53-2).

Niacin is often considered a first-line therapy to lower LDL and raise HDL (through an unknown mechanism). However, this drug is limited by its side effects, most notably flushing. This unpleasant warm feeling can affect patients at any time, although it most often occurs with higher doses. To avoid these side effects, begin with low-dose niacin (100 mg tid), use prophylactic aspirin (325 mg) to counteract flushing for the first few weeks, and advance the dose slowly, doubling every 2 weeks until reaching 500 to 1000 mg tid. Even with these efforts, up to 50% of patients will discontinue the medication. Other side effects include aggravating peptic ulcer disease, gout, and hyperglycemia (in diabetics).

TABLE 53-1

Levels of LDL to Begin Treatment

Risk Factors	Dietary Rx	Drug Rx
0–1	>160	>190
2 or more	>130	>160
Known CAD	>100	>130

Values are based on patient's CAD risk.

TABLE 53-2

Drug Effects on Lipid Profiles

	LDL	HDL	Triglycerides
Niacin	↓	↑↑	↓
HMG-CoA reductase inhibitors	↓↓	±	±
Bile acid resins	↓	—	↑
Fibric acid derivatives	↑↓	↑	↓↓
Hormone replacement therapy	↓	↑	↓

The **HMG-CoA reductase inhibitors** include all the statins (atorvastatin, fluvastatin, lovastatin, pravastatin, simvastatin) and inhibit the rate-limiting step in cholesterol synthesis. They are the most successful in reducing LDL levels (20 to 30% reduction) and are easy to administer (once daily). Important side effects include myositis (especially when taken with niacin or fibric acid derivatives) and elevated liver function tests. Patients who complain of muscle pain or cramping on these medications should be examined and creatine kinase levels checked.

Bile acid sequestrants (cholestyramine, colestipol) are nonabsorbable drugs that bind bile acids and prevent enterohepatic circulation of cholesterol. Side effects include bloating and constipation and binding certain drugs (e.g., digoxin, thyroxine, warfarin). These agents are administered in scoops of powder twice daily.

Fibric acid derivatives (gemfibrozil) are reserved for lowering triglycerides by increasing VLDL metabolism. HDL cholesterol may increase as well if triglycerides are lowered. Gemfibrozil (300 to 600 mg bid) is also limited by gastrointestinal side effects and may increase the risk of gallstones.

Estrogen replacement therapy is a reasonable option in all postmenopausal women. Because unopposed estrogen increases the risk of endometrial cancer, progestin should be added (unless patient has undergone hysterectomy).

Patients should have a fasting lipid analysis 1 to 3 months after a change of therapy. Failure to achieve LDL goal leads to increasing dietary restrictions and adding or increasing medication. Given the risk of myositis with niacin and fibrates, the statins are best combined with bile acid resins.

▶ KEY POINTS

1. Screening for hyperlipidemia consists of a nonfasting cholesterol and high-density lipoprotein; desirable values are less than 200 mg/dL and greater than 35 mg/dL, respectively.

2. Secondary causes of hyperlipidemia include nephrotic syndrome, diabetes, liver disease, and hypothyroidism.

3. Treatment is initially dietary restriction.

4. Drug treatment includes niacin (inexpensive but flushing problematic) and the statin drugs; the LDL goal is based on CAD risk.

5. Patients with known CAD have a goal of LDL < 100 mg/dL.

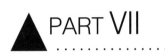

PART VII

Rheumatology

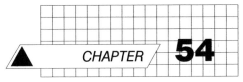

CHAPTER 54

Acute Monoarticular Arthritis

*A*cute monoarticular arthritis is an inflammatory process that develops in a single joint, usually over several days. Rapid assessment is required to rule out bacterial infection, which quickly leads to irreversible joint damage if not treated. Accurate diagnosis requires joint aspiration and examination of synovial fluid.

▶ DIFFERENTIAL DIAGNOSIS

The differential diagnosis can be divided into several categories:

Infection

▲ gonococcal

▲ nongonococcal bacterial (most commonly *Staphylococcus aureus*)

▲ Lyme disease

Crystalline disease

▲ gout

▲ pseudogout

Trauma

▲ cruciate ligament or meniscal tear (knee)

▲ osteoarthritis

▲ hemarthrosis

Rheumatologic disease

▲ rheumatoid arthritis

▲ seronegative spondyloarthropathy

▲ systemic lupus erythematosus

Rheumatologic disease is often polyarticular but may present with solitary joint involvement in atypical cases. These diseases are discussed in detail in Chapters 56, 57, and 58.

▶ CLINICAL MANIFESTATIONS
History

Duration of symptoms assists in differentiating the likely cause of joint inflammation. Extremely rapid onset, especially when associated with a "pop" or "snap," implies torn menisci or ligaments. Gout and bacterial infection usually develop over hours to days, whereas pseudogout may take several days to develop. Rheumatologic causes are often more subacute, occurring over weeks.

A past history of monoarticular arthritis may suggest a crystalline or rheumatologic disease; a history of a tick bite strongly raises the suspicion of Lyme disease. Bacterial infection is more common in diabetics and intravenous drug users. Swelling of a prosthetic joint is of great concern for infection. Patients on anticoagulation drugs (heparin, warfarin) or with an inherited defect in coagulation (hemophilia) are at increased risk for hemarthrosis with minor trauma.

Risk factors for gout include diabetes, hypertension, obesity, hyperlipidemia, alcohol intake, and thiazide use.

Physical Examination

The presence of **fever** is an important sign because most patients with bacterial infection are febrile. However, gout and rheumatologic disease may also cause an increase in temperature.

Skin examination should concentrate on searching for the typical rashes of gonococcal (GC) infection or Lyme disease. **Skin lesions in GC** are found on the extremities, begin as small papules, and then quickly become pustular with a necrotic center. **Erythema migrans** (Lyme disease) is a round or oval lesion, well demarcated, and usually has central clearing. The diameter of the lesion is greater than 5 cm and median size is 15 cm. Other findings to look for on skin examination include gouty tophi (subcutaneous nodules found on extensor surfaces), needle track marks (risk for septic arthritis), and psoriatic plaques (spondyloarthropathy).

Joint examination reveals a warm and tender joint. Painful limitation of motion is almost always present with articular involvement but may sometimes be present in nonarticular causes of joint pain (e.g., cellulitis, tendinitis). The **knee joint** is the most common joint affected in bacterial infection, Lyme disease, pseudogout, and traumatic causes. Gout primarily affects the **first metatarsal joint** or **ankle joint** but may involve the knee as well.

► DIAGNOSTIC EVALUATION

Arthrocentesis is the definitive diagnostic procedure. Septic arthritis has a predilection for damaged joints; therefore, joint aspiration still needs to be performed in patients with a past history of osteoarthritis or crystalline-induced arthritis. Aspiration of some joints (e.g., hip) requires fluoroscopic or ultrasonographic guidance and should be performed by a specialist. Fluid appearance is sometimes helpful in determining etiology. The presence of frank blood on aspiration confirms hemarthrosis; cloudy or turbulent fluid is likely to be secondary to infection or crystalline disease.

Leukocyte count should be performed to determine the inflammatory nature of the effusion. Table 54-1 shows general guidelines in interpreting the leukocyte count. **Fluid culture** and **Gram's stain** are mandatory when infection is a possibility. Gram-positive cocci are seen in 80% of *S. aureus* infected joints. *Neisseria gonorrhea* are rarely seen.

Crystal examination should be performed on synovial fluid to rule out gout (needle-shaped, negatively birefringent crystals) or pseudogout (rhomboid, weakly positive birefringence). Figure 54-1 shows examples of these crystals. The presence of crystals does not exclude infection because damaged joints are more susceptible to infection.

Urethral, pharyngeal, cervical (in women), and rectal cultures should be sent on all patients with suspected GC infection. Partial thromboplastin time is elevated in patients with hemophilia. X-rays of the affected joint may show chondrocalcinosis in pseudogout or an associated fracture in traumatic causes. The presence of osteoarthritis may be seen, but this does not rule out other causes, such as crystalline disease or infection.

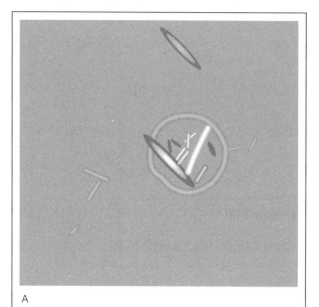

A

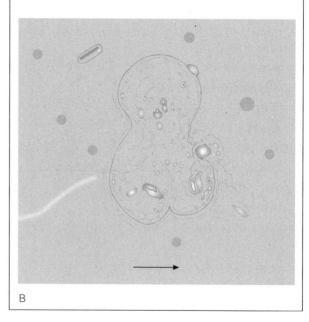

B

Figure 54-1 A. Urate crystal (gout). B. Calcium pyrophosphate (pseudogout).

Uric acid level is **not** useful to rule out gout because it is normal in 30% of patients with acute gouty arthritis. Lyme antibody is neither sensitive nor specific and **should not** be relied on for diagnosis.

► TREATMENT
Infection

Patients with suspected or confirmed bacterial infection should be receive parenteral antibiotic therapy as

TABLE 54-1
General Guidelines to Interpret Leukocyte Count

WBC Count (cells/mm³)	Interpretation
<200	Normal fluid
<2000	Noninflammatory (e.g., osteoarthritis)
2000–50,000	Mild to moderate inflammation (rheumatologic, crystalline)
50,000–100,000	Severe inflammation (sepsis or gout)
>100,000	Sepsis until proven otherwise

soon as cultures are sent. **Vancomycin** (1 g every 12 hours) is the drug of choice for most patients to cover *S. aureus*. Intravenous drug users or diabetic patients should be covered for gram-negative organisms as well. In the patient with suspected gonococcal infection (especially a young patient with rash or tenosynovitis), ceftriaxone is the drug of choice, although most disseminated GC is sensitive to penicillin. Repeated drainage is needed in all patients with confirmed septic arthritis to avoid joint damage. Acute Lyme disease is treated with doxycycline 100 mg twice daily for 2 to 3 weeks.

Crystalline Disease

Gout and pseudogout should be treated with a **nonsteroidal anti-inflammatory drug** (NSAID; such as indocin 50 mg three times daily). **Colchicine** may also be used but is limited by its side effects (diarrhea and myelosuppression). It may be used in patients unable to take NSAIDs (e.g., peptic ulcer disease) but should be avoided in patients with hepatic or renal disease. Intra-articular steroid injection is an alternative if oral therapy is contraindicated and infection has been excluded.

Traumatic Causes

General principles include rest, ice, elevation, and anti-inflammatory agents. Osteoarthritis may be treated with acetaminophen or NSAIDs. Active patients with possible ligament or meniscal tears should be referred to an orthopedic surgeon to consider arthroscopic repair.

▶ KEY POINTS

1. Acute monoarticular arthritis should be promptly evaluated because history and physical are unable to definitively rule out bacterial infection, which will lead to irreversible damage if untreated.

2. Gout often occurs in the first metatarsal or ankle joint. Diabetes, hypertension, obesity, and alcohol intake increase risk for gout. Treatment consists of NSAIDs or colchicine.

3. Gonococcal infection is a common cause of monoarticular arthritis in young individuals. Associated findings include pustular rash and tenosynovitis. Fluid Gram stain and synovial cultures are often negative. Treatment is ceftriaxone.

4. Bacterial infection should be ruled out by Gram stain and culture. Suspicion is high when fluid leukocyte count is >100,000 cells/mm^3.

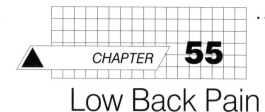

CHAPTER 55

Low Back Pain

*L*ow back pain affects about 80% of people at some time in their lives. Evaluation may not result in a specific diagnosis, but because most patients have resolution of the symptoms in 2 to 6 weeks, diagnostic testing can be limited to those patients with worrisome historical or physical findings.

▶ DIFFERENTIAL DIAGNOSIS

Differential diagnosis can be divided into several categories:

Musculoskeletal causes

▲ musculoskeletal (or ligamentous) injury

▲ herniated intervertebral disk

▲ spinal stenosis

▲ vertebral compression fracture

▲ spondylosis or spondylolisthesis

Systemic causes

▲ malignancy (breast, lung, prostate, multiple myeloma)

▲ vertebral osteomyelitis

▲ epidural abscess

▲ spondyloarthropathy

Referred pain

▲ aortic dissection

▲ pyelonephritis

▲ prostatitis

▲ pancreatic malignancy

▶ CLINICAL MANIFESTATIONS

The evaluation of low back pain is focused on two key aspects: evidence of systemic disease and evidence of nerve compression.

History

Although many patients with musculoskeletal injury will have pain radiating to buttocks or thighs, only true **sciatica** from nerve root compression radiates below the knee to the foot. Back pain without sciatica is rarely due to disk herniation. A history of low back pain with morning stiffness in a younger person raises the question of **ankylosing spondylitis**. The patient with **spinal stenosis** often presents with back or leg pain that worsens with walking (pseudoclaudication) and with prolonged standing.

Important "**red flags**" to obtain from the history are past history of malignancy, fever, weight loss, bladder or bowel dysfunction, and "saddle anesthesia." Patients with a previous diagnosis of cancer should be presumed to have back pain secondary to malignancy until proven otherwise. **Fever** and back pain raises the suspicion of osteomyelitis or epidural abscess.

Age is an important risk factor for worrisome etiologies of back pain. Compression fractures, malignancy, and spinal stenosis increase in incidence with age. Additional information to obtain includes relation of the back pain to litigation or worker's compensation. These nonmedical factors may influence the patient's desire for testing and recovery.

Physical Examination

Physical examination focuses on elucidating signs of **nerve root compression**. Disk herniation occurs at the L4–L5 level or L5–S1 level in 95% of all disk herniations. Weakness of dorsiflexion occurs in L5 root compression, and weakness of plantar flexion occurs in S1 root compression. Cauda equina syndrome is an extremely uncommon occurrence in disk herniation but is a "must-not-miss" diagnosis. Sensory examination in these patients may reveal saddle anesthesia (decreased sensation over buttocks, perineum, and posterior thighs). Table 55-1 lists these syndromes associated with disk herniation.

Straight leg raising should also be performed in patients with suspected disk herniation. With the patient supine, the extended leg is raised off the table. A positive sign reproduces back pain or sciatica at 30 to 60 degrees of elevation. A more specific (but less sensitive) sign is pain that is reproduced when the contralateral leg is raised.

Paraspinal tenderness is often seen in musculoskeletal strain but is difficult to reproduce. Osteomyelitis or epidural abscess may cause focal vertebral tenderness. Although pain may limit range of motion in many cases of back pain, limited flexion is also seen in ankylosing spondylitis.

TABLE 55-1

Findings of Herniated Disks

Disk	Nerve Root			
Location	Involved	Pain Radiation	Neuro Deficits	Additional Features
L4–L5	L5	Anterolateral leg and great toe	Dorsiflexion (ankle and great toe)	
L5–S1	S1	Posterior leg and lateral toes	Plantar flexion (ankle)	Decreased ankle reflex
Midline disk herniation	Cauda equina	Bilateral leg numbness	Saddle anesthesia	Urinary retention

Over-reaction during the examination, superficial tenderness, and back pain with "axial loading" (pressing on patient's head) all suggest a psychological component to the back pain.

▶ DIAGNOSTIC EVALUATION

Most patients with low back pain and no worrisome clinical features need no further evaluation beyond history and physical examination and most patients improve in less than 4 weeks. Unnecessary testing may demonstrate radiologic findings such as spondylolisthesis or disk protrusion that are common in asymptomatic individuals and may mislead the physician.

Patients older than 50 or patients with a history of weight loss, malignancy, or chronic steroid use should have a **lumbar spine film** to look for compression fractures or malignant lesions. An erythrocyte sedimentation rate, although not specific or sensitive, may be elevated in infections or malignancies that cause back pain.

Further testing up depends on the response to treatment. **Treatment strategy** for nonworrisome low back pain consists of the following:

▲ Nonsteroidal anti-inflammatory drugs (NSAIDs), such as ibuprofen or naproxen;

▲ Bedrest for only 1 to 3 days because prolonged bedrest may lead to deconditioning and worse outcomes;

▲ Ice to affected area for first 24 hours, followed by warm compresses;

▲ Back exercises that extend and flex back muscles.

Magnetic resonance imaging and **surgical referral** should be considered for sciatica that fails to im-prove after 4 to 6 weeks, progressive neurologic deficit, findings suspicious for epidural abscess, and bilateral neurologic deficits or urinary retention (suggesting cauda equina syndrome). The cauda equina syndrome requires urgent evaluation.

Patients with a history or physical worrisome for malignancy should have **routine screening tests** performed for common malignancies that metastasize to the vertebrae (lung, prostate, breast). A new compression fracture without risks such as steroid use should raise the suspicion of multiple myeloma; **immunoelectrophoresis** may be performed to rule out this diagnosis. **Bone scans** are useful when searching for osteomyelitis or malignancy when plain films are unrevealing.

▶ KEY POINTS

1. Most patients with back pain do not receive a definitive diagnosis and are labeled with musculoskeletal strain; 80% of these patients improve with conservative treatment in less than 6 weeks.

2. Systemic causes of back pain include malignancy, infection, and spondyloarthropathy.

3. Patients at risk for compression fractures or malignancy should receive an initial lumbar spine film; magnetic resonance imaging should be reserved for selected patients with neurologic findings.

4. Treatment consists of short-term rest, ice, NSAIDs, and back exercises. Psychologic factors may impede the patient's recovery.

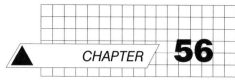

Rheumatoid Arthritis

Rheumatoid arthritis (RA) is an inflammatory arthritis characterized by lymphocytic infiltration of the synovial joints and granulomatous extra-articular nodules. RA affects 1% of the adult population with a peak onset most often between the ages of 25 and 40. Women are more affected than men (3:1).

There appears to be a genetic predisposition to RA, with a strong linkage to certain HLA-DR alleles. First-degree relatives of RA patients have a fourfold higher risk of developing the disease. Theories about infectious agents precipitating RA have not been proven.

▶ CLINICAL MANIFESTATIONS

History

Patients often present with **pain** and **swelling** in joints, usually a polyarticular symmetric arthritis. **Morning stiffness** (>1 hour) is a key feature. Constitutional symptoms such as weight loss, fatigue, and anorexia may also occur and even precede onset of joint symptoms.

Physical Examination

PIP

MCP

Most often involved are the **proximal interphalangeal**, **metacarpophalangeal**, and **wrist joints**. Examination of the joints reveals an inflammatory synovitis (warmth, tenderness, swelling). Late presentations include joint deformities such as ulnar deviation of the phalanges, swan neck, or boutonniere deformities (Fig. 56-1).

Subcutaneous **rheumatoid nodules** may be found on the extensor surfaces of the forearm and elbow or Achilles tendon. Splenomegaly may be found in RA and when also associated with leukopenia is known as **Felty's syndrome**. **Baker's cysts**, located in the popliteal fossa, may develop and mimic deep venous thrombosis by causing pain and swelling when they rupture.

RA may also be associated with a severe **vasculitis**, presenting with digital infarcts, palpable purpura, and mononeuritis multiplex.

▶ DIFFERENTIAL DIAGNOSIS

The differential diagnosis involves other etiologies of **arthritis** or joint pain, including:

▲ osteoarthritis

▲ psoriatic arthritis

▲ gout or pseudogout

▲ connective tissue diseases (lupus)

▲ septic arthritis

▲ Lyme disease

Diagnostic Evaluation

Table 56-1 shows the diagnostic criterion for RA. Most criteria are achieved through clinical examination and history. The two additional criteria are **rheumatoid factor** (RF) and **plain films**. RF is an autoimmune antibody to IgG and is positive in 70 to 80% of patients with RA. However, it is not specific for RA and by itself does not confirm the diagnosis. The following conditions may contain a positive RF in the absence of RA:

▲ older age

▲ other autoimmune diseases (systemic lupus erythematosus, sarcoid, etc.)

▲ infective endocarditis

▲ liver disease

▲ chronic infections (syphilis, leprosy, parasites)

▲ hyperglobulinemic states

Plain films of the hands may demonstrate periarticular osteopenia or erosions, usually in more advanced disease.

Other laboratory findings suggest the inflammatory nature of the disease, such as an increased erythrocyte sedimentation rate (ESR) or C-reactive protein. Joint aspiration is usually performed to rule out other causes, such as infection or gout. See Chapter 54 for joint fluid examination.

Chest x-ray may reveal extra-articular disease such as rheumatoid nodules, interstitial lung disease, or pleural effusions. Pulmonary nodules should be tested in the usual manner (see Chapter 18). Effusions that are tapped will show an exudative pattern, usually with a **low fluid glucose**.

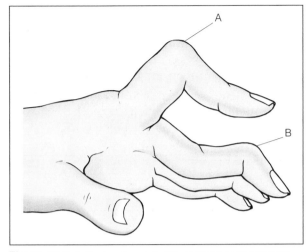

Figure 56-1 A. Boutonniere deformity. B. Swan neck deformity.

Patients with RA may also have **atlantoaxial subluxation** discovered on cervical spine films. This must be ruled out before manipulation of the patient's neck, as in endotracheal intubation.

▶ TREATMENT

The primary goal of treatment in RA is to achieve a complete remission, defined as absence of symptoms, no radiographic progression, and a normal ESR. For most patients, second-line drugs (so called **disease modifying agents**) are required to accomplish this goal. When remission is unable to be achieved, management focuses on pain control, maintenance of function, and slowing irreversible joint destruction. Patients with positive RF, erosions on hand films, or extra-articular manifestations tend to have a more severe disease course; however, there is no reliable way to predict poor prognosis.

Nonsteroidal anti-inflammatory drugs (NSAIDs) are the first-line therapy for RA. Examples include

---

TABLE 56-1

Criteria for Diagnosis of Rheumatoid Arthritis*

Morning stiffness of joints >1 hr
Arthritis (soft tissue swelling) of 3 or more joints
Arthritis of wrist, metacarpophalangeal, or proximal intraphalangeal joints
Symmetric arthritis
Rhematoid nodules
Elevated rheumatoid factor
Hand or wrist films showing erosions or periarticular osteopenia

*Four or more criteria necessary for definite diagnosis.

---

ibuprofen, ketoprofen, and naproxen. NSAIDs provide symptom relief for mild cases but do not significantly influence synovial inflammation or joint destruction. **Side effects of NSAIDs** are numerous and include:

▲ peptic ulcers/gastritis

▲ renal dysfunction

▲ increased liver enzymes

▲ rash

Corticosteroids remain controversial in RA. Low-dose prednisone may be effective, but the numerous side effects (osteoporosis, immunosuppression, hyperglycemia) make this choice less desirable.

Disease-modifying drugs (DMDs) have the added benefit of slowing disease progression in RA. Although once reserved for moderate to severe cases, these drugs are now started sooner because joint destruction may occur early if inflammation is uncontrolled. Typical DMDs and their common side effects are:

▲ sulfasalazine (rash)

▲ antimalarials, such as hydroxychloroquine (retinopathy)

▲ gold (bone marrow toxicity, proteinuria, rash)

▲ penicillamine (same as gold)

▲ azathioprine (immunosuppression)

▲ methotrexate (bone marrow toxicity, hepatic fibrosis, pneumonitis, stomatitis)

Methotrexate has recently gained increased popularity as a DMD. It is given in low dose (7.5–15 mg) in weekly intervals. A unique feature of methotrexate is that rheumatoid nodules may increase with initiation of treatment. Liver biopsy for cirrhosis was once recommended in all patients on treatment but now is reserved for persistent liver function abnormalities. Alcohol should certainly be avoided because this greatly increases risk of liver damage. Gastrointestinal symptoms may be decreased with oral folate supplements.

Monitoring in RA consists of following the patient's symptoms and joint examination for improvement. Other monitoring includes hand and/or foot films for disease progression, ESR, liver and renal function (especially patients on NSAIDs or methotrexate), and regular retinal evaluation (if on hydroxychloroquine).

▶ KEY POINTS

1. Rheumatoid arthritis is an inflammatory disease characterized by symmetric arthritis, most commonly affecting the wrist, metacarpophalangeal,

and proximal interphalangeal joints. Morning stiffness is a key feature.

2. Rheumatoid factor is positive in 70 to 80% of patients with RA. This is not a specific test, however. RF may be positive in older age, other autoimmune diseases, infective endocarditis, liver disease, chronic infections, and hyperglobulinemic states.

3. Extra-articular manifestations of RA include rheumatoid nodules, pleural effusions, vasculitis, and Felty's syndrome (associated splenomegaly and leukopenia). Associated conditions include atlantoaxial subluxation and Baker's cysts.

4. Treatment consists of NSAIDs followed by early institution of second-line agents such as sulfasalazine, methotrexate, or chloroquine.

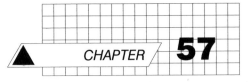
Seronegative Spondyloarthropathies

The seronegative spondyloarthropathies are an inter-related group of inflammatory disorders affecting the spine, joints, and periarticular structures. The **spondyloarthropathies** include:

▲ ankylosing spondylitis (AS)

▲ psoriatic arthritis

▲ enteropathic arthritis (associated with inflammatory bowel disease [IBD])

▲ reactive arthritis — Reiter's

Reiter's syndrome is a special type of reactive arthritis characterized by conjunctivitis, urethritis, and arthritis. Unless otherwise mentioned, statements concerning reactive arthritis apply to Reiter's as well.

▶ EPIDEMIOLOGY

Reactive arthritis and AS are **more common in men** than women (two of the few rheumatologic diseases showing a male predominance). The other disorders (the arthritis of IBD and psoriatic arthritis) are equally prevalent in men and women. Spondyloarthropathies usually occur in patients younger than 40 years old.

▶ ETIOLOGY

The spondyloarthropathies have varying degrees of association with **HLA B-27**. The strongest is AS, where 90% of patients are HLA B-27 positive. Family members positive for B-27 who have a first-degree relative with AS have a 10 to 20% chance of developing the disease.

Reactive arthritis (including Reiter's syndrome) appears to be precipitated by **infectious diarrhea** (due to salmonella, shigella, campylobacter, or yersinia) or **genitourinary infection** (chlamydia). Arthritis usually occurs 1 to 3 weeks after infection.

▶ CLINICAL MANIFESTATIONS
History

Chronic **low back pain,** with morning stiffness, in a young adult is the typical presenting symptom for AS. The subacute nature (worsening over several months) of the pain and its improvement with exercise distinguishes AS from the more common mechanical etiologies of back pain.

Enthesopathy (inflammation of ligaments and tendons) is a key feature of all spondyloarthropathies, often affecting the Achilles tendon or plantar fascia. Heel pain may be the presenting symptom in reactive arthritis.

Eye involvement occurs in about 20% of spondyloarthropathy cases. Conjunctivitis is a defining feature of Reiter's syndrome but also occurs in the other diseases. Uveitis (inflammation of pigmented structures: iris, ciliary body) can present as pain, photophobia, or decreased vision.

Physical Examination

Sacroileal involvement in AS may show pain on compression of pelvis, limitation of lumbar spine extension and lateral flexion, loss of normal lumbar lordosis, and tenderness to palpation around spinous processes and iliac crests.

Inflammation of tendons in reactive and psoriatic arthritis cause diffuse swelling of fingers or toes, leading to the typical "**sausage digit**" appearance. Peripheral arthritis is often asymmetric and localized to lower extremities (knees, ankles, metatarsophalangeal joints). Peripheral arthritis in IBD flares around the same time as the bowel symptoms and often improves with resection of diseased bowel. Spinal disease in IBD does not show this correlation.

In addition, certain **skin lesions** are helpful (although not always present) in differentiating the spondyloarthropathies. Psoriasis is characterized by erythematous scaly lesions, usually seen on extensor surfaces of the extremities, and nails may show pitting or oncolysis. The classic skin lesion of Reiter's syndrome is **keratoderma blenorrhagica**. This is a hyperkeratotic papular rash on the soles of the feet that mimics pustular psoriasis. Reiter's syndrome also is associated with **balanitis circinata**, which appears as shallow painless ulcers on the penis.

▶ DIFFERENTIAL DIAGNOSIS

In the patient who presents with **low back pain,** the differential includes:

▲ lumbar strain

▲ herniated vertebral disk

▲ spinal stenosis

▲ malignancy

In the patient with **inflammatory peripheral arthritis,** consider:

▲ septic arthritis (including gonococcal arthritis)

▲ gout

▲ Lyme disease

▲ rheumatoid arthritis

▲ connective tissue disease (e.g., lupus)

▲ sarcoidosis

▶ DIAGNOSTIC EVALUATION

Blood tests show signs typical of an inflammatory process, including **elevated ESR.** In addition, these diseases are seronegative for rheumatoid factor and antinuclear antibody, the reason for the name **sero-negative** spondyloarthropathies.

HLA typing for B-27 may be useful in cases that are atypical and the diagnosis is uncertain. Because 5% of caucasians are positive for B-27, this is not specific for spondyloarthropathies and not recommended as a screening test.

Spine and pelvic films may be normal in early disease but are often helpful. **X-ray features of anky-losing spondylitis** include:

▲ sacroilitis (erosions of iliac bone lead to "pseudo-widening" of joint, followed by sclerosis and obliteration)

▲ squaring of vertebrae on lateral view of spine

▲ ossification of ligaments between vertebral bodies ("bamboo spine")

Hand films in advanced psoriatic arthritis may reveal erosion of the distal interphalangeal joint, giving the "pencil in cup" appearance on x-ray.

In cases of suspected reactive arthritis, **stool cultures** for pathogens or **urethral chlamydial DNA probe** should be performed to rule out underlying infection. In cases of urethritis, gonococcal culture or probe should be performed as well, because this is an important distinction to make. Urinalysis may show a sterile pyuria.

▶ TREATMENT

The **natural history** of the spondyloarthropathies varies for each specific disease. AS is a lifelong disease and may remain localized or may ascend to the thoracic and cervical spine. The lifespan of patients with AS is usually normal.

Reactive arthritis is often self-limited but may become chronic or relapsing in 20 to 40% of patients and in severe cases resembles AS. Reactive arthritis (especially Reiter's) that is associated with chlamydial infection may benefit from prolonged treatment (3 months) with tetracycline.

Psoriatic arthritis and enteropathic arthritis may regress with treatment of the underlying disease. IBD-associated arthritis has improved with sulfasalazine or bowel resection (in ulcerative colitis). Psoriatic arthritis has been reported to respond to methotrexate or psoralen ultraviolet therapy. Otherwise, treatment is directed at symptoms. Anti-inflammatory medications are effective in most patients. Back extension exercises appear useful in maintaining mobility with sacroilitis.

First-line therapy in the spondyloarthropathies remains **nonsteroidal anti-inflammatory drugs** (NSAIDs), usually indomethacin 50 mg **tid** (see Chapter 56 for side effects). In refractory cases, **sulfasala-zine** 1 g **tid** has been tried with some success, even in absence of known IBD.

Glucocorticoids have not been effective and are generally not recommended. However, topical steroids may be used to treat associated uveitis.

Patients with chronic disease (such as AS) are at risk for complications many years after diagnosis. **Spinal fractures** may occur with minor trauma and should be suspected in the previously stable patient with an increase in back pain. Atlantoaxial subluxation may also occur, presenting as occipital pain with or without signs of cord compression.

About 10% of patients with AS may have **cardiac complications**, such as aortic insufficiency or conduction disease.

In patients with reactive arthritis due to chlamydial infection, prevention of recurrence by education and use of condoms is important. Recurrent attacks may be more severe than the primary occurrence.

▶ KEY POINTS

1. Spondyloarthropathy should be suspected in younger individuals complaining of back pain with stiffness or asymmetric lower extremity arthritis. Eye involvement (conjunctivitis or uveitis) is also a key feature.

2. Reiter's syndrome is a reactive arthritis occurring after infectious diarrhea or urethritis consisting of the classic triad of conjunctivitis, urethritis, and arthritis.

3. Patients with spondyloarthropathies have an increased incidence of HLA B-27 and are negative for rheumatoid factor and antinuclear antibodies.

4. Complications in ankylosing spondylitis include spinal fractures, atlantoaxial subluxation, aortic insufficiency, and cardiac conduction disease.

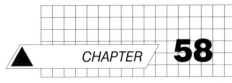
Connective Tissue Disease

*T*he term connective tissue disease (CTD) refers to one of a heterogeneous group of diseases that are characterized by alterations in immune function, often leading to the production of autoantibodies. Autoantibodies are immunoglobulins that are specific for self-antigens, often components of the cell nucleus.

A number of different clinical entities are classified as CTDs:

▲ systemic lupus erythematosus (SLE)

▲ rheumatoid arthritis (RA)

▲ systemic sclerosis (SSc), also known as scleroderma

▲ polymyositis/dermatomyositis (PM/DM)

▲ Sjögren's syndrome

▲ the spondyloarthropathies

▲ mixed connective tissue disorder (MCTD)

Both RA and the spondyloarthropathies are discussed in separate chapters (56 and 57, respectively) and are not the focus of this chapter.

▶ EPIDEMIOLOGY

Each CTD has particular **epidemiologic associations**:

▲ SLE: 90% of cases occur in women of childbearing age and is more common in blacks than whites.

▲ SSc: 75% of cases occur in women, disease onset generally between ages 40 and 60, and all races are affected.

▲ PM/DM: approximately one-third of cases occur in the setting of another CTD and about 10% of cases are associated with an underlying malignancy.

▲ Sjögren's syndrome: 90% of cases occur in women and, like PM/DM, a portion of cases occur in the setting of another CTD.

▲ MCTD: 80% of cases occur in women with a mean age of about 40 years old.

In addition, there are **genetic predispositions** to the development of a CTD. Many of these predispositions are related to inheritance of particular alleles of genes in the major histocompatibility complex (MHC), often MHC class II alleles.

▶ ETIOLOGY AND PATHOGENESIS

The etiology and pathogenesis of the CTDs are poorly understood. As mentioned above, many CTDs are associated with inheritance of particular MHC class II alleles. Because the MHC class II gene products are important in the **presentation of antigens** to the immune system, abnormalities in this function may result in the production of autoantibodies. It is not entirely clear if the specific autoantibodies are the cause of the disease manifestations rather than just a marker for altered immune function. Clinical disease can occur in the absence of specific autoantibodies.

The **pathology** that is encountered in CTD is diverse:

▲ Immune complex deposition: most often seen in SLE. Circulating immune complexes can be found in many forms of CTD, but deposition in tissues (e.g., the glomeruli) can result in tissue destruction.

▲ Vascular damage: damage to the blood vessels can be seen in many CTDs and may resemble that seen in the primary vasculitides (see Chapter 59). Abnormal immune responses (ranging from unregulated cytotoxic T-cell responses to antibody-mediated inflammation) are believed to be responsible.

▲ Overproduction and accumulation of extracellular matrix (ECM) components: after vascular damage occurs, deposition of collagen and other components of the ECM can occur. This is the outstanding pathologic feature of SSc and results in fibrosis of the skin and other organs.

▲ Altered immune responses: the widespread disturbances in immune function can lead to an immunosuppressed state where agents that normally engender a brisk immune response (e.g., viruses and encapsulated bacteria) may escape immune surveillance. This is compounded by the fact that many of the treatments for CTD involve immunosuppressive agents.

► CLINICAL MANIFESTATIONS

The **signs and symptoms** associated with CTDs vary and can involve almost any organ system:

▲ Systemic—fever, fatigue, anorexia, weight loss;

▲ Musculoskeletal—arthralgias, arthritis (erosive and nonerosive), myopathy, myositis;

▲ Dermatologic—rash (see below), Raynaud's phenomenon, mucosal ulcers, cutaneous ulcers, alopecia, skin thickening;

▲ Hematologic—anemia, thrombocytopenia, leukopenia, hypercoagulability, lymphadenopathy, vasculitis;

▲ Cardiac—pericarditis, myocarditis, hypertension, heart failure;

▲ Pulmonary—pleural effusions, pleurisy, pneumonitis, interstitial fibrosis, pulmonary hypertension, pulmonary hemorrhage;

▲ Renal—proteinuria, renal failure, nephrotic syndrome;

▲ Gastrointestinal—dysphagia, xerostomia, nausea, bleeding, ascites;

▲ Neurologic—seizures, mental status changes, peripheral neuropathy;

▲ Ocular—conjunctivitis/episcleritis, conjunctival dryness (sicca syndrome).

Rashes and other dermatologic signs are common in many CTDs:

▲ Erythematous rashes—malar ("butterfly") rash can be seen in lupus and dermatomyositis (in DM, the rash is a deeper lilac color, the so-called **helio-trope rash**);

▲ Vasculitic rashes—palpable purpura can be seen in many CTDs, often heralding a flare of disease;

▲ Ulcers—can be cutaneous or mucosal;

▲ Skin thickening—this is the hallmark of systemic sclerosis but can be seen in other CTDs;

▲ Calcinosis—calcific deposits in the intracutaneous and subcutaneous tissues;

▲ Raynaud's phenomenon—episodic vasoconstriction of small arteries/arterioles of the fingers and toes that is triggered by cold exposure, vibration, and emotional stress. The classic "tricolor" changes are initial pallor with cyanosis and rubor on rewarming.

Particular symptom complexes are characteristic for each CTD (Table 58-1) but **extensive overlap** is encountered. The clinical entity of mixed connective tissue disorder is defined by clinical features that can be seen in SLE, SSc, polymyositis, RA, and Sjögren's syndrome, accompanied by a particular autoantibody (anti-RNP). Other overlap syndromes cannot be formally defined and often are referred to as **undifferentiated connected tissue disorders**.

As a group, CTDs are notable for their **episodic nature**; patients may have relatively long periods without symptoms punctuated by acute flares of disease.

► DIFFERENTIAL DIAGNOSIS

The connective tissue disorders can mimic a wide variety of disease because of their extensive symptom complexes:

▲ Systemic diseases—cancer, primary vasculitis, allergic/hypersensitivity reactions;

▲ Musculoskeletal diseases—infectious myositis, degenerative joint disease, myasthenia gravis, motor neuron disease, primary muscular dystrophies;

▲ Dermatologic diseases—primary vasculitis, hypersensitivity reactions;

▲ Hematologic diseases—leukemia/lymphoma, myelodysplastic syndrome, hypercoagulability syndromes;

▲ Cardiac diseases—infectious pericarditis, secondary (e.g., uremic) pericarditis, amyloidosis;

▲ Pulmonary diseases—primary pulmonary hypertension, interstitial lung disease;

▲ Renal diseases—chronic renal failure from other causes, acute/chronic glomerular disease;

▲ Gastrointestinal diseases—malabsorption syndromes (e.g., gluten intolerance), achalasia, hepatic disease (cirrhosis, chronic hepatitis);

▲ Neurologic diseases—stroke, primary/secondary neuropathies.

► DIAGNOSTIC EVALUATION

The diagnosis of collagen vascular disease is usually initially suspected when a patient presents with a constellation of suggestive symptoms and signs. For example, when a young woman presents with several months of arthralgias, fatigue, and a suggestive facial rash, the diagnosis of SLE can be entertained. A preliminary laboratory workup is initiated, consisting of electrolytes, serum creatinine, complete blood count, liver function tests, ESR, and a screening antinuclear

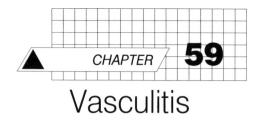
Vasculitis

The vasculitides, diseases involving inflammation of blood vessels, are syndromes characterized by the size of the blood vessel involved and the predominant organs that are affected. These **vasculitides** include:

▲ polyarteritis nodosa (PAN)

▲ Churg-Strauss disease (allergic angiitis and granulomatosis)

▲ Wegener's granulomatosis (WG)

▲ Takayasu's arteritis

▲ temporal arteritis

▲ hypersensitivity vasculitis (including Henoch-Schönlein purpura)

▶ EPIDEMIOLOGY

Most vasculitides occur in middle-aged individuals (mean age 40 to 45 years), with men affected slightly more often (ratio 1.3:1). Exceptions include temporal arteritis (elderly), Henoch-Schönlein purpura (mostly children), and Takayasu's arteritis (adolescent and young women). As a group, however, the vasculitides are rare.

▶ ETIOLOGY

Many cases of vasculitis such as PAN and hypersensitivity vasculitis may be associated with immune complex deposition. Other diseases (WG, Churg-Strauss) have a more prominent granulomatous involvement, suggesting cell-mediated pathology.

▶ CLINICAL MANIFESTATIONS
History

Many patients with vasculitis present with nonspecific findings such as **fever, weight loss, malaise,** and **arthralgias.** Organ-specific manifestations are more common in certain diseases. PAN affects the visceral arteries and may present with abdominal pain. Churg-Strauss disease presents as **recurrent asthma** attacks. WG often involves the lungs and upper airways, presenting as **recurrent sinusitis, dyspnea, cough,** and/or **hemoptysis. New onset headache, scalp tenderness, jaw claudication** in the elderly are seen in temporal arteritis. Takayasu's arteritis, which affects large vessels such as the carotid arteries, may cause **syncope** and **stroke.**

Hypersensitivity vasculitis may involve an offending drug or associated disease. Certain drugs may cause "serum sickness" occurring 7 to 10 days after primary exposure. Diseases associated with hypersensitivity vasculitis include **systemic lupus erythematosus** and **rheumatoid arthritis.** Finally, **chronic hepatitis C** may lead to essential mixed cryoglobulinemia, which also causes a hypersensitivity vasculitis.

Physical Examination

Physical examination may often reveal skin changes, most notably **palpable purpura.** These lesions are red to purple, raised, do not blanch, and usually appear on the lower extremities. Skin involvement is predominant in hypersensitivity vasculitis (and often the only organ affected). Purpura can be seen in the other vasculitides as well, although it is most common in Churg-Strauss disease.

Hypertension is seen in those diseases involving the renal vasculature: PAN, WG, Takayasu's arteritis, and Henoch-Schönlein purpura. Involvement of the subclavian arteries in Takayasu's arteritis (a.k.a., "pulseless disease") leads to diminished peripheral pulses. Temporal arteries may be tender to palpation and thickened in temporal arteritis.

Eye examination may reveal episcleritis or uveitis; nasal ulceration may be seen in WG. Neurologic manifestations include **mononeuritis multiplex** and **cranial nerve palsies.**

▶ DIFFERENTIAL DIAGNOSIS

Vasculitis presenting with fever, skin lesions, and weight loss must be differentiated from **subacute bacterial endocarditis.** Other causes of palpable purpura include **disseminated meningococcal** or **gonococcal infection** and **Rocky Mountain spotted fever.**

Eosinophilia with pulmonary infiltrates (as in Churg-Strauss disease) is also seen in **allergic bronchopulmonary** aspergillosis, **Loeffler's syndrome** (often parasitic in nature), and **chronic eosinophilic pneumonia.**

In the patient with WG presenting with pulmonary and renal disease, one must consider Goodpasture's syndrome (anti-GBM disease).

▶ DIAGNOSTIC EVALUATION

Elevated erythrocyte sedimentation rate is almost always seen with active vasculitis, often greater than 100 mm. Other signs of inflammation include a normochromic, normocytic anemia and thrombocytosis. Leukocytosis can also be seen, leading to a search for an infectious etiology. Eosinophilia is the hallmark of Churg-Strauss disease. Although hypersensitivity vasculitis may also have increased eosinophils in the blood, the history of recurrent asthma is not present.

Chest x-ray may reveal pulmonary infiltrates in both WG and Churg-Strauss disease; the former may also show cavitary lesions or nodules. A widened aorta may be seen in Takayasu's arteritis.

Antineutrophil cytoplasmic antibody, specifically the cytoplasmic type (c-ANCA), is diagnostic for WG in the setting of a compatible clinical picture. High titers of rheumatoid factor (RF) may be seen in rheumatoid vasculitis, although RF is also positive in mixed cryoglobulinemia. Hepatitis C antibody is often found in patients with mixed cryoglobulinemia, and hepatitis B surface antigen is seen in 30% of patients with PAN.

Renal disease may occur with all vasculitides but is most notable in WG and Henoch-Schönlein purpura. Glomerulonephritis and its manifestations are discussed in Chapter 24.

Biopsy remains the definitive test to document inflammation and destruction of the vessels. Table 59-1 shows the size and type of blood vessels affected and the predominant microscopic appearance. However, because vasculitis tends to be segmental and focal, biopsy may miss an affected area.

In cases where biopsy may be difficult to perform, angiography is used to confirm the diagnosis. Angiography of the mesenteric arteries in PAN shows a "beaded" appearance of aneurysms and segmental stenosis. In Takayasu's arteritis, the aorta and subclavian arteries can show irregular vessel walls, stenosis, and poststenotic dilatation.

▶ TREATMENT

Treatment is directed at the underlying disease for those vasculitides with known causes. Withdrawal of the offending drug in serum sickness and treatment of hepatitis C with interferon in mixed cryoglobulinemia are two such strategies. Henoch-Schönlein purpura often remits on its own. In the other diseases, immunosuppression is the mainstay of treatment. These treatments have led to major improvements in survival for PAN and WG, which previously had 5-year mortality rates of 85 to 100%.

Prednisone (1 mg/kg/d) and cyclophosphamide (2 mg/kg/d) are the first-line therapy for WG and PAN. Prednisone is usually continued for about 6 months and then tapered off to avoid long-term side effects such as cataracts and osteoporosis. Cyclophosphamide is continued for about 1 year. Complications of cyclophosphamide include hemorrhagic cystitis, bladder cancer, myelodysplasia, and infertility.

Prednisone (1 mg/kg) is required for temporal arteritis and Churg-Strauss disease. After improvement, a steroid taper may be attempted. Prednisone is also used for severe cases of Henoch-Schönlein purpura.

Takayasu's arteritis is treated with steroids and, in more severe cases, methotrexate. Aggressive surgical repair with grafting of affected arteries has markedly improved survival.

TABLE 59-1

Biopsy Results in the Vasculitides

Vasculitis	Vessels Involved	Appearance
PAN	Small to medium arteries	Mononuclear or PMNs, necrotizing
Churg-Strauss disease	Various sizes, including venules	Granulomas with eosinophils
Wegener's granulomatosis	Small arteries and veins	Granulomas
Takayasu's arteritis	Large arteries (aorta, subclavian)	Usually not biopsied
Temporal arteritis	Medium arteries (temporal)	Granulomas
Hypersensitivity vasculitis	Arterioles and venules	Leukocytoclastic vasculitis, IgA present in Henoch-Schönlein purpura

► KEY POINTS

1. Vasculitis may often present as fever, weight loss, and malaise. Accompanying symptoms specific to an organ system may help narrow the differential.

2. Palpable purpura is a common finding in the vasculitides, especially hypersensitivity vasculitis (including Henoch-Schönlein purpura) and Churg-Strauss disease. Purpura are also seen in life-threatening infections.

3. Pulmonary involvement occurs in both Wegener's granulomatosis and Churg-Strauss disease. The latter is also characterized by eosinophilia.

4. c-ANCA is highly specific for WG, although it may be negative in diseases limited to the lungs.

5. Treatment consists of prednisone and in some cases cyclophosphamide (WG and PAN).

Palpable purpura
- HSP
- churg-Strauss

Pulmonary sympts.
- Wegner's
- churg-strauss
  (eosinophilia)

C-ANCA
- wegner's

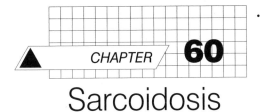

CHAPTER 60

Sarcoidosis

Sarcoidosis is a chronic, systemic, idiopathic granulomatous disease, primarily affecting the lungs. Although it can lead to progressive restrictive lung disease, most patients have a benign course, often with spontaneous remission.

▶ EPIDEMIOLOGY

Sarcoidosis is more prevalent in blacks than in whites in the United States. It is usually diagnosed in individuals aged 20 to 40 years; women are affected more than men.

▶ ETIOLOGY

The precipitating factor in sarcoidosis remains unknown. Atypical mycobacteria have been suspected because of the granulomatous nature of the disease, but this remains unproved. The central pulmonary granulomas are comprised mostly of helper (CD4+) cells, resulting in a deficiency of CD4 cells in the peripheral blood. This relative CD4 deficiency results in most sarcoid patients being anergic to skin testing.

▶ CLINICAL MANIFESTATIONS
History

Patients may have one of the following **presentations**:

▲ pulmonary complaints (dry cough, dyspnea)

▲ constitutional symptoms (fever, weight loss, fatigue)

▲ arthralgias (usually bilateral ankle pain)

However, another common presentation (5 to 10% of all cases) is the asymptomatic patient with hilar adenopathy on routine chest x-ray.

An occupational history should be obtained to rule out berylliosis, which may mimic the pulmonary findings of sarcoid. Beryllium exposure can occur in the aerospace, computer, and electronic industries. Beryllium exposure also occurred in fluorescent light manufacturing before the 1950s.

Physical Examination

Skin examination may reveal erythema nodosum, which are erythematous nodules often located on the lower extremities. Patients with this skin manifestation have an excellent prognosis.

Pulmonary examination is usually unrevealing. Periarticular swelling occurs in setting of joint involvement, and adenopathy (usually cervical) is often present. Involvement of the lacrimal and parotid glands may result in their enlargement. Uveitis and cranial nerve palsies (especially VII) are other manifestations of sarcoidosis.

▶ DIFFERENTIAL DIAGNOSIS

In the patient with hilar adenopathy and nonproductive cough, consider:

▲ tuberculosis

▲ lymphoma

▲ fungal infections (coccidiomycosis, histoplasmosis)

▲ berylliosis

In the patient with diffuse lung disease, consider:

▲ hypersensitivity pneumonitis

▲ Wegener's granulomatosis

▲ pneumoconiosis

▶ DIAGNOSTIC EVALUATION

Chest x-ray is almost always abnormal (even if asymptomatic) and is classified as follows:

▲ Stage 1: hilar adenopathy ± right paratracheal adenopathy;

▲ Stage 2: adenopathy as above with pulmonary infiltrates;

▲ Stage 3: pulmonary infiltrates without adenopathy.

A fourth stage, characterized by honeycombing, is sometimes distinguished from stage 3. Most individuals with stage 1 improve in the next 2 years, whereas less than 20% of those with stage 3 will improve.

Alkaline phosphatase may be elevated and is often due to hepatic granulomas. Hypercalcemia is occasionally seen. Granulomatous cells produce the vitamin D 1-hydroxylase, which is usually under tight regulation, resulting in increased activation of vitamin D and elevated calcium.

The angiotensin-converting enzyme (ACE) level is elevated in 60% of patients with sarcoidosis. Although other conditions may increase ACE levels, values more than two times the upper limit of normal are almost always due to sarcoidosis.

Pulmonary function tests show restrictive lung disease, with decreased forced expiratory volume in 1 second and forced vital capacity. Decreased diffusing capacity (DLCO) may occur earlier in the disease.

In the asymptomatic case of sarcoidosis, biopsy is often not necessary because many of these individuals improve in a short time. However, if other diseases, such as tuberculosis or lymphoma, are considered, further workup is required. Transbronchial biopsy should confirm the diagnosis. The histology of the affected node reveals noncaseating granulomas with multinucleated giant cells.

▶ TREATMENT

Most patients with sarcoidosis do well. However, about 25% will have progressive lung disease and 10% will die from sarcoidosis. Patients with asymptomatic hilar adenopathy require no therapy. Corticosteroids should be considered for:

- ▲ severe or progressive lung disease
- ▲ hypercalcemia
- ▲ cardiac involvement
- ▲ uveitis
- ▲ neurosarcoidosis

If used, prednisone should be started at 40 mg daily. Over the next few months, the drug can be ta-

pered slowly. Many patients will need to remain on 10–15 mg of prednisone for years.

Patients should be monitored for progression of pulmonary disease by following pulmonary function testing. If on chronic steroids, complications such as cataracts and osteoporosis should be expected. Additional organ systems may be affected in sarcoidosis, including posterior pituitary dysfunction (leading to diabetes insipidus) and cardiac involvement (leading to arrhythmias, often ventricular). Ventricular arrhythmias due to cardiac sarcoid are often difficult to treat, even if the disease is well controlled. Cardiac disease may also manifest as a restrictive heart disease. Signs of restrictive heart disease are found in Chapter 61.

▶ KEY POINTS

1. Sarcoidosis is an idiopathic granulomatous disease affecting primarily the lungs. It should be suspected in all patients with bilateral hilar adenopathy.

2. Systemic manifestations such as uveitis, arthritis, cranial nerve palsies, and hypercalcemia often occur.

3. Biopsy reveals noncaseating granulomas. Fungal diseases, tuberculosis, and lymphoma should be ruled out.

4. Prognosis is excellent in most patients, especially those who present with erythema nodosum. Remission occurs spontaneously in most patients.

5. Patients with severe lung disease, cardiac or neurologic involvement, or hypercalcemia can be treated with prednisone.

Prednisone for:
severe LUNG
& CARDIAC
NEURO
HYPER Ca²⁺

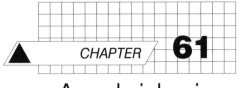

CHAPTER 61

Amyloidosis

*A*myloidosis is a systemic disorder characterized by extracellular deposition of amyloid, a fibrous protein, in one or more sites of the body. Although the etiologies are numerous, all types of amyloid share the following common characteristics on **pathologic** examination:

▲ amorphous, eosinophilic, extracellular deposition

▲ staining with Congo Red dye, and green birefringence under polarized light

▲ protein structure is a beta-pleated sheet

▶ EPIDEMIOLOGY

Amyloidosis tends to be a disease of older individuals; less than 1% of patients are under the age of 40. It occurs in equal frequency in men and women.

▶ ETIOLOGY

Amyloid may either be primary (i.e., no apparent cause) or secondary to an ongoing disease. Amyloidosis is often classified by the specific **protein type**, and the major types are as follows:

▲ immunoglobulin light chain (primary amyloidosis, multiple myeloma)

▲ serum protein SAA (amyloidosis due to chronic infection or inflammation, familial Mediterranean fever)

▲ β2 Microglobulin (hemodialysis)

▲ transthyretin (familial amyloid polyneuropathy)

▶ CLINICAL MANIFESTATIONS

Clinical findings in amyloidosis are dependent on the numerous organ systems the disease affects. The major syndromes seen in amyloidosis are listed by organ system in Table 61-1.

History

Amyloidosis often presents with generalized nonspecific symptoms, such as **fatigue** and **weight loss**. The weight loss is often marked, and averages around 15 to 20 pounds. Other symptoms may signify specific organ damage from amyloid. These include the edema and dyspnea of heart involvement or the paresthesias and light-headedness of neurologic involvement.

TABLE 61-1

Organ Involvement in Amyloidosis

Organ Systems	Syndromes
Neurologic	Autonomic dysfunction
	Carpal tunnel syndrome
	Distal polyneuropathy
Cardiac	Restrictive cardiomyopathy
	Conduction disturbance
Renal	Nephrotic syndrome
	Renal tubular acidosis
Gastrointestinal	Malabsorption
	Motility disorders
	Macroglossia
Hepatic	Intrahepatic cholestasis
Rheumatologic	Symmetric arthritis
Hematologic	Acquired factor X deficiency

Physical Examination

Vitals signs may reveal an orthostatic drop in blood pressure or bradycardia from cardiac conduction disturbances. Fever suggests an underlying infectious etiology, such as osteomyelitis, leading to secondary amyloidosis.

Neurologic involvement may be manifested by orthostatic hypotension, carpal tunnel syndrome, and distal polyneuropathy.

Cardiac amyloidosis will appear as a **restrictive cardiomyopathy** on physical examination. Increased jugular venous pressure will be present along with Kussmaul's sign (jugular venous pressure increases instead of decreases with inspiration) or rapid Y descent (Fig. 61-1). ↑ JVP c̄ inspiration

Skin examination may show signs of easy bruising, including periorbital ecchymoses. Amyloid deposition in the skin appears as **raised waxy papules**. Gastrointestinal involvement may be indicated by macroglossia or hepatomegaly.

▶ DIFFERENTIAL DIAGNOSIS

Amyloidosis is often considered when the patient presents with fatigue and weight loss, suggesting a chronic wasting illness. Other etiologies, such as malignancy or chronic infections, may resemble amyloidosis or may cause amyloidosis. Amyloidosis should be

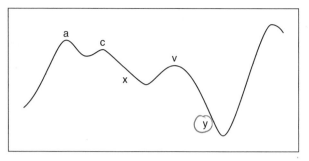

Figure 61-1 Rapid y descent in restrictive cardiomyopathy.

suspected when additional systemic features (nephrotic syndrome, orthostatic hypotension, or restrictive cardiomyopathy) are present.

▶ DIAGNOSTIC EVALUATION

Infiltration of the heart can lead to conduction disturbances (atrioventricular block) and low voltage QRS. On echocardiogram, there is a characteristic "sparkling" of the myocardium and the ventricle wall is often thickened (especially compared with the low voltage on the electrocardiogram).

Urinalysis will often show proteinuria from nephrotic syndrome. Of note, light chain excretion will not be detected by a dipstick, which only detects albuminuria. Immunoelectrophoresis of the urine or serum often reveals a monoclonal spike in primary amyloidosis or multiple myeloma.

Other nonspecific laboratory findings may include increased alkaline phosphatase (cholestasis from liver infiltration), decreased albumin (malabsorption and nephrotic syndrome), and increased prothrombin time (acquired factor X deficiency).

Diagnosis of amyloidosis requires a biopsy that shows the characteristic Congo Red staining. Although affected organs, such as liver or kidney, will often show amyloid on pathology, biopsy may be dangerous from the high rate of bleeding. Therefore, diagnosis is preferentially made by abdominal fat pad or rectal biopsy. The fat pad biopsy is a newer technique but is reported to be more sensitive. Amyloidosis is also detected in bone marrow biopsies, which are often performed to rule out multiple myeloma.

▶ TREATMENT

Once the diagnosis of amyloidosis is made, treatment focuses on supportive care. There is no effective treatment for amyloidosis itself, although treatment aimed at the underlying etiology may be effective (see below). Diuretics may be used for symptomatic relief of

heart failure and edema, but digoxin is often avoided because of increased cardiotoxicity in these patients. Dialysis has been used in certain patients who have progressed to end-stage renal disease.

The prognosis in amyloidosis remains poor (average, 1 year) and is dependent on the extent of organ involvement. Patients presenting with congestive heart failure survive a median of 6 months, whereas patients presenting with peripheral neuropathy alone have median survivals around 56 months.

Treatment directed at the underlying etiology may improve survival in amyloidosis. The most dramatic example is familial Mediterranean fever, which is successfully treated with colchicine. Prophylactic colchicine not only reduces symptomatic episodes in familial Mediterranean fever but seems to prevent the development of amyloidosis. If multiple myeloma is present, melphalan and prednisone may be used and prolong survival several months. Treatment with any of the above agents has been used with primary (idiopathic) amyloidosis, but the benefit remains unclear.

▶ KEY POINTS

1. Amyloidosis is a systemic disorder characterized by extracellular deposition of an amorphous eosinophilic protein that shows apple-green birefringence on Congo Red stain.

2. Diagnosis may be made by biopsy of any affected organ but is easiest and safest with an abdominal fat pad biopsy.

3. Cardiac involvement appears as a conduction disturbance and/or restrictive cardiomyopathy. Echocardiogram reveals a classic "sparkling" pattern. Patients may be extremely sensitive to digoxin toxicity.

4. Development of signs of amyloidosis (such as carpal tunnel syndrome or polyneuropathy) in a patient on long-term hemodialysis should raise the suspicion of β2 microglobulin-mediated amyloidosis.

5. Amyloidosis should be included in the differential diagnosis of elderly patients with fatigue and weight loss.

6. Treatment is supportive with the exception of colchicine for amyloidosis secondary to familial Mediterranean fever and chemotherapy for multiple myeloma.

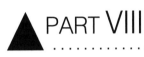

PART VIII

Hematology/Oncology

CHAPTER 62

Evaluation of Anemia

$\mathbf{\mathcal{A}}$nemia is a **reduction in the total red blood cell mass**, as defined by the number of red blood cells, hemoglobin level in the blood, or percentage of red cell volume (hematocrit). Lower limits of normal hemoglobin vary between laboratories, but general criteria for anemia are a hemoglobin level less than 13 g/dL in men and 12 g/dL in women.

Anemia is not itself considered a disease, but rather it is a sign of an underlying disease. Anemia is the result of one of the following mechanisms:

▲ decreased red blood cell production

▲ increased red cell destruction (hemolysis)

▲ blood loss

Red cell destruction and blood loss result in an increased production of immature red cells, known as **reticulocytes**. Thus, these two causes of anemia, which have a high reticulocyte count, are differentiated from decreased production, which has a low reticulocyte count (see diagnostic strategy below). Hemolytic anemias will be discussed in Chapter 64.

▶ DIFFERENTIAL DIAGNOSIS

The differential diagnosis of anemia is classified by its mechanism as well as the size of the red blood cells. Microcytosis is defined by a mean corpuscular volume (MCV) of $<80\ \mu m^3$ and macrocytosis is an MCV of $>100\ \mu m^3$.

High reticulocyte count:

▲ acute blood loss (trauma, gastrointestinal bleeding)

▲ hemolysis

Low reticulocyte count (decreased production):

▲ Microcytic
  iron deficiency
  thalassemia
  anemia of chronic disease
  sideroblastic anemia

▲ Macrocytic
  B12 deficiency
  folate deficiency
  alcohol abuse
  liver disease

  myelodysplastic syndrome
  hypothyroidism, severe
  drug effects

▲ Normocytic
  anemia of chronic disease
  anemia of renal failure
  aplastic anemia
  myelophthisis
  hypothyroidism

Anemia of chronic disease (ACD) is caused by the trapping of iron in the reticuloendothelial system and suppression of erythropoiesis, perhaps mediated by cytokines such as interleukin-1. The three major categories of disease associated with ACD are **infection, malignancy**, and **inflammatory disease** (e.g., rheumatoid arthritis).

Sideroblastic anemia has multiple etiologies including alcohol abuse, lead poisoning, isoniazid use, and pyridoxine deficiency. The characteristic feature is the presence of **ringed sideroblasts** in the bone marrow, which represents abnormal iron accumulation in the mitochondria.

Chemotherapy of any type can cause an anemia through myelosuppression. Folate antagonists, such as methotrexate and trimethoprim, may cause anemia in susceptible individuals.

Myelodysplastic syndrome (MDS) is a disorder characterized by an arrest in maturation of all blood cells, usually presenting as a pancytopenia. It occurs most often in the elderly.

▶ CLINICAL FINDINGS
History

Patients with anemia are usually asymptomatic, unless the decrease in hematocrit is sudden or severe. General symptoms include:

▲ fatigue

▲ dyspnea

▲ dizziness

Patients who are of Mediterranean descent are at increased risk for beta-thalassemia; alpha-thalassemia is seen in African-Americans.

Alcohol consumption should be determined in all patients. There are multiple causes of anemia in alcoholic patients: folate deficiency, liver disease, and alcohol itself cause macrocytic anemias; sideroblastic anemia tends to be microcytic.

Patients should be assessed for potential sites of blood loss. In premenopausal women, menstrual bleeding is the most common cause of anemia. Gastrointestinal bleeding may present with a history of dark, tarry stools or bright red blood from the rectum.

Physical Examination

Most patients with mild anemia have a normal physical examination. However, when hemoglobin is < 11 g/dL, patients may have **pallor** of the nail beds, palmar creases, and conjunctiva. Fever raises the suspicion of a hemolytic anemia.

Findings seen in marked **iron deficiency anemia** include:

▲ atrophic glossitis

▲ angular chelitis (scaling at corners of mouth)

▲ koilonychia ("spoon nails")

Peripheral neuropathy may be seen in B12 deficiency. The posterior columns of the spinal cord are involved, affecting position and vibratory sense. Almost all patients should be evaluated for occult blood loss from the gastrointestinal tract with **stool guaiac testing**.

Diagnostic Test Strategy

The key to the diagnostic workup is to classify the anemia by the **red cell indices** (micro-, macro-, or normocytic) and **reticulocyte count**. The reticulocyte count must be corrected for the level of anemia:

Corrected reticulocyte count = retic count $\times$ $\dfrac{\text{patient's Hct}}{\text{expected Hct}}$

A correct reticulocyte count of 2% or less suggests the diagnosis of decreased red blood cell production, while a value of > 3% indicates hemolysis or blood loss.

The next important step is to examine the **peripheral smear**. The blood smear is used to decide if there is a single morphology of cells or two different populations (dimorphic). An anemia that has a dimorphic population also has a high **red cell distribution width** (RDW). This automated measure of red cell variation may assist in distinguishing two common types of microcytic anemia: iron deficiency (high RDW) and thalassemia (low RDW).

Table 62-1 lists classic findings on peripheral smear (see Figs. 62-1–62-3 as well).

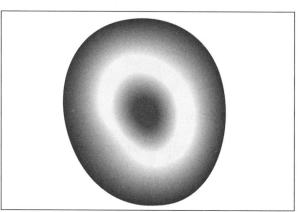

Figure 62-1 Target cell.

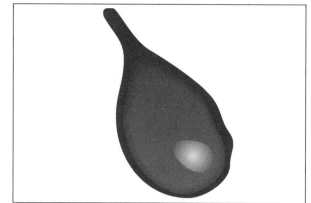

Figure 62-2 Hypersegmented PMN.

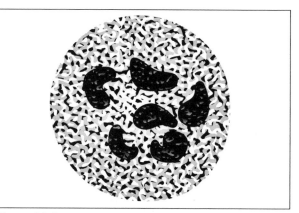

Figure 62-3 Teardrop cell.

Microcytic Anemia

All pure microcytic anemias are associated with a low reticulocyte count. The most useful initial tests are **iron studies**. Ferritin is the storage form of iron; transferrin is the transport protein and the main determinant of the total iron binding capacity (TIBC). Table 62-2 lists the common patterns.

TABLE 62-1
Peripheral Smear Findings

Finding on Smear	Likely Etiologies
hypersegmented PMNs ovalocytes	megaloblastic anemia
target cells	liver disease, thalassemia, hemolysis
bilobed PMNs	myelodysplastic syndrome
teardrop cells	myelophthisis
schistocytes	microangiopathic hemolytic anemia

PMN = polymorphonuclear cell.

It is often difficult to distinguish between anemia of chronic disease and iron deficiency anemia because both can lower iron levels. Since ferritin (an acute phase reactant) may be elevated with inflammation, some state that a normal ferritin level does not rule out iron deficiency in the presence of chronic disease. However, iron deficiency is **extremely uncommon** when ferritin is >150 μg/L. Finally, the diagnosis of beta-thalassemia is confirmed by an elevated level of **hemoglobin A2** (an alternative form of hemoglobin).

Macrocytic Anemia

A high reticulocyte count should be ruled out in these patients. Macrocytic anemias are then subclassified into those with **impaired DNA synthesis** (megaloblastic anemias) and those without impairment. Megaloblastic anemias include B12 and folate deficiency, myelodysplastic syndrome, and drug effects. Characteristics of megaloblastosis are listed in Table 62-1.

Folate and **B12 levels** should be checked in all patients with a megaloblastic picture. Low levels confirm deficiency. Drug effects from chemotherapy and folate antagonists should be excluded as well. Patients with myelodysplasia often have extremely high B12 levels. **Lactate dehydrogenase** (LDH) may be elevated in all megaloblastic anemias due to ineffective erythropoiesis.

TABLE 62-2
Common Patterns in Microcytic Anemias

	Iron	TIBC	Ferritin
Iron deficiency	↓	↑	↓
Thalassemia	N	N	N
Anemia of chronic disease	↓	↓	↑
Sideroblastic anemia	↑	N	N/↑

↑ = increased; ↓ = decreased; N = normal.

Liver function tests and thyroid function tests should be sent as well. The MCV is rarely >110 in patients with hypothyroidism or liver disease.

Normocytic Anemia

A high reticulocyte count should be ruled out in these patients. Anemias of chronic disease is the most common cause of normocytic anemia. Aplastic anemia is characterized by pancytopenia and a zero reticulocyte count. The anemia of renal failure may be present in patients with creatinine levels >2 mg/dl. Patients with no known chronic disease and no apparent cause of the anemia are candidates for bone **marrow biopsy** to rule out myelophthisis.

Diagnostic Test Strategy
Iron Deficiency

Menstruating or pregnant women have known losses of iron, and therapy is empirically begun in these patients. However, in postmenopausal women and men, iron deficiency should be further investigated. The most worrisome cause of iron deficiency in the elderly is gastrointestinal cancer, particularly colon cancer. These patients should be evaluated for an etiology of bleeding, preferably by endoscopy. Symptoms, such as constipation or heartburn, may direct the initial endoscopic evaluation.

B12 Deficiency

The body stores enough B12 to last for years, so most causes of B12 deficiency are not from poor diet. **Pernicious anemia** is due to lack of intrinsic factor, produced by the stomach and necessary for B12 absorption. Achlorhydria may also hamper absorption in these patients. B12 is absorbed by the terminal ileum, so patients with **ileal disease** (e.g., Crohn's disease) are at risk for B12 deficiency. Bacterial overgrowth, as seen in the **blind loop syndrome**, reduces the B12 available for absorption.

A **Schilling test** helps differentiate between these etiologies of B12 deficiency. After loading the body with intramuscular B12, a radioactive dose of B12 is ingested and excretion through the kidney is measured. Failure to excrete the radioactive B12 indicates lack of absorption. The next part of the test (part 2) involves administering B12 and intrinsic factor together; excretion of B12 during this part confirms that the deficiency is due to lack of intrinsic factor (pernicious anemia). Failure to absorb and the excrete B12/intrinsic factor complex suggests malabsorption as a

TABLE 62-3

Schilling Test Results

Able to Absorb B12 After Oral Administration of:	Likely Etiology
B12 only	Inadequate diet
B12 and intrinsic factor	Pernicious anemia
B12 after administration of antibiotics	Blind loop syndrome
Failure to absorb B12 in all above tests	Ileal disease

cause. Correction of this malabsorption after antibiotics suggests blind loop syndrome. Table 62-3 summarizes these results.

Bone Marrow Biopsy

A bone marrow biopsy is an invasive and painful procedure, but it is occasionally necessary to determine the etiology of the anemia. Some indications for bone marrow biopsy are:

▲ pancytopenia (suggesting aplastic anemia or marrow infiltration)

▲ macrocytic anemia of unknown etiology (to rule out myelodysplasia)

▲ findings suggestive of sideroblastic anemia or myelophthisis

► KEY POINTS

1. Anemia is caused by increased RBC destruction, blood loss, or decreased production. A reticulocyte is a useful initial test to determine the underlying mechanism.

2. Iron deficiency is a common cause of microcytic anemia. Although usually a benign condition in premenopausal women, it may be due to occult gastrointestinal malignancy in men and post-menopausal women.

3. In healthy patients, a normal ferritin almost always excludes iron deficiency. Although ferritin may be elevated in inflammatory conditions, it rarely rises higher than 150 µg/L with associated iron deficiency.

4. B12 deficiency may present with a macrocytic anemia and peripheral neuropathy. The most common cause of B12 deficiency is pernicious anemia, which may be confirmed with a Schilling test.

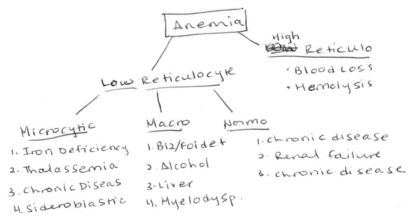

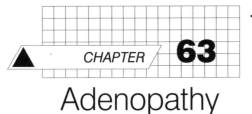

CHAPTER 63

Adenopathy

*A*denopathy often represents a benign self-limited process. However, more serious diseases such as lymphoma or human immunodeficiency virus (HIV) infection may also present with enlarged lymph nodes. In normal individuals, lymph nodes range from 0.5 to 2 cm in size. Lymph nodes greater than 1 cm in size are often evaluated further; the age of patient and the characteristics of the node should be considered in this decision.

▶ CLINICAL MANIFESTATIONS
History
Adenopathy that persists after a few weeks is less likely to be infectious in origin. **Associated symptoms** may suggest certain etiologies:

▲ weight loss, night sweats (lymphoma, metastatic cancer, tuberculosis)

▲ sore throat (mononucleosis, pharyngitis)

▲ genital lesion (syphilis, chancroid)

▲ pets, especially cats (cat-scratch disease, toxoplasmosis)

▲ history of travel to southwestern United States (coccidioidomycosis) or midwestern United States (histoplasmosis)

▲ history of intravenous drug use or high-risk sexual behavior (HIV)

Age is also an important consideration. Individuals greater than 50 years old have a malignant etiology 50% of the time; those younger than 30 years old have a benign etiology 80% of the time. When considering lymphoma as a cause of adenopathy, inquire about **phenytoin** (Dilantin) use, which may cause a pseudolymphoma syndrome.

Physical Examination
The **location** of the adenopathy often leads to the diagnosis (see Differential Diagnosis). Tender erythematous nodes are consistent with lymphadenitis, whereas firm rubbery adenopathy may be found in lymphoma. Metastatic disease tends to present with hard fixed nodes.

▶ DIFFERENTIAL DIAGNOSIS
The evaluation of adenopathy is best categorized by the location of the adenopathy.
Generalized
▲ HIV infection

▲ lymphoma

▲ hypersensitivity reaction (including phenytoin)

▲ toxoplasmosis

▲ secondary syphilis

Cervical
▲ mononucleosis

▲ lymphoma

▲ pharyngitis

▲ toxoplasmosis

▲ sarcoidosis

Inguinal
▲ syphilis

▲ herpes simplex

▲ lymphogranuloma venereum

▲ chancroid

Supraclavicular
▲ mediastinal or pulmonary malignancy (right)

▲ abdominal malignancy (left)

Hilar adenopathy
▲ sarcoidosis (bilateral)

▲ lymphoma

▲ tuberculosis

▲ bronchogenic carcinoma (unilateral)

▲ fungal infection (bilateral)

Two additional clinical scenarios deserve mention. **Secondary syphilis** may present with bilateral epitrochlear adenopathy; **cat-scratch disease** presents with unilateral adenopathy proximal to the cat bite or scratch (usually epitrochlear or axillary).

▶ DIAGNOSTIC EVALUATION
In the young patient with cervical adenopathy, infectious mononucleosis is the primary consideration. A

▲ **217**

complete blood count with differential should be sent. Lymphocytosis, with atypical lymphocytes, is almost always seen. A **heterophile antibody** confirms the diagnosis of mononucleosis, although it may be negative early in the disease.

If inguinal adenopathy is present, urethral or cervical cultures should be obtained to rule out sexually transmitted disease (see Chapter 28).

In the older patient with supraclavicular adenopathy, a **chest x-ray** should be obtained to rule out bronchogenic carcinoma or lymphoma. However, these patients are likely to proceed to biopsy given the concern for malignancy. A **mammogram** should be obtained in all women with axillary adenopathy (if not infectious in origin).

Asymptomatic hilar adenopathy with symptoms consistent with sarcoidosis (see Chapter 59) may be observed if tuberculosis and fungal disease are not considerations. Patients with hilar adenopathy due to lymphoma or bronchogenic cancer usually have associated symptoms. If the adenopathy is associated with a mass or effusion, it must be investigated further.

Lymph node biopsy remains the definitive diagnostic test. Often the adenopathy resolves after a **period of observation**, making biopsy unnecessary. **Early biopsy** should be considered when the following features are present:

▲ Lymph node greater than 2 to 3 cm in diameter without symptoms or laboratory findings suggestive of mononucleosis;

▲ Adenopathy in association with an abnormal chest x-ray (hilar adenopathy, pulmonary mass or cavity);

▲ Supraclavicular adenopathy (especially in the older patient);

▲ Axillary adenopathy without signs of upper extremity infection (consider breast malignancy in women and non-Hodgkin's lymphoma in both sexes).

Additional tests that may be performed to assist in diagnosis if indicated include:

▲ purified protein derivative (PPD) skin test to rule out tuberculosis

▲ toxoplasma titers

▲ HIV antibody testing

▲ rapid plasma reagin (RPR) to rule out syphilis

Biopsy may be nondiagnostic in about 30% of patients who eventually undergo biopsy. These patients should be carefully followed as some will eventually prove to have lymphoma.

▶ KEY POINTS

1. Location of the adenopathy is a key feature in determining etiology. Cervical adenopathy in a young patient is often mononucleosis; asymptomatic hilar adenopathy is often due to sarcoidosis.

2. A period of observation is often indicated in the young patient with adenopathy; many of these patients have a reactive adenopathy that will resolve.

3. Supraclavicular adenopathy may represent malignancy. The left supraclavicular node (Virchow's node) drains the abdominal cavity and therefore may be enlarged in gastric, colon, or ovarian cancer.

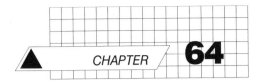
Evaluation of Hemolytic Anemia

*H*emolysis is the premature destruction of red blood cells (RBCs). The decreased survival of the RBCs results in an increase in the production of immature RBCs (reticulocytes). Thus, hemolytic anemia is characterized by a decreased hemoglobin level and an increase in reticulocyte count. Acute blood loss may mimic this pattern, but an obvious site of bleeding is usually identified.

Hemolysis may be caused by **intravascular factors** (usually acquired) or **intrinsic defects** in the RBC (often inherited). In addition, hemolysis can occur in the intravascular space or in the extravascular space (mainly the spleen and liver). **Intravascular hemolysis** results in release of hemoglobin, which is quickly bound to the serum protein **haptoglobin.** Next, the hemoglobin–haptoglobin complex is cleared by the reticuloendothelial (RE) system, and the haptoglobin level rapidly falls to low or undetectable levels. Once intravascular hemoglobin overloads the haptoglobin capacity, it is filtered by the kidney and reabsorbed in the proximal tubule. These tubular cells when sloughed off into the urine can be detected as urine **hemosiderin.** Finally, when proximal tubular reabsorption is overwhelmed (only in severe hemolysis), **hemoglobinuria** can be detected. This is suggested by a positive occult blood reading on urine dipstick but no RBCs seen on urinalysis. In **extravascular hemolysis**, RBCs are removed by the spleen and RE system; therefore, little hemoglobin is released into the bloodstream. Haptoglobin may be low, but urine hemosiderin and hemoglobin uria are usually not present.

▶ DIFFERENTIAL DIAGNOSIS

Causes are classified as causing intravascular (I) or extravascular (E)hemolysis.

Intravascular factors
Microangiopathic hemolyticanemia—(I)

▲ disseminated intravascular coagulation (DIC)

▲ hemolyticuremic syndrome (HUS)

▲ thrombotic thrombocytopenic purpura (TTP)

▲ cardiac valve hemolysis

Immune-mediated hemolyticanemia

▲ warm antibody (hematologic malignancy, connective tissue disorders, drugs)—(E)

▲ cold antibody (lymphoma, mycoplasma, mononucleosis)—(I)

Infections—(I/E)

▲ malaria

▲ babesiosis

▲ clostridial toxin

Splenomegaly—(E)

▲ infiltrative diseases

▲ portal hypertension

Red blood cell defects
Hemoglobinopathies—(E)

▲ sickle cell disease

Enzyme defects—(I)

▲ pyruvate kinase deficiency

▲ glucose-6-phosphate dehydrogenase (G6PD) deficiency

Membrane defects

▲ hereditary spherocytosis (E)

▲ paroxysmal nocturnal hemoglobinuria (I)*

▶ CLINICAL FINDINGS
History
There are no specific symptoms associated with hemolytic anemia. However, the history may lead to a suspected etiology of the hemolysis. A **history of travel** to Africa, Asia, or Central America may suggest malaria. A **family history** of hemolytic anemia may be found in any patient with an RBC defect (see above). Sickle cell disease and G6PD deficiency occurs in African-Americans; G6PD deficiency can also occur in people of Mediterranean descent.

*Paroxysmal nocturnal hemoglobinuria (PNH) is a unique RBC defect because it is acquired. It is a stem cell disorder that results in RBCs with an increased sensitivity to complement-mediated hemolysis.

Certain **drugs** are associated with **warm-antibody** hemolytic anemia:

▲   methyldopa

▲   quinine

▲   sulfonamides

▲   penicillin

Drugs that can induce hemolysis in persons with **G6PD deficiency** include:

▲   sulfa drugs

▲   nitrofurantoin

▲   methylene blue

▲   primaquine

Physical Examination

Fever suggests the presence of an infectious or microangiopathic etiology. Scleral icterus (from hyperbilirubinemia) may be seen in all cases. Splenomegaly may be the cause of the hemolysis or a result of the hemolysis (in extravascular cases). It is not helpful in distinguishing etiologies.

Diagnostic Test Strategy

The key **laboratory features of hemolysis** include:

▲   elevated indirect bilirubin

▲   elevated lactate dehydrogenase (LDH)

▲   increased reticulocyte count

▲   decreased haptoglobin

Note that elevated LDH and indirect bilirubin may also be seen in patients with ineffective hematopoiesis (e.g., B12 deficiency). However, the reticulocyte count is low in these patients.

   Thrombocytopenia may be seen in many causes, but is most prominent in the microangiopathic etiologies (TTP, HUS, DIC). **Prothrombin time** is elevated in DIC, but is normal in TTP and HUS. Renal failure is an important feature of HUS, but is also seen in other microangiopathic etiologies.

   The next important step is examination of the **peripheral smear.** Figures 64-1–64-3 demonstrate examples of abnormal smears in hemolysis. The hemolysis itself commonly results in target cells and spherocytes. However, large numbers of spherocytes are limited to hereditary spherocytosis and warm-antibody hemolysis.

   Once examination of the smear eliminates microangiopathic hemolysis or infections, a **Coombs' test** should be performed to evaluate for immune-mediated hemolysis. An **indirect** Coombs' test looks for an antibody in the patient's serum that can agglu-

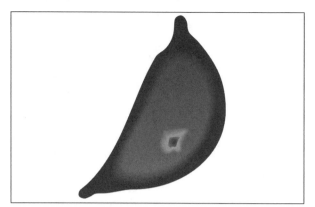

Figure 64-1 Schistocyte.

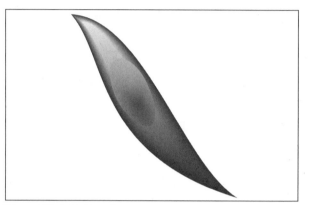

Figure 64-2 Sickle cell.

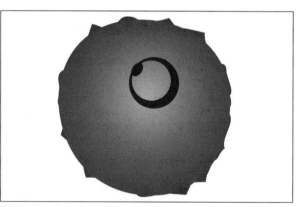

Figure 64-3 RBC with malaria.

tinate normal RBCs. However, a **direct** Coombs' test is the definitive test for immune-mediated hemolysis, searching for the presence of the antibody directly on the patient's own RBCs.

   A direct Coombs' test may be further classified by the type of antibody associated with the hemolysis. Most warm-antibody hemolysis is mediated by immunoglobulin (Ig)G and therefore IgG and C3 will be detected on the RBC surface. Cold-antibody hemolysis is mostly IgM mediated. IgM binds to the RBC and fixes complement at lower temperatures, but then dissociates from the RBC. Therefore, only C3 will be detected on the cell surface.

Further Diagnostic Tests

The **osmotic fragility test** is used to look for membrane defects, such as a hereditary spherocytosis. The abnormal cells will lyse more easily compared with normal RBCs. The **sucrose lysis test** and the **acidified serum lysis test** are two methods used to detect paroxysmal nocturnal hemoglobinuria by activating the complement pathway.

Enzyme deficiencies may be diagnosed by testing for the specific enzyme in the patient's RBCs. However, screening tests, such as the fluorescent spot test, are reliable measures for G6PD deficiency. In cases of severe hemolysis, the most deficient cells will already be destroyed, resulting in a falsely normal test. The assay should be repeated at a later time.

▶ KEY POINTS

1. Hemolytic anemia is characterized by an indirect hyperbilirubinemia, elevated LDH, and decreased haptoglobin. Urine hemosiderin may be present (especially with intravascular hemolysis).

2. Schistocytes and thrombocytopenia indicate microangiopathic hemolytic anemia. Causes include disseminated intravascular coagulation, hemo- DIC lytic uremic syndrome, and thrombotic thrombo- HUS cytopenic purpura. TTP

3. Immune-mediated hemolysis may be due to warm antibodies (IgG) or cold antibodies (IgM). A direct Coombs' test will be positive.

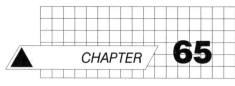

CHAPTER 65

Coagulation Disorders

*H*emostasis is maintained via the action of the cellular and protein components of the clotting cascade. Once formed, blood clots are removed via the action of the thrombolytic system. Defects in coagulation or thrombolysis can lead either to **hypercoagulability** or **bleeding disorders**.

A complete discussion of the coagulation and thrombolytic systems is beyond the scope of this chapter. Instead, the focus is on the clinical presentation of the major bleeding disorders and the diagnostic workup of these problems.

▶ ETIOLOGY AND PATHOGENESIS

Hemostasis is accomplished after vascular injury via the interplay of the proteins comprising the clotting cascades and a variety of cells, including platelets, leukocytes, and endothelial cells. Normal function of these elements after vascular injury leads to the **formation of a clot**, composed of the **fibrin** and **platelets**. Fibrin is produced by the cleavage of **fibrinogen** by the protease **thrombin**.

There are **tight controls on the activation of the clotting cascades** that prevent generalized coagulation. The **thrombolytic system**, in which the fibrin-cleaving protein **plasmin** is a central component, is responsible for remodeling and removing existing fibrin clots. The thrombolytic system is activated from the time the coagulation system begins clot formation, providing close regulation of hemostatis.

The balance between coagulation and clot formation on one hand and thrombolysis on the other can be disturbed in a number of ways:

▲ Defects in the coagulation proteins;

▲ Abnormal platelet function;

▲ Abnormal initiation of the clotting cascades leading to consumption of coagulation factors;

▲ Interference with the action of activated coagulation factors;

▲ Disturbances in the thrombolytic pathway.

These defects shift the balance of hemostasis, resulting in a tendency toward abnormal bleeding. The most common **hemorrhagic disorders in adults** are acquired rather than hereditary:

▲ vitamin K deficiency/anticoagulant therapy

▲ liver failure–associated coagulopathy

▲ disseminated intravascular coagulation

Vitamin K deficiency leads to decrease of the coagulation factors II, VII, IX, and X and the coagulation regulators protein C and protein S. Vitamin K is required for the proper synthesis of these factors. The anticoagulant drug warfarin interferes with the action of vitamin K, leading to a similar defect.

The liver plays an important role in the production and metabolism of coagulation factors. Severe liver failure can therefore result in a bleeding tendency due to factor deficiency.

Disseminated intravascular coagulation (DIC) is a condition in which a number of diseases (including sepsis, trauma/tissue injury, neoplasms, and obstetric catastrophes) can trigger **accelerated, unregulated activation of the coagulation cascades**. There is formation of small thrombi and emboli throughout the vascular tree that eventually leads to depletion of coagulation factors and platelets. A severe coagulation defect can result.

The deliberate manipulation of the coagulation and thrombolytic systems is used in the therapy of a number of disorders. The therapeutic index of these drugs is low because abnormal bleeding can have catastrophic consequences. The most feared complication of therapeutic anticoagulation or thrombolysis is **intracerebral hemorrhage**. Most other bleeding (e.g., gastrointestinal, severe epistaxis) can be dealt with in a timely fashion with minimal long-term sequelae.

▶ CLINICAL MANIFESTATIONS
History

Disorders in coagulation may present as overt spontaneous **bleeding**. The classic disorder of coagulation is the inherited disease hemophilia, in which defective clotting factors lead to abnormal bleeding at an early age. Other inherited diseases (e.g., type I von Willebrand disease) cause less severe disturbances and the coagulopathy is apparent only under times of significant hemostatic stress, such as trauma, surgery, dental extraction, and childbirth. A **family history** of abnormal bleeding is also an important clue to an inherited disorder.

A careful drug history may reveal the use of anticoagulants such as warfarin and aspirin (the latter may be ingested unknowingly in combination "cold remedies" and "headache remedies"). Certain drugs (e.g., sulfa and beta-lactam antibiotics) are associated with **immune-mediated platelet destruction.**

Other coagulation defects can be totally asymptomatic and only suspected by the presence of abnormal laboratory tests of coagulation (see below).

Physical Examination

The nature and site of abnormal bleeding can give clues to the nature of the coagulation defect. **Platelet disorders** usually manifest as **superficial bleeding** involving the skin, mucous membranes, and gastrointestinal and urinary tracts. Typical skin findings include **petechiae** and **ecchymoses.** Epistaxis is a common manifestation. Bleeding occurs immediately after trauma because of the inability to form a platelet plug.

Disorders involving plasma **coagulation factor defects** generally manifest as **deeper bleeding,** affecting joints and body cavities (e.g., peritoneum). Chronic bleeding into joints, as is seen in hemophilia, can lead to joint deformity. Because platelet function is unaffected, abnormal bleeding does not manifest immediately after trauma but can be delayed hours to days.

▶ DIFFERENTIAL DIAGNOSIS

The differential diagnosis of bleeding disorders can be divided based on the primary abnormality.

Platelet disorders

▲ Abnormal function (decreased cyclooxygenase activity due to aspirin and nonsteroidal anti-inflammatory agents, uremia, von Willebrand disease);

▲ Thrombocytopenia (immune destruction, DIC, splenic sequestration, marrow failure).

Coagulation factor disorders

▲ Defective factors (hemophilia, dysfibrinogenemia);

▲ Consumption of coagulation factors (DIC);

▲ Vitamin K deficiency (insufficient dietary intake, intestinal malabsorption, chronic liver disease);

▲ Interference with vitamin K activity (warfarin administration);

▲ Interference with activated coagulation factors (heparin administration, circulating anticoagulants).

Abnormal activity of the fibrinolytic pathway

▲ Exogenous plasminogen activator (tissue plasminogen activator or streptokinase administration during acute myocardial infarction);

▲ Abnormal regulation of fibrinolysis (plasmin inhibitor deficiency).

▶ DIAGNOSTIC EVALUATION

The definitive diagnosis and characterization of a hemostatic defect is generally made via a number of laboratory tests. A **platelet count** gives a rapid assessment of the quantitative state of the primary hemostatic system. Assessing the functional capacity of platelets is more difficult. The **template bleeding time** is often used to assess platelet function, but subtle as well as significant abnormalities may be missed. Direct assessment of platelet function is possible using a **platelet aggregometer,** but this is generally a research tool and not widely available in the clinical setting.

The **state of the coagulation cascade** is assessed grossly by the partial thromboplastin time (PTT), prothrombin time (PT), and the thrombin time (TT). The PTT assesses the so-called **intrinsic limb** of the coagulation pathway (factors VIII, IX, XI, and XII, high molecular weight kininogen and prekallikrein), whereas the PT assesses the **extrinsic** (factor II and tissue factor-dependent) **limb.** Both tests assess the adequacy of the final steps of the coagulation cascade, leading to thrombin-mediated cleavage of fibrinogen (factors II, V, and X and fibrinogen). The **cleavage of fibrinogen to fibrin** can be specifically tested by the TT. A possible defect in a coagulation factor that leads to an abnormal PT or PTT can be screened for by the addition of normal plasma to the patient's plasma and repeating the test. Normalization by the addition of normal serum indicates a factor deficiency, whereas a continued prolongation indicates the presence of a **coagulation inhibitor.** Specific assays are available for the various coagulation factors that can pinpoint a particular factor deficiency.

Abnormal results of these screening tests can narrow the differential diagnosis:

▲ Prolonged PTT: heparin administration, classic hemophilia (factors VIII, IX, and XII deficiency);

▲ Prolonged PT: warfarin administration, vitamin K deficiency, factor VII deficiency;

▲ Prolonged PTT and PT: factor II, V, and X deficiency, prolonged vitamin K deficiency, higher dose warfarin administration;

▲ Prolonged TT: dysfibrinogenemia.

▶ TREATMENT

Once the diagnosis is made of a coagulation defect, attempt must be made to correct the underlying etiology if possible. Supportive care with red blood cell transfusion and factor/platelet replacement (see below) can be initiated if indicated.

The treatment of **specific factor deficiencies** (hemophilia) is accomplished by the replacement of the missing factors. Traditionally, this has been via the administration of **plasma products** containing the missing factors (fresh-frozen plasma, cryoprecipitate, factor VIII concentrate). The transmission viral infection (hepatitis, human immunodeficiency virus) using these preparations has prompted additional virus-neutralizing steps during preparation. **Recombinant coagulation factors** that will obviate the need to expose these patients to pooled blood products are being developed and tested.

Thrombocytopenia or qualitative platelet defects that cause significant hemorrhage can be managed with **platelet transfusions**. In the case of immune mediated thrombocytopenia, infused platelets are often consumed rapidly. The administration of intravenous immune globulin can reduce consumption.

Vitamin K deficiency and excessive anticoagulation with warfarin can be treated by administration of intramuscular vitamin K. If a more rapid reversal of the defect is required because of clinically significant bleeding or the need for immediate surgery, fresh-frozen plasma can be administered.

The management of patients on **chronic oral anticoagulation** (warfarin administration) requires close patient follow-up. This is particularly true in the period immediately after the initiation of anticoagulant therapy, when most problems occur. The **level of anticoagulation** is determined by calculating the International Normalized Ratio (INR), which compares the intensity of anticoagulation at a recognized standard. Particular INR values are recommended for various indications of anticoagulation.

In patients who have a strong indication for anticoagulation (e.g., a prosthetic heart valve) and who are overanticoagulated, it may be reasonable to simply hold warfarin therapy and allow the PT to drift down into a therapeutic range. The caveats are that there is not significant clinical bleeding and the PT elevation is not excessive (empirically determined as a particular INR, usually 20). In other cases, partial reversal or complete reversal followed by the institution of heparin therapy may be necessary.

▶ KEY POINTS

1. Hemostasis is maintained by the opposing actions of the coagulation and thrombolytic systems.

2. Defects in the coagulation system or abnormal activation/augmentation of the thrombolytic system can lead to a bleeding tendency.

3. The diagnosis of a coagulation disorder is confirmed and characterized by laboratory tests, including the partial thromboplastin time, prothrombin time, thrombin time, bleeding time, and platelet count.

4. Treatment of coagulation disorders involves correcting the underlying etiology and reversing the coagulation defect by the administration of missing/defective elements when there is clinically significant hemorrhage.

5. The therapeutic administration of anticoagulants requires close monitoring to avoid bleeding complications.

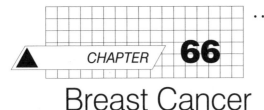

CHAPTER **66**

Breast Cancer

▶ EPIDEMIOLOGY

Breast cancer is the most common cancer in women and the second most common cause of cancer deaths. About 12% of women will develop breast cancer and 3.5% will die from it. Although the incidence of breast cancer in recent years has increased 1 to 2% per year, the mortality rate has been stable.

▶ RISK FACTORS

The risk of breast cancer increases with increasing age; the median age for breast cancer is 54 years. Family history is also important, with a relative risk of 1.5 to 2 for patients with a first-degree relative with breast cancer. The risk from family history is increased if the relative had an early diagnosis (premenopausal) or bilateral breast cancer.

Patients with a previous breast biopsy showing benign proliferative changes appear to be at higher risk, especially those biopsies that show atypical hyperplasia.

Other risk factors are not as strong and appear to have a hormonal basis. These include:

▲ early menarche

▲ late menopause

▲ late age of first pregnancy

▲ nulliparity

A controversial risk factor is estrogen replacement therapy; some studies suggest long-term treatment (>10 years) may be associated with a modest increased risk (relative risk = 1.5).

Dietary factors, such as fat intake and alcohol consumption, have not been consistently related to increased risk. Despite the emphasis on the above, most patients (70 to 80%) with breast cancer do not have any identifiable risk factor.

▶ CLINICAL MANIFESTATIONS
History

An asymptomatic breast mass is the most common complaint of the patient with breast cancer. Approximately 20% of the masses will prove to be malignant. Important historical points include risk factors (see above), duration of mass, change in size, and relation to menses. Patients with intraductal cancer may present with unilateral nipple discharge. Bloody discharge increases the concern for malignancy. Breast pain without an associated mass is an uncommon presenting sign; less than 5% of these women will have cancer.

Physical Examination

Physical examination should concentrate on finding an underlying breast mass. Although benign masses are often mobile, soft, or cystic, these features are not specific enough to rule out malignancy. The breasts should be examined for asymmetry or skin changes, such as thickening or dimpling. Lymphadenopathy, particularly axillary, suggests malignancy.

▶ DIFFERENTIAL DIAGNOSIS

In the patient presenting with a breast mass the following diagnoses should be considered in addition to malignancy:

▲ cyst

▲ fibroadenoma

▲ fibrocystic changes

In the patient with nipple discharge, the differential includes:

▲ ductal papilloma

▲ ductal ectasia

▲ endocrinopathies, such as prolactinoma (especially if discharge is bilateral)

▶ DIAGNOSTIC EVALUATION

Ultrasonography can be used to differentiate cystic from solid masses. This is helpful for young women who have a high rate of cystic disease relative to cancer. The ultrasound may then be used to guide aspiration of the cyst.

Mammography is useful in identifying suspicious lesions or concurrent nonpalpable lesions. An irregular spiculated mass or cluster of microcalcifications suggests carcinoma. However, because of the high false-negative rate (8 to 20%), a normal mammogram does not rule out malignancy.

Mammograms have also proven useful to screen asymptomatic women. Annual or biannual mammograms have been shown to decrease breast cancer mortality in women aged 50 to 74. To date, no conclusive evidence has been demonstrated in younger women, and therefore screening is not universally recommended in this group. Screening should be started earlier for women with a family history of breast cancer.

Although some serum markers (such as CA 15-3) may correlate with breast cancer, there are no accepted blood tests for early detection. After the diagnosis of breast cancer, a chest x-ray, serum calcium level, and alkaline phosphatase should be obtained to screen for advanced disease.

In evaluating a patient with a breast complaint, one must consider the underlying risk of breast cancer. A mammogram is a reasonable start for all women over the age of 35. For younger women or those with findings that suggest cystic disease, an ultrasound may identify cysts and guide aspiration. A cyst may be followed closely if the fluid is nonbloody and the cyst resolves completely. Bloody fluid or a nonresolving mass necessitate further workup.

As mentioned above, a normal mammogram does not rule out cancer. Fine-needle aspiration may yield a diagnosis, but it also has a high false-negative rate. Excisional biopsy remains the definitive diagnostic procedure. Positive biopsies should be sent for estrogen and progesterone receptor testing, because these tumors respond better to hormonal therapy.

▶ TREATMENT

Prognosis in breast cancer is highly correlated with size of the tumor and the number of involved lymph nodes. If the biopsy shows malignancy, patients should undergo axillary dissection and lymph node sampling. This will likely guide the decision regarding adjunctive therapy.

Until recently, all patients with localized breast cancer underwent a modified radical mastectomy. Recent studies indicate that for some tumors, lumpectomy (breast-conserving surgery) with primary radiation therapy is equivalent in 5- and 10-year survival benefits to mastectomy. The choice of therapy should be discussed with the patient after the biopsy-proven diagnosis of breast cancer. Important factors in the decision include size of tumor, size of breast, expected cosmetic result, and patient preference. Local recurrence rate is high after lumpectomy if radiation treatment is omitted.

Adjuvant therapy for breast cancer includes chemotherapy and hormonal therapy (tamoxifen, ovarian ablation). The overall benefit of adjuvant therapy in patients with positive nodes is approximately a 20 to 30% reduction in odds of death; the following are some treatment recommendations in node-positive women:

▲ Tamoxifen, in women over 50 years old. Estrogen receptor-positive tumors respond better than estrogen receptor-negative tumors. Treatment for 2 or more years appears superior to 1 year. Treatment greater than 5 years seems to offer little additional benefit.

▲ Chemotherapy, in women less than 50 years old. Multiple drugs (such as cyclophosphamide, methotrexate, 5-FU) are superior to single-drug regimens. Four to 6 months appears to be an adequate duration.

▲ Ovarian ablation is only beneficial in premenopausal women.

In women without lymph node involvement, the decision is more complex, because about 70% of these women will have no recurrence of their cancer. Discussions regarding adjuvant therapy should be held with the patient and her oncologist to weigh the individual risk/benefit profile. Large or poorly differentiated tumors may have a significant risk of recurrence despite negative lymph nodes.

Patients on adjuvant therapy should be monitored for side effects. Tamoxifen can cause nausea, menopausal symptoms (e.g., hot flashes), and a small increase in uterine cancer (uterine bleeding must be worked up). Chemotherapy can cause nausea and vomiting and bone marrow suppression. Daunorubicin can cause cardiomyopathy at cumulative doses greater than 450 mg/m^2. Cyclophosphamide (an alkylating agent) can cause hemorrhagic cystitis and carries an increased risk of leukemia many years after treatment.

Follow-up involves monitoring the patient for recurrence of breast cancer. These women have five times the baseline risk for cancer in the contralateral breast. Physical examination and mammography should be conducted at regular intervals.

Although there is no evidence that early detection of metastatic disease will improve survival, patients should be evaluated for complaints that may indicate metastatic disease. Common sites of spread and clinical scenarios include:

- ▲ bone (back pain)
- ▲ brain (seizures, headache)
- ▲ lung (dyspnea, cough)
- ▲ liver (abdominal complaints)

Patients with these symptoms should be worked up with the appropriate tests since systemic treatment or radiation often palliates symptoms.

► KEY POINTS

1. The asymptomatic breast mass is the most common presentation of breast cancer. A normal mammogram does not rule out malignancy.

2. Breast conserving surgery combined with radiation is equivalent in efficacy to modified radical mastectomy.

3. Adjuvant therapy, such as tamoxifen or chemotherapy, is indicated in node-positive patients; it may be considered in node-negative patients based on individualized risks and benefits.

4. Symptoms such as headaches, seizures, or back pain in the patient with a history of breast cancer may represent metastatic disease.

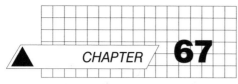
Leukemia and Lymphoma

Leukemias and lymphomas are neoplasms of hematopoietic cells. In the case of **leukemia**, the neoplastic cells **arise in the bone marrow** and then spread to the peripheral blood and the rest of the body. **Lymphomas arise in peripheral lymphoid tissue** (usually lymph nodes) and may eventually spread to the peripheral blood and eventually the bone marrow. This bloodstream stage of lymphomas is referred to as the "leukemia phase."

Leukemias can be broadly classified according to the cell of origin and their clinical course:

▲ acute lymphocytic leukemia (ALL)

▲ acute myelogenous leukemia (AML)

▲ chronic lymphocytic leukemia (CLL)

▲ chronic myelogenous leukemia (CML)

Lymphomas can be broadly divided into:

▲ Hodgkin's disease (HD)

▲ non-Hodgkin's lymphoma (NHL)

The leukemias and NHL can be further divided by histologic, biochemical (e.g., cell surface markers and enzyme production) and genetic (e.g., chromosomal rearrangements) means, giving rise to numerous subtypes. A full discussion of the common subtypes is beyond the scope of this chapter.

▶ EPIDEMIOLOGY

There are approximately 40,000 new cases of leukemia diagnosed each year in the United States. There are a similar number of new diagnoses of NHL each year, whereas about 7500 new cases of HD are diagnosed yearly.

Men have a slightly higher incidence of leukemia and lymphoma than women. ALL is most commonly seen in children and young adults. HD has two peaks of incidence, the first in the second and third decade and another in the sixth. AML, CLL, CML, and NHL all generally have increased incidence with increasing age.

▶ ETIOLOGY AND PATHOPHYSIOLOGY

In most cases, a specific etiology for a leukemia or lymphoma is not known. As with most neoplasms, genetic alterations are believed to be important in their development. As such, both **genetic and environmental factors** have been linked to the development of leukemia and lymphoma:

▲ Radiation exposure: appears to be dose related (as seen in the survivors of the atomic bomb in Japan) and has peak incidence of about 5 to 10 years after exposure;

▲ Chemotherapy: particularly when combined with radiotherapy is associated with subsequent development of a myeloid leukemia;

▲ Immunosuppression: both human immunodeficiency virus infection and immunosuppression for conditions such as organ transplantation are associated with a significantly increased risk of NHL;

▲ Viral infection: human T-cell leukemia virus type-1 has been linked to the development of adult T-cell leukemia, a form of CLL. Epstein-Barr virus infection has been linked to the development of a form of ALL and also Burkitt's lymphoma.

The **pathophysiology** of leukemias and lymphomas is complex. Leukemias, as well as lymphomas that spread to the marrow, can lead to significant **bone marrow abnormalities**. Replacement of the normal marrow elements can lead to **cytopenia**, which has a number of consequences including bleeding and immune suppression. Leukemic cells can cause problems by **accumulation in extramedullary sites** such as the spleen, liver, meninges, and lymph nodes. **Leukostasis** in the microvasculature can result from significant leukemic tumor burden. This is most often seen in CML when the white cell count can exceed 150,000/μL. Lymphomas can produce symptoms due to local **mass effect**. The metabolic products of certain leukemias and lymphomas can lead to other problems. Immunoglobulins produced by these neoplasms can result in conditions such as **amyloidosis, renal failure**, and **cryoglobulinemia. Hyperuricemia** can result from the rapid turnover of neoplastic cells and purine release, a complication of therapy that increases cell death.

▶ **CLINICAL MANIFESTATIONS**
History

Patients with a **leukemia**, particularly an acute leuke-mia (ALL, AML), may present with:

▲ constitutional symptoms—fever, malaise, dyspnea

▲ bleeding—usually related to thrombocytopenia

▲ infection—can be as dramatic as overwhelming sepsis

▲ bone pain—from the expanding leukemic cell mass within the marrow

▲ neurologic symptoms—ranging from headache to seizures and cranial nerve palsies and caused by leukemic cell infiltration of the meninges

The **chronic leukemias** CLL and CML are often clinically silent. Diagnosis may occur when a complete blood count is done for another reason and an inciden-tal leukocytosis is found. CML is characterized by a clinically mild phase, followed after a so-called "blast crisis" when the clinical picture resembles that seen in the acute leukemias. CLL can be much more indolent, and in the most benign forms, patient life span can be greater than 10 years after diagnosis.

Patients with **lymphoma** generally present with painless **lymphadenopathy** and/or a mass. Common locations include the axillary, supraclavicular, and cer-vical nodes. Lymphadenopathy can cause symptoms due to **mass effect**. For example, mediastinal adenop-athy can cause cough and respiratory compromise.

The so-called B symptoms (named for their use in staging of lymphomas) include fever, night sweats, and weight loss. Other constitutional symptoms, such as malaise and anorexia, may be present.

Physical Examination

On physical examination, a patient with **leukemia** may exhibit:

▲ Signs of thrombocytopenia, such as bleeding from gums, ecchymoses, petechiae;

▲ Lymphadenopathy, most often with ALL, CLL;

▲ Splenomegaly, which may be the only physical finding in patients with CML and also commonly seen in ALL and CLL;

▲ Hepatomegaly, most often seen in ALL but also in about 50% of cases of CLL.

Other physical examination findings generally relate to specific organ involvement with leukemic cells (e.g., neurologic signs from meningeal involvement).

As mentioned, patients with lymphoma generally present with persistent peripheral adenopathy. They are usually firm, freely mobile, and nontender. Sple-nomegaly may be present.

▶ **DIFFERENTIAL DIAGNOSIS**

The differential diagnosis of the history and physical findings described above includes entities such as in-fection, idiopathic thrombocytopenic purpura, and col-lagen vascular disease. Once a peripheral white blood cell count is obtained, the differential diagnosis is then generally between the different leukemias themselves. One important exception is the differential between CLL and a reactive lymphocytosis (e.g., from viral in-fection). This distinction is generally made by further laboratory tests (see below). Additionally, intense stim-ulation of white cell production (e.g., from overwhelm-ing bacterial infection) can result in extremely high white cell counts, a so-called **leukemoid reaction**.

The differential diagnosis of lymphoma includes conditions that can lead to lymphadenopathy and is discussed in detail in Chapter 63.

▶ **DIAGNOSTIC EVALUATION**

An **elevated white blood cell count** is the hallmark of leukemia. Examination of the peripheral smear may reveal normal mature-looking white cells (particularly in CLL), but more immature forms are often seen. Morphologic features (e.g., Auer rods in AML, Phila-delphia chromosome in CML), biochemical studies (e.g., nonspecific esterase, terminal deoxynucleotidyl transferase), and determination of specific cell surface markers (e.g., immunoglobulin, T-cell receptor) can be used to determine the type and subtype of the leukemia.

These special studies are usually done in consul-tation with a hematologist. **Bone marrow biopsy** is the definitive study, useful in making the specific diagno-sis of a leukemic subtype and also in providing some indication of the clinical stage of the disease.

The diagnosis of lymphoma is generally made by **biopsy** of suspicious lymph nodes or masses (see Chapter 63). Similar tests are done on the biopsy sam-ple as are done on leukemic cells in peripheral blood.

Computed tomography is often performed in the case of suspected lymphoma to determine the ana-tomic stage of the disease.

▶ **TREATMENT**

The treatment of leukemia and lymphoma is deter-mined by the specific type, subtype, and clinical stage of disease. Consultation by a hematologist/oncologist who specializes in the treatment of these diseases is generally requested.

Specific therapy for leukemia and lymphoma is constantly undergoing revision secondary to results of clinical trials and is beyond the scope of this discussion. However, **several generalizations** can be made. Chemotherapy has traditionally been the mainstay of management of the acute leukemias, CML, and lymphomas that are beyond limited (local) stage and used alone is often successful in the curative treatment of ALL. CML and AML generally respond to chemotherapy alone with a clinical remission, but relapse is common, leading to use of bone marrow transplant (see below) as the curative treatment.

CLL, because of its relatively benign course, is generally not treated unless there are complications (e.g., clinically significant cytopenia, anatomically significant adenopathy or organomegaly, severe systemic symptoms). In these cases, chemotherapy is administered with the goal of disease control rather than cure.

Limited-stage HD can be successfully treated with radiotherapy alone. Radiation with chemotherapy is generally used in more advanced HD. NHL is generally treated with radiation and chemotherapy, except in extremely limited local disease.

Bone marrow transplantation (BMT) is used with curative intent in most cases of AML, CML, and relapsed ALL. Allogeneic BMT (using bone marrow harvested from a human lymphocyte antigen-matched relative or unrelated donor) has lower relapse rates than autologous BMT (where the patient's marrow is harvested and treated to try to remove leukemic cells and then reinfused after intensive chemotherapy). This is at the cost of significantly increased risk of complications (graft-versus-host disease, severe immunosuppression leading to infection) in allogeneic BMT. BMT is invested as salvage therapy in patients with NHL but appears to benefit only a small subgroup of patients.

Modern therapy has significantly increased the life span of patients diagnosed with leukemia or lymphoma. In certain subgroups, there is a significant fraction of patients who can be cured of their disease. **Current research** in the treatment of these disorders is proceeding along a number of pathways:

▲ Developing better chemotherapies for recurrences;

▲ Expanding the role of BMT, both allogeneic and autologous, in both primary and salvage treatment regimens;

▲ Use of immune therapies, for example, tumor-specific monoclonal antibodies linked to toxins;

▲ Use of growth factors in an attempt to modulate the biology of these neoplasms, in the hope that chemotherapy or radiotherapy will be more effective.

▶ KEY POINTS

1. Leukemias are neoplasms of hematopoietic cells that arise in the bone marrow and then spread to the periphery.

2. Lymphomas are hematopoietic neoplasms that arise in peripheral lymphoid tissue.

3. Leukemias can be divided according to the cell of origin (lymphoid or myeloid) and the clinical course (acute or chronic).

4. Lymphomas can be divided into Hodgkin's and non-Hodgkin's.

5. Acute leukemias can present with constitutional signs, bleeding, infection, and complications of peripheral leukostasis. Chronic leukemias are generally more indolent.

6. Lymphomas generally present as painless adenopathy or a mass.

7. The therapy of these neoplasms can involve various combinations of chemotherapy, radiation, and bone marrow transplant.

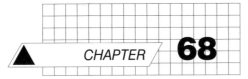

CHAPTER 68

Acute Complications of Cancer Therapy

*7*he therapeutic modalities of chemotherapy, radiation therapy, and bone marrow transplantation have improved the survival rates of many forms of cancer. However, these therapies are associated with a number of serious and potentially fatal acute **complications**.

▶ MUCOSITIS

A number of chemotherapeutic agents and local radiation can induce **inflammation of the mucous membranes**. The oral cavity is commonly involved (stomatitis). Inflammation can be quite painful, interfering with oral intake and leading to dehydration and malnutrition. In addition, the inflamed mucosa can predispose to the development of infections.

Patients who develop stomatitis need to maintain strict oral hygiene to reduce the risk of infections. Oral rinses with **hydrogen peroxide** solutions are generally sufficient.

Topical therapy with a local anesthetic such as lidocaine gel can relieve the discomfort associated with stomatitis. In extremely severe cases, dose modification of chemotherapy is needed to limit recurrences.

▶ NEUTROPENIA

Many modern chemotherapeutic regimens will cause **transient neutropenia**, because the granulocyte fraction contains a high percentage of rapidly dividing cells.

Neutropenia increases the likelihood of **serious infections**; this risk is proportional to the degree of neutropenia. The **absolute neutrophil count** (ANC) provides an objective measure of the degree of risk of infection. An ANC > 1000/mm^3 does not significantly increase the risk of infection, whereas the risk begins to rise linearly between ANCs of 500 and 1000/mm^3. Below an ANC of 500/mm^3, the risk of a serious infection rises significantly.

An important consideration is that many of the cardinal features of infection are diminished in the neutropenic patient. Signs of inflammation such as **erythema, pain, purulence, warmth,** and **swelling** can be completely absent. In many cases, the only initial indication of infection in a neutropenic patient may be **fever**.

When a patient presents with **fever and neutropenia** the following procedure for workup and therapy should be taken:

▲ Place the patient on **reverse isolation precautions** (positive pressure room; masks for visitors; strict handwashing before visiting patient; no fresh fruits, vegetables, or flowers).

▲ Perform a thorough physical examination, paying particular attention to the mucous membranes (mouth, genitalia, perianal area).

▲ Draw blood cultures and also redraw for continued fevers.

▲ Obtain a chest radiograph.

▲ Start empiric antibiotic therapy after cultures are drawn, usually using agents that have activity against gram-negative organisms (including *Pseudomonas*). If the patient has an indwelling venous catheter, expanded gram-positive coverage with an antibiotic such as vancomycin should be added.

▲ Monitor cultures and ANC daily. Antibiotics and reverse precautions are generally continued until the patient is afebrile and the ANC is >500/mm^3, provided no source of infection is found. The ANC nadir generally occurs 7 to 14 days after the administration of chemotherapy, with recovery occurring at about days 21 to 28.

▲ For continued fevers after 4 to 5 days of broad antibacterial coverage, consider broadening antibiotic therapy via the initiation of antifungal therapy.

▲ The use of colony stimulating factors (G-CSF and GM-CSF) is being investigated as a specific treatment for chemotherapy-induced neutropenia.

▲ Future rounds of chemotherapy may require dose adjustment to avoid recurrent severe neutropenia.

▶ ANEMIA AND THROMBOCYTOPENIA

In addition to neutropenia, many chemotherapeutic regimens also affect the production of red blood cells and platelets. Because of their more rapid turnover, **thrombocytopenia** is more likely to be significant than anemia. When coupled with the development of **sto-matitis**, thrombocytopenia can lead to significant oral hemorrhage.

The clinical signs of chemotherapy-induced anemia and thrombocytopenia do not differ significantly from those seen in cytopenias from other causes (see Chapters 62 and 65).

Chemotherapy-induced anemia rarely requires transfusion of red blood cells. Thrombocytopenia that results in clinically significant bleeding can be treated by the infusion of platelets while waiting for production to return to normal levels. As with neutropenia, the platelet count nadir occurs 1 to 2 weeks after the administration of chemotherapy; normal production returns by 3 to 4 weeks.

▶ NAUSEA AND VOMITING

Although seldom life-threatening, nausea and vomiting are among the most disturbing side effects of cancer therapy for patients. Most chemotherapeutic regimens can induce nausea and vomiting, but regimens containing **cisplatin** are among the most emetogenic.

The proper **control of nausea and vomiting** uses several principles. First, **prophylactic** antiemetic therapy should be administered on a **scheduled basis** to patients receiving emetogenic therapy. Second, aggressive antiemetic therapy during the initial administration of chemotherapy can significantly reduce **anticipatory nausea and vomiting** before subsequent doses. Finally, certain **dietary maneuvers** can limit nausea and vomiting: limit intake to clear liquids during periods of severe nausea and vomiting, eat more frequent small meals, avoid overly fatty or sweet foods, and avoid lying down immediately after eating.

The treatment of chemotherapy-induced nausea and vomiting has been improved by the recent development of the **serotonin-blocking antiemetics** (ondansetron and granisetron). When coupled with **corticosteroids** (dexamethasone), they are often quite effective in limiting side effects from highly emetogenic chemotherapy.

Older antiemetics, including metoclopramide (Reglan), prochlorperazine (Compazine), and dimenhydrinate (Dramamine), are less effective but are sometimes used for treatment of less emetogenic chemotherapy regimens. **Benzodiazepines** (e.g., lorazepam) can be useful in relaxing an anxious patient before chemotherapy and may limit subsequent development of anticipatory nausea.

▶ GRAFT-VERSUS-HOST DISEASE

GVHD is a potentially fatal side effect of **allogeneic bone marrow transplantation** (BMT). GVHD is a **multisystem disease** that appears to be the result of immunologic attack of the host tissues by T cells in the donated bone marrow. Both **acute** and **chronic** forms of GVHD exist. Moderate to severe acute GVHD occurs in about half of patients receiving an allogeneic BMT. Approximately a third of patients who develop moderate to severe GVHD will die from it.

In **acute GVHD**, the following abnormalities are commonly encountered:

▲ Skin rash: may be a maculopapular eruption or vasculitic-appearing rash with ulcers, ecchymosis, and petechiae. This is generally the first manifestation of acute GVHD.

▲ Gastrointestinal disturbances: diarrhea (which can be bloody) is the most common manifestation, but severe abdominal pain and ileus can result.

▲ Hepatic abnormalities: elevated liver transaminases and hyperbilirubinemia are common.

▲ Immunosuppression: infection is common in GVHD and is a common cause of death in patients who develop GVHD. In addition to the breakdown in primary immune barriers in the gastrointestinal tract and skin, severe functional immune defects result from GVHD. Additionally, the preferred treatment for GVHD uses immunosuppressive drugs (see below) that further increases the infection risk.

The **treatment of acute GVHD** involves immunosuppression to try to limit the immune-mediated damage to host tissues. **Cyclosporin glucocorticoids, methotrexate,** and **antithymocyte globulin** have all been used to treat acute GVHD. Additionally, some of these agents are used **prophylactically** immediately after BMT to prevent the development of GVHD. Another technique that is being studied is the depletion of T cells from donor marrow by treatment of the graft with T-cell specific antibodies before infusion into the patient.

Chronic GVHD affects the same organs as acute GVHD, with additional involvement of the mucous membranes. A chronic inflammatory state, similar to that seen in collagen vascular diseases (see Chapter 58) develops. The clinical course in chronic GVHD is generally more indolent, but once again, infection is a major cause of morbidity and mortality in these patients. Immunosuppression is also the treatment of choice for chronic GVHD.

► KEY POINTS

1. Modern cancer therapy is associated with potentially fatal acute side effects, including mucositis, neutropenia, anemia, thrombocytopenia, nausea/vomiting, and graft-versus-host disease.

2. Neutropenia increases the likelihood of infection, with a risk that is proportional to the degree of neutropenia.

3. Nausea and vomiting associated with certain chemotherapy regimens can be effectively treated with prophylactic antiemetic drugs.

4. Graft-versus-host disease is caused by T cells in transplanted bone marrow that cause tissue damage.

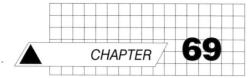
Paraneoplastic Disorders

*P*araneoplastic disorders are generally defined as effects of cancer that occur at sites that are remote from the primary tumor and any metastases. The effects can be quite dramatic, and at times more disabling than the tumor itself. Paraneoplastic disorders can precede, coexist, or follow the primary tumor by months or years.

Paraneoplastic disorders are estimated to occur in about 10% of all malignancies. They are most commonly associated with lung (particularly small cell), stomach (and other gastrointestinal malignancies), and breast cancers.

▶ PATHOGENESIS AND CLINICAL PRESENTATION

The most common paraneoplastic disorders can be divided into four major groups: endocrine, neurologic, hematologic, and dermatologic.

Endocrine Disorders

These disorders are the result of ectopic peptide hormone production. Particular hormones are commonly associated with specific tumors. **Ectopic adrenocorticotropic hormone** (ACTH) secretion, is associated with **small cell lung cancer, carcinoid tumors**, and **thyroid cancer**. This ectopic ACTH can result in Cushing's syndrome (see Chapter 50). Clinically apparent Cushing's syndrome is estimated to occur in ~5% of patients with small cell lung cancer.

Parathyroid hormone-related polypeptide (PTHrP) is similar, but not identical, to parathyroid hormone (PTH) and is the product of a distinct gene. Ectopic PTHrP can be secreted by breast cancer, squamous cell lung cancer, head and neck cancer, esophageal cancer, and ovarian cancer. Excess PTHrP secretion results in hypercalcemia (see Chapter 49). Diagnosis can be made by commercial assays for serum PTHrP, which is undetectable in normal individuals and in cancer patients without malignancy-associated hypercalcemia.

Osteoclast activating factor (OAF) is associated with hematologic disorders such as multiple myeloma and lymphoma as well as some breast cancers. OAF has not been identified precisely (there is evidence that in myeloma, it is tumor necrosis factor-beta) but it acts locally to stimulate osteoclast-mediated bone resorption, resulting in hypercalcemia. Diagnosis is generally one of exclusion, made in a patient with hypercalcemia, appropriate malignancy, and normal PTH and PTHrP levels.

Antidiuretic hormone is associated with small cell lung cancers that may produce the syndrome of inappropriate antidiuretic hormone secretion (SIADH). SIADH is characterized by serum hyponatremia and hypoosmolarity. When making the diagnosis, it is important to consider other causes of hyponatremia, including edematous states, diuretic therapy, hypovolemia, adrenal deficiency, thyroid deficiency, and hypolipidemia (see Chapter 20). A critical feature that suggests SIADH is the production of an abnormally concentrated urine (>300 mOsmol/kg) in the setting of hyponatremia and hypoosmolality. If the diagnosis is not clear, a **water-load test** may be performed, testing the ability of a patient to excrete a water load by production of dilute urine. Care must be taken to avoid causing dangerous hyponatremia during this test.

Ectopic **erythropoietin** production has been described in the setting of renal cell cancers, hepatomas, and cerebellar hemangiomas. This results in an increase in red cell mass.

Neurologic Disorders

These disorders are characterized by the production of autoantibodies. The mechanism by which autoantibody production is triggered by the malignancy as well as the specific role of these antibodies in pathogenesis are not completely understood. Pathologically, inflammation results in demyelination, neuronal and muscular degeneration, and damage to the neuromuscular junction.

Cerebellar degeneration is associated with breast, ovarian, and lung cancers. The key pathologic finding is degeneration of the cerebellar Purkinje cells. The autoantibody called anti-Yo is detected in many cases. This disorder presents with ataxia, nystagmus, dysarthria, and vertigo. Examination of the cerebrospinal fluid (CSF) reveals mild pleocytosis and elevated protein. Electrophoresis of the CSF may reveal oligoclonal bands.

Encephalomyelitis is associated with small cell lung cancer and the presence of the anti-Hu autoantibody. Inflammation and neuronal loss occurs in varied regions of the central nervous system. Clinical manifestations depend on the anatomic location of the lesion and includes cerebellar and cerebral dysfunction and motor neuron disease.

Lambert-Eaton myasthenic syndrome occurs with small cell lung cancer and is characterized by weakness, myalgia, and fatigability. A key feature is reduction in muscle strength at rest that transiently improves with repeated muscle stimulation. The primary defect appears to be impaired release of the neurotransmitter acetylcholine from the presynaptic nerve terminal due to antibody-mediated destruction of a calcium channel.

Guillain-Barré syndrome (acute inflammatory demyelinating polyneuropathy) is seen in lymphoma (both Hodgkin's and non-Hodgkin's) and is characterized by an ascending paralysis, areflexia, and elevated CSF protein.

Hematologic Disorders

Hematologic changes in cancer are usually due to direct bone marrow involvement, but there are a number of paraneoplastic disorders as well. **Hypercoagulability** is common and may present as migratory thrombophlebitis, also known as Trousseau's syndrome. Classically, Trousseau's syndrome has been associated with adenocarcinomas of the lung and gastrointestinal tract.

Leukocytosis is seen in many nonhematologic malignancies. A less common finding is the leukemoid reaction, in which the leukocyte count can approach 100,000/mm^3.

Red blood cell disorders include malignancy-associated anemia that may take one of several forms (see Chapter 61):

▲ Anemia of chronic disease (erythropoietin deficiency);

▲ Autoimmune hemolytic anemia (particularly in lymphomas, chronic lymphocytic leukemia, and certain solid tumors);

▲ Pure red cell aplasia (depletion of erythroid elements in bone marrow, seen in the setting of a thymoma);

▲ Microangiopathic hemolytic anemia (may be associated with disseminated intravascular coagulation and is generally in the setting of mucinous adenocarcinomas).

Certain tumors can result in erythrocytosis due to ectopic secretion of erythropoietin (see above).

Dermatologic Disorders

There is a wide variety of dermatologic disorders that occur in the setting of malignancy, but only a few are commonly associated with cancer. **Acanthosis nigricans** is characterized by the appearance of brown velvety areas appearing in the skin folds of the neck, axillae, and groin. More than half of patients with this finding have an underlying malignancy, most often of the gastrointestinal tract. Acanthosis nigricans is often associated with another lesion called "tripe palms" for the characteristic velvety appearance of the palms and palmar surfaces of the fingers.

Erythroderma may be seen with cutaneous T-cell lymphoma (Sézary syndrome). A lesion called neurolytic migratory erythema (characterized by erosive migratory erythema of the face and girdle area) is pathognomonic of a glucagonoma.

Dermatomyositis and **polymyositis** may be a harbinger of malignancy. About 10% of cases are due to cancer of the breast, lung, ovaries, or stomach. The clinical disorder consists of progressive weakness with elevated serum muscle enzymes and characteristic findings on muscle biopsy.

Sweet's syndrome is characterized by fever, neutrophilia, and the appearance of tender erythematous plaques on the skin. It is a rare disorder, but about 20% of cases are associated with an underlying cancer, most often hematologic.

▶ DIAGNOSIS

The recognition of a paraneoplastic disorder, particularly in a patient who does not have a known diagnosis of cancer, is difficult. Many paraneoplastic disorders have counterparts that are encountered in patients without a known malignancy. A high degree of clinical suspicion is required to make the diagnosis of a paraneoplastic condition in a previously healthy individual.

The occurrence of a paraneoplastic condition may be a tipoff to a previously occult malignancy. In the case of deep venous thrombosis (DVTs), patients with **recurrent** DVTs are more likely to have a subsequent diagnosis of a malignancy. However, the malignancies were of quite varied types (ranging from brain tumors to ovarian carcinomas), making it difficult to recommend a detailed head-to-toe search for a malignancy in the setting of recurrent DVTs.

▶ **TREATMENT**

The treatment of paraneoplastic disorders is generally supportive; the principal treatment is of the underlying malignancy. Unfortunately, the presence of a paraneoplastic disorder generally carries a worse prognosis than a similar stage malignancy without one.

▶ **KEY POINTS**

1. Paraneoplastic disorders are effects of cancer that occur at sites that are remote from the primary tumor and any metastases.

2. The most common cancers associated with paraneoplastic disorders are lung (small cell), breast, and gastrointestinal tract malignancies.

3. The most common paraneoplastic disorders are those that affect the endocrine, nervous, hematologic, and dermatologic systems.

4. The presence of a paraneoplastic disorder with a given tumor generally predicts a worse prognosis.

Index